The Business of Medicine

J. K. Silver, MD

Medical Director
Spaulding Neighborhood Rehabilitation Center
Framingham, Massachusetts

Instructor
Department of Physical Medicine and Rehabilitation
Harvard Medical School
Boston, Massachusetts

Associate in Physiatry
Massachusetts General Hospital
Boston, Massachusetts

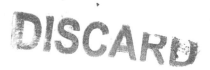

Hanley & Belfus, Inc. Philadelphia

Publisher: HANLEY & BELFUS, INC.
              Medical Publishers
              210 South 13th Street
              Philadelphia, PA 19107
              215-546-7293; 800-962-1892
              FAX 215-790-9330
              Web site: http://www.hanleyandbelfus.com

Library of Congress Cataloging-in-Publication Data

The business of medicine / [edited by] Julie K. Silver.
       p.   cm.
     Includes bibliographical references and index.
     ISBN 1-56053-254-8 (alk. paper)
     1. Medicine—Practice.   I. Silver, Julie K., 1965–
     [DNLM: 1. Practice Management, Medical—organization &
     administration.   2. Career Mobility.   3. Marketing of Health
     Services.   W 80 B9788 1998]
     R728.B883   1998
     610'.68—DC21
     DNLM/DLC
     for Library of Congress   98-12942
                                                              CIP

THE BUSINESS OF MEDICINE   ISBN 1-56053-254-8

Last digit is the print number: 9 8 7 6 5 4 3 2 1

CONTENTS

W. Michael Alberts, MD, MBA was graduated from medical school at the University of Illinois and received his Master of Business Administration degree from the University of South Florida. He is currently a Professor of Medicine and Associate Chair for Clinical Affairs in the Department of Internal Medicine at the University of South Florida College of Medicine in Tampa, Florida. Dr. Alberts also serves as the medical director of quality management for the USF Physicians Group.

Gerald M. Aronoff, MD is a graduate of the New Jersey College of Medicine. He completed his psychiatric residency at Harvard Medical School, McLean Hospital, followed by a fellowship in consultation psychiatry at Boston University Medical Center. Currently, Dr. Aronoff is Medical Director of the Presbyterian Center for Pain Medicine in Charlotte, North Carolina. He is an Assistant Professor at Tufts Medical School and serves as President of both the North Carolina Pain Society and the American Academy of Pain Medicine (AAPM). Dr. Aronoff's work includes chairing a committee at the AAPM that is evaluating pain care at the end of life to establish guidelines for euthanasia and physician-assisted suicide. Previously, he served as President of the New England Pain Association and the Eastern Pain Association. Dr. Aronoff is the author/editor of five books on chronic pain and numerous scientific publications on pain, the prevention of disability, and pharmacologic management. Formerly, Dr. Aronoff was Editor-in-Chief of the *Clinical Journal of Pain*, and he is currently Co-Editor of *Current Review of Pain*.

Barry Beder, MSW, LICSW is a graduate of the University of Michigan School of Social Work and is a Licensed Independent Clinical Social Worker. He has designed health promotion interventions for the major teaching hospitals of Harvard Medical School.

Gail P. Bender, MD, MS received her bachelor's degree from Cornell University and a master's degree from Stanford University prior to obtaining her medical degree from the University of Minnesota in 1975. She performed her internal medicine residency at the University of Minnesota Hospitals and Ohio State University Hospitals. She completed her fellowship in medical oncology in 1980. Dr. Bender is board certified by the American Board of Internal Medicine in both internal medicine and medical oncology. She is a fellow of the American College of Physicians. Dr. Bender has served on the boards of directors of the Methodist Hospital Foundation, the Minnesota Medical Foundation, Medica Health Plan, HealthSystem Minnesota, and the Midwest Medical Insurance Company. She is currently a solo medical oncologist in Minneapolis, where she has practiced since 1982.

Jill Berger-Fiffy, MS, MHA is a licensed Speech Language Pathologist who has a Master of Science degree in Communication Disorders from Boston University and a Master of Health Administration from Suffolk University, where she received commendation for Outstanding Academic Achievement. Her experience in health care administration includes sales and marketing, program development, practice management, and health care planning. Ms. Berger-Fiffy is also the physician recruiter for Spaulding Rehabilitation Hospital, which is one of the largest rehabilitation hospitals in the country. Additionally, she serves as the Business Manager for the Physician Group Practices at Spaulding Rehabilitation Hospital and is a member of the Medical Group Management Association and the Healthcare Financial Management Association.

David T. Burke, MD, MA received his medical degree from the University of South Carolina and his Master of Arts in Clinical Psychology at Wichita State University in Kansas. He completed his residency training in physical medicine and rehabilitation at Louisiana State University in New Orleans. Dr. Burke is the Editor-in-Chief and founder of *Rehab in Review*, a surveillance journal of current literature focused on the continuing education of PM&R physicians. He is also the Residency Program Director of the Harvard Department of PM&R and Director of the brain injury program at Spaulding Rehabilitation Hospital in Boston, Massachusetts.

Michael P. Burke, MA has a Bachelor of Arts degree in Business Management from Ottawa University and a Master of Arts degree in Gerontology from Wichita State University. Mr. Burke has a federal and state license as a Nursing Home Administrator and is board certified by the American College of Health Care Administrators. Currently, he is very active in developing and presenting seminars to health care professionals on business-related topics such as marketing, understanding Medicare within the nursing home industry, and time management for medical professionals.

Francis X. Campion, MD is a graduate of Harvard Medical School and a board certified internist who is currently the Vice President for Clinical Integration of the Caritas Christi Health Care System. Dr. Campion maintains a clinical practice at St. Elizabeth's Medical Center in Boston. He is the former Medical Director for Quality Resources and Risk Management at the Lahey-Hitchcock Clinic in Burlington, Massachusetts. Dr. Campion is also the author of the book *Grand Rounds on Medical Malpractice*, which is published by the American Medical Association.

John S. Cook, DPhil holds a doctorate in mathematics from Oxford University. He is an independent health care consultant who specializes in prospective payment system design and implementation for state governments, provider groups, and private health plans. He was instrumental in the design of the public utility model regulatory system in Maryland, the Medicare demonstrations sponsored by the Hospital Consortium of Greater Rochester, and the payment arrangements of several private sector insurance companies, including Blue Cross and Blue Shield of Massachusetts.

Melinda B. Everett, AB, MS, APR is accredited in public relations by the Public Relations Society of America and has more than 20 years experience in the field of health care, public relations, and marketing communications. She is currently the Director of Public and Professional Relations at Seidler Bernstein, Inc., in Cambridge, Massachusetts. Ms. Everett is the recipient of the Gold Touchstone Award, one of the highest honors conferred in the field of health care marketing and public relations.

Kenneth M. Fine, MD is an Assistant Professor of Orthopaedic Surgery and the Director of Sports Medicine at the George Washington University. He is the team physician for the George Washington University varsity teams as well as for many of the high school teams in the Washington, DC, area. Dr. Fine has served as team physician for the Washington Mustangs of the U.S. Inter-regional Soccer League and has participated in the care of the U.S. Diving Team and the Joffrey Ballet for events in the Washington, DC, area. Dr. Fine also provided medical coverage for visiting soccer teams during the 1996 Summer Olympics and is the medical director for the Race for the Cure and the Cherry Blossom road races in Washington, DC.

Wendy W. Fink, BA is a health educator specializing in behavioral approaches to lifestyle change. Her Boston-based firm, wfa Incorporated, designed continuing education programs for physicians, nurses, and patients before moving into corporate settings where the firm has created and managed wellness initiatives for more than 300 employers. Ms. Fink is CEO of the Institute for Wellness Education, a national collaborative of 15 companies specializing in disease management. She has published more than 40 articles in health care journals, including the *New England Journal of Medicine*.

James S. Hamrock, Jr., JD is a graduate of Boston College Law School. He is a former Assistant District Attorney for Suffolk County in Boston, Massachusetts. Currently, he is a partner in the law firm of Rafferty, Hamrock & Tocci located in Cambridge, Massachusetts Attorney Hamrock represents physicians, hospitals, and other medical professionals and institutions in medical malpractice litigation.

William B. Howard, Jr., BBA, ChFC, CFP is President of William Howard & Co. Financial Advisors, Inc., a fee-only financial planning and investment advisory firm in Memphis, Tennessee. Mr. Howard is recognized by *Worth* magazine as one of the 60 best financial advisors in America. He has more than 18 years of experience in advising physicians on financial matters and is the author of a financial planning column for the Memphis and Shelby County Medical Society. Mr. Howard has been interviewed for his expertise by such prestigious publications as the *Wall Street Journal*, *USA Today*, *Money*, *Morning Star Investor*, *Medical Economics*, *American Medical News*, and *Physicians Management*. Mr. Howard also serves on the editorial review board of the *Journal of Financial Planning*.

Richard T. Katz, MD completed his residency training in physical medicine and rehabilitation at the Rehabilitation Institute of Chicago. Currently, Dr. Katz is Associate Professor of Clinical Internal Medicine at St. Louis University as well as vice president of medical affairs and medical director of the SSM Rehabilitation Institute. He is on the editorial board of *Neuro Rehabilitation* and the *AMA Guides Newsletter*. Dr. Katz is also a primary reviewer for the *Archives of Physical Medicine and Rehabilitation* and the *American Journal of Physical Medicine and Rehabilitation*. Additionally, he has served as a grant reviewer for the National Institute of Disability and Rehabilitation Research and for Paralyzed Veterans of America. He is a member of the research committee of the Association of Academic Physiatrists and has served as the chairman of several committees within the American Academy of Physical Medicine and Rehabilitation and the American Academy of Electrodiagnostic Medicine. Dr. Katz is the author of more than 75 scientific publications related to spinal cord injury, traumatic brain injury, electrophysiology, and spastic hypertonia.

Jack C. Keane, MS, MBA has a Master of Science degree in Health Services Administration from Harvard University. He currently works as an independent health care consultant providing data analysis, contract negotiation, and payment system design services to various clients including several Blue Cross/Blue Shield plans, hospitals, and physician groups. Mr. Keane has helped establish PTO or HMO programs in approximately 60 markets throughout the United States.

Charles M. Key, BA, JD was graduated cum laude from Arkansas State University with an undergraduate degree in philosophy. He received his law degree from the University of

Missouri—Columbia in 1984. Mr. Key is a partner in the Bogatin Law Firm, PLC, in Memphis, Tennessee, where he specializes in health care law. Mr. Key is a member of the American Medical Association Doctors Advisory Network, the National Health Lawyers Association, the American Bar Association Health Law Section, and State Bar Associations of Missouri and Tennessee. The Bogatin Law Firm, PLC, represents health care providers and related organizations in a wide range of areas including tax, business, regulatory, employment, trademark, and immigration law, as well as civil and criminal litigation. Mr. Key focuses his practice primarily on business and regulatory matters such as service contracting, managed care systems, provider networks, faculty practice plans, Medicare reimbursement, antitrust, insurance, risk management, peer review, and licensing.

Michael D. Kneeland, MD, MPH is a graduate of Tufts Medical School and a board certified internist. He received his Master of Public Health degree from the Harvard School of Public Health. Dr. Kneeland is Vice President of Performance Improvement in the Caritas Christi Health Care System in Massachusetts, where he also manages the Caritas Christi Insurance Program. Dr. Kneeland teaches epidemiology and biostatistics at Tufts Medical School.

Sung J. Liao, MD, MPH, DPH, Dip. Bact. is a Clinical Professor of Surgical Sciences at the New York University College of Dentistry. He is also a consultant at the Rusk Institute of Rehabilitation Medicine at the New York University College of Medicine and Honorary Consultant at the China Rehabilitation Research Centre in Beijing, China. Dr. Liao is a senior fellow of the American College of Physicians and a senior fellow of the Royal Society of Medicine in England. He has done extensive clinical and academic work in alternative medicine and is currently the Chairman of the American College of Acupuncture, Inc., Honorary Chairman of the Society for Acupuncture Research, and a member of the Board of Directors for the Medical Acupuncture Research Foundation. Dr. Liao is also co-author of the book *Principles and Practice of Contemporary Acupuncture*.

John S. Lloyd, MBA, MSPH is Vice Chairman of Witt/Kieffer, Ford, Hadelman & Lloyd, which is a leading executive search firm. Mr. Lloyd has more than 25 years of consulting and executive search experience, and he is a frequent speaker to trustees, physician executives, and top management groups in the United States and abroad. He has published numerous articles and book chapters on issues relating to executive leadership and has been named one of the top 10 executive search consultants in the health care industry. In addition to being listed in Faulkner and Gray's 1500, he has served on the board of the Association of Executive Search Consultants and the National Advisory Board of the Health Care Forum.

Mary Frances Lyons, MD is a diplomate of the American Board of Internal Medicine and a fellow of the American College of Cardiology. Dr. Lyons is also a search consultant with Witt/Kieffer, Ford, Hadelman & Lloyd and has extensive experience as a specialist in physician executive search engagements. In addition to authoring a column in the American College of Physician Executive's magazine titled "Career Rx," she is a featured speaker on physician executive career development at regional and national meetings and has led a recent national survey on the role of the physician executive and hospitals, systems, and managed care organizations.

Robert Naparstek, MD is the Medical Director of Occupational and Environmental Medicine at the Good Samaritan Medical Center in Brockton, Massachusetts.

Lorenz K. Y. Ng, MD received his bachelor's degree from Stanford University and medical degree from the Columbia University College of Physicians and Surgeons. He is a Clinical

Professor of Neurology at the George Washington University School of Medicine in Washington, DC, and is also Director of the Outpatient Pain Clinic at the National Rehabilitation Hospital in Washington, DC. He is a member of the Alternative Medicine Program Advisory Council of the National Institutes of Health in Bethesda, Maryland. He is recipient of the S. Weir Mitchell Award of the American Academy of Neurology, the A. E. Bennet Award for the Society of Biological Psychiatry, and the Commendation Medal from the United States Public Health Service for development of federal programs on pain research and treatment. He has authored or co-authored more than 70 scientific publications and is co-author of the book *Principles and Practice of Contemporary Acupuncture.*

Jerry C. Parker, PhD is a graduate of the doctorate program in psychology from the University of Missouri—Columbia. He is Director of the Mental Health Service Line at the Harry S. Truman Memorial Veterans Hospital in Columbia, Missouri. He is also a Clinical Professor of Internal Medicine at the University of Missouri—Columbia School of Medicine. Dr. Parker is the co-director of the Missouri Arthritis Rehabilitation Research and Training Center, and he is the director of the Research Enrichment Program for Physiatrists, which is a research training grant sponsored by the National Institute on Disability and Rehabilitation and Research. Dr. Parker has published extensively in the areas of neuropsychology and health psychology.

Kenneth H. Paulus is the Chief Operating Officer of Partners Community Health Care, Inc., the network created by Partners Health Care System. Partners Health Care System is the corporate holding company that is representing the merger of the Massachusetts General Hospital and Brigham and Women's Hospital. Mr. Paulus has over 15 years of senior group practice administrative experience at some of the nation's leading health care delivery organizations.

Edward M. Phillips, MD is an instructor in the Department of Physical Medicine and Rehabilitation at Harvard Medical School and is the director of outpatient medical services at Spaulding Rehabilitation Hospital in Boston. Dr. Phillips is also a clinical associate at Massachusetts General Hospital and works for Vencor, Inc., as the physician director of rehabilitation programs at five subacute and long-term care facilities in eastern Massachusetts. Dr. Phillips has extensive experience in both written and oral presentations for physicians and other health care providers in the field of subacute and long-term care.

Walter E. Schuler, BBA, JD received a Bachelor of Business Administration degree (magna cum laude) from the University of Memphis and a law degree (cum laude) with a Certificate in Health Law (cum laude) from Saint Louis University. Mr. Schuler is an associate of the Bogatin Law Firm, PLC, in Memphis, Tennessee, and is a member of the National Health Lawyers Association, the American Bar Association Health Law Section, and the State Bar Association of Tennessee. The Bogatin Law Firm, PLC, represents health care providers and related organizations in a wide range of areas including tax, business, regulatory, employment, trademark, and immigration law, as well as civil and criminal litigation. Mr. Schuler focuses his practice primarily on business and regulatory matters such as service contracting, managed care systems, provider networks, faculty practice plans, Medicare reimbursement, antitrust, insurance, risk management, peer review, and licensing.

Julie K. Silver, MD graduated from the Georgetown University School of Medicine and completed a residency in physical medicine and rehabilitation at the National Rehabilitation Hospital in Washington, DC. Dr. Silver is currently the Medical Director of the Spaulding

Neighborhood Rehabilitation Center in Framingham, Massachusetts, which is a comprehensive outpatient rehabilitation facility. She is also a clinical consultant in physiatry at Massachusetts General Hospital, on the staff at MetroWest Medical Center in Framingham, and an instructor in the Department of PM&R at Harvard Medical School. Dr. Silver has extensive experience in writing for local and national publications and peer-reviewed medical journals and frequently speaks professionally on business-related topics.

James M. Slayton, MD, MBA is a graduate of the Stanford University School of Medicine and Harvard Business School. He is currently Director of Ambulatory Services in the Department of Psychiatry at the Cambridge Public Health Commission in Massachusetts and Clinical Instructor in Psychiatry at Harvard Medical School. Dr. Slayton's professional interests include the study of medical delivery systems in the public sector and the evaluation of cost-effective care for under-served populations.

Dorothy R. Sweeney is Vice President of The Health Care Group, President of Health Care Consulting, Inc., and editor and publisher of *On Managing*, a monthly newsletter for practice managers. Ms. Sweeney has lectured and written extensively for physician and non-physician audiences and has been a frequent contributor to health care publications such as *Medical Economics*, *Group Practice Journal*, *Physicians Management*, *Pennsylvania Medicine*, *The North Carolina Medical Society Journal*, and *Connecticut Medicine*. She has also contributed to the books *How to Recruit and Hire Staff* and *Managing Your Medical Practice*. Ms. Sweeney is also a former president of the Society of Medical-Dental Management Consultants and is currently active with the National Association of Health Care Consultants.

Barry S. Taylor, ND is a naturopathic physician who graduated from the National College of Naturopathic Medicine in Portland, Oregon. Dr. Taylor trained in both modern and traditional approaches to holistic healing and is co-founder of the New England Family Health Center in Boston, Massachusetts.

J. Gray Tuttle, Jr., CPBC is a mathematics and economics graduate of Hampden-Sydney College in Virginia and did postgraduate work in accounting and taxation at Georgia State University and Pfeiffer College. Mr. Tuttle is currently a principal in Professional Consultants, Inc., in Lansing, Michigan, where he has provided business management and consulting services to physicians and medical groups since 1976. He is also the president of the Institute of Certified Professional Business Consultants and the director of the National Association of Health Care Consultants. Mr Tuttle is a past president of the Society of Professional Business Consultants. He is a longtime member of the Medical Group Management Association and is a contributing editor to *Medical Economics*. Mr. Tuttle also served as an editorial consultant for *OBG Management* and *Pediatric Management* magazines.

In a time of drastic change it is the learners who inherit the future. The learned usually find themselves equipped to live in a world that no longer exists.

—Eric Hoffer from *Reflections on the Human Condition*

The field of medicine is drastically changing, and, like it or not, business influences are dominating how we deliver health care services. While it is imperative to learn and maintain superb clinical skills, it is also important to learn the business of medicine. Without this knowledge, health care providers are unable to negotiate managed and capitated care contracts, understand billing procedures in order to avoid government audits, advocate for patients with insurers, increase productivity and decrease expenses in the office and hospital environments, or decide which practice opportunities are financially viable; and the list goes on. In short, health care providers who do not understand business principles as they relate to medical practice are in danger of becoming ineffective healers. In contrast, those providers who maintain a high level of clinical skill and business acumen truly find themselves equipped to practice medicine in an ever-changing environment.

J. K. Silver, MD

This book is dedicated to all health care providers who appreciate the value of a physiatry consult.

1

Introduction

THE LATEST REVOLUTION IN THE BUSINESS OF MEDICINE: ITS IMPACT ON YOU

Many Americans are amazed by the transformation of health care from what it was just ten years ago. Both providers and patients may not fully realize that the business of medicine has undergone revolutionary changes in each generation. The most recent revolution has been the establishment of "managed" health care and the consolidation of hospitals and clinics into vertically integrated health delivery systems. Solo and group practitioners have begun to learn how contracting changes with insurers will require them to take on the financial risk of caring for groups of patients under a system called capitation. This book is designed to acquaint physicians with the various aspects of those changes in the business of medicine and how they can prosper professionally with a basic knowledge of the health industry environment.

My father, a medical oncologist who retired in 1986, was trained in the "Golden Era" of American medicine, just after the discovery of penicillin ushered in the antibiotic era after World War II. It was an exciting time for physicians, other care providers, and the hospitals and clinics where they practiced. The Great Depression had generated Blue Cross and employer-based insurance to support the health care of millions of Americans. Physicians and hospitals no longer needed to rely on direct payment from patients for the care they received—a fact that had previously bankrupted many providers and organizations during the hard economic times of the 1930s and 1940s. Fee-for-service reimbursement by insurers was routine, and few barriers hindered new physicians from entering the health marketplace, "hanging their shingle," and creating a successful practice with little or no business experience or training.

American medicine expanded greatly after the advent of Medicare and Medicaid in the 1960s. For the first time, the elderly and many of the poorest Americans were entitled to health insurance, administered by the federal or state government. Health expenditures rose rapidly after the establishment of these programs, increasing from $27.1 billion in 1960 and $74.4 billion in 1970 to $666 billion in 1990.[5] Congress provided for the funding of new medical schools designated to train physicians devoted to primary care in underserved rural and urban areas. Treatment of preventable infectious disease was revolutionized with widespread vaccination programs, effectively bringing an end to diseases such as polio and smallpox in the United States.

In the 1980s and 1990s, cost containment in the growth of health care expenditures became a critical development in the national battle against inflation. Economists estimated that uncontrolled increases in health expenditures would consume up to 26% of the gross domestic product in the year 2030, up from 7% in 1970 and 12% in 1990.[7] In response, the Health Care Financing Administration (HCFA) created "diagnostic related groups" (DRGs), the reimbursement of hospitals on a per-case rate for each diagnosis of a given illness. DRGs were instituted in 1983 to control Medicare expenses[6] and were quickly adopted by the health insurance industry.

Health maintenance organizations (HMOs), which initially had been authorized by federal law in 1973 to encourage preventive health care and to constrain insurance costs through a prepaid plan, quickly became populated with healthier people who were not as likely to get sick. HMO members typically were younger and paid a comprehensive fee for their care, typically lower than the traditional fee-for-service indemnity insurance plans, which demanded a copayment of up to 20% and reimbursed the other 80%. Such HMO plans grew from an enrollment of 31 million Americans in 1987 to 67.6 million in 1995.[2]

One more recent method to reduce health resource utilization has been to "manage" care actively. Prior approval of patients entering the hospital, or even the emergency department, has become commonplace. Utilization management of patients has increasingly been carried throughout the hospital course. Insurance plans that did not actively manage care declined from 41% in 1987 to only 5% of all plans in 1990.[3] These innovations have changed practice patterns for care providers in notable ways. For example, routine postoperative care for cesarean sections was pushed down from four to three days at the hospital where I performed my medical internship in 1992. Further changes in the practice of obstetrics and gynecology have occurred since the hospital, formerly a nonprofit institution, merged with the neighboring community hospital, then was acquired by the nation's largest for-profit hospital chain.

In 1996, President Clinton garnered political support for his disapproval of "drive-by deliveries," in which managed care reviewers essentially required new mothers to leave the hospital within 24 hours of giving birth. Such reaction against managed care by the public is increasing, although the implementation of utilization reviews allowed HMO plans to hold their premium rate increases to an average of 3.6% in 1995, essentially matching the inflation rate for the rest of the economy.[3] For now, it appears that at least some utilization management of care is allowing medical inflation to return to a less superheated level.

WHY THE REVOLUTION IN THE BUSINESS
OF MEDICINE MATTERS TO PHYSICIANS

Physicians and other health care providers have largely lost control over many aspects of the practice of medicine during the most recent revolution, described by some as the "corporatization of health care." As health economist John Iglehart explains, managed care programs "which circumscribe the freedom of physicians to practice medicine autonomously . . . receive decidedly mixed reviews from doctors."[4] Iglehart adds that many providers have reluctantly accepted lower fees with the prospect of a larger volume of patients guaranteed through such plans. Still other providers have organized into groups to lower their practice overhead costs and to gain bargaining leverage with insurance plans or self-insured organizations (e.g., General Electric, John Deere) that contract directly with providers, effectively shutting out the health plan as a "middle man." Yet other providers are getting advanced training or degrees in the business of medicine so that they can "speak the language" and integrate Hippocratic values of patient care in a more competitive business environment. This book provides a description of all these strategies, which aim to allow physicians to face proactively the emerging challenges in the health care system instead of reacting to such changes with fear and disappointment. The book also describes activities typically considered "outside" a traditional medical practice, such as expert testimony, subacute and long-term care consultations, alternative medical activities (e.g., acupuncture), and television, radio, and print media opportunities—activities that can realize considerable additional income. Finally, the book offers a nuts-and-bolts approach on how to develop, market, and run a practice successfully and how to translate one's practice into personal financial success.

WHY A FUND OF BUSINESS KNOWLEDGE
IS ESSENTIAL FOR ANY PHYSICIAN

The business of medicine has changed in ways that require physicians to manage their career development and financial well-being much more closely. For instance, as a medical oncologist, my father worked for the same hospital for 30 years, which provided him a defined benefit pension at retirement. Such arrangements have become uncommon in the 1990s, as large companies and health organizations have attempted to shed their pension burden. In a medical career anticipated to stretch to the year 2030, I am likely to work for myself, along with several employers, during that period, if I am like most of my medical colleagues. In Boston, where I live, I am likely to work with one of the four major health systems instead of one of the dozen independent hospitals in existence when I moved here just six years ago. Instead of getting a defined benefit pension, I will guide my retirement savings through choosing any of several mutual funds in a 403(b) or 401(k) plan. If any job of mine carries significant clinical responsibilities, my contract is likely to include productivity measures that require me to achieve a minimal level of billable patient hours, or my salary will be docked accordingly. If I choose to have a private practice, I will receive a discounted fee for service or carry some financial risk for patients under capitated reimbursement. All of these differences require me to be better informed about the business of medicine than my father and his generation of colleagues.

Moreover, physicians who choose to pursue business training beyond that offered in a clinical residency have the opportunity to lead their department, field, or medical discipline or to create new health ventures of their own. In a profession more and more dominated by health activists who demand "convenience and mastery"[1] from their health providers, as Regina Herzlinger postulates in her recent book about market-driven health care, it is likely that the medical field will face even greater challenges, both from macroeconomic forces and from individual consumers. Flexible providers who are capable of understanding and responding to changing business dynamics are likely to survive and prosper in the ongoing revolution in the business of medicine.

REFERENCES

1. Herzlinger RE: Market-Driven Health Care: Who Wins, Who Loses in the Transformation of America's Largest Service Industry. New York, Addison Wesley, 1997.
2. HMO-PPO Digest: Managed Care Digest Series. Indianapolis, Hoechst Marion Roussell, 1996.
3. Hoy EW, Curtis RE, Rice T: Changes and growth in managed care. Health Affairs (Millwood), 10(4):18–36, 1991.
4. Iglehart JK: The American health care system: Introduction. N Engl J Med 326:962–967, 1992.
5. Iglehart JK: The American health care system: Managed care. N Engl J Med 327:742–745, 1992.
6. Iglehart JK: The American health care system: Medicare. N Engl J Med 327:1467–1472, 1992.
7. Waldo DR, Sonnefled ST, Lemieux JA, McKusick DR: Health spending through 2030: Three scenarios. Health Affairs (Millwood) 10(4):231–242, 1991.

2

Solo Practice

The key words describing the business of American medicine in the past two decades of the twentieth century are managed care, integration, and consolidation. The marketplace is characterized by competition among health plans, physician groups, and hospitals, all of which battle in the marketplace for covered lives. It is a marketplace in which patients will change their doctor, their hospital system, and their health plan to save less than $20 in premiums each month.

In this environment, why would any practitioner wish to provide care in a solo practice setting? The answer to this question is easy. In a solo private practice, physicians have an opportunity to build a practice that provides superior quality to patients and at the same time allows them the freedom to design a work environment compatible with their personal and family needs. Furthermore, the freedom to design one's own practice style, the challenge of building and marketing a practice, and the financial rewards of independent ownership continue to make the work fun and fulfilling.

This chapter provides some insight into the way I have grown my own private practice of medical oncology in Minneapolis since 1982. It describes some of the techniques that I have used to develop my medical practice, manage my business, market my services for growth, and integrate with other health care providers in the Minneapolis-St. Paul metropolitan area. Although these strategies are not the only "right" strategies, they have worked for me.

BUILDING A SOLO PRACTICE

PROVIDE HIGH-QUALITY CARE

To become a successful solo practitioner, the most important practice builder is to provide high-quality patient care. Quality of care has many meanings to different consumers of health care. In my practice it includes offering state of the-art standard care as well as cutting-edge oncology treatment options, patient advocacy, availability and accessibility, personalized care, continuity of care, and cost-effective care.

High-quality patient care must not only be state of the art but also provide patients and families with superior clinical outcome and personalized service. I use many strategies. For example, I keep up to date by reading the most important journals in my field. I demand of myself that I attend at least three oncologic conferences yearly. My favorite conferences address new ways to use old drugs or introduce me to new drugs or new drug combinations. My attendance at oncology meetings provides opportunities to introduce myself to nationally recognized academic oncologists who have special expertise with various diagnoses or treatment modalities. When a patient's situation is applicable, I often phone an expert for advice in patient management or refer outside the Minneapolis-St. Paul area for treatment not available locally.

I take advantage of my associations with various oncology study groups to gain access for my patients to investigational treatment modalities. The Minneapolis-St. Paul metropolitan area is fortunate to have a National Cancer Institute-sponsored Community Clinical Oncology Program with access to Eastern Cooperative Oncology Group and National Surgical Adjuvant Breast and Bowel Project protocols. In addition, the major health care systems, such as HealthSystem Minnesota and Allina, also have their own designated cancer centers, which may have local protocols or studies organized by drug companies.

This cutting-edge perspective allows me to offer a wider range of treatment options to my patients. Often the options that I offer may still be under study. Unfortunately, many oncology patients do not have the 5–10 years required to test the efficacy of a certain drug regimen or treatment strategy. They appreciate the opportunity to consider newer and perhaps more aggressive treatment regimens before we inevitably run out of the standard list of options. The fact that I attend conferences and provide cutting-edge treatment options in their fight against cancer boosts their confidence that all opportunities for improved quantity and quality of life are considered.

BE A PATIENT ADVOCATE

Delivery of care that is superior in outcome requires being an outspoken patient advocate. I make it a point to ensure that my patients get state-of-the-art care whether their insurance will pay for it or not. This often involves telephone calls to HMOs and letters to medical directors. It may require enlisting the assistance of an attorney to help my patients get what I believe is state-of-the-art and appropriate care. If my use of a drug or a therapeutic technique is questioned, I depend on my journal reading to point out a referenced publication that describes utilization of the drug or technique in a similar situation. Thus, despite the intervention of managed care in the physician–patient relationship,

HIRE THE RIGHT PEOPLE

The most important person in a solo d
was lucky enough to find an office ma
extremely caring but also an honest, lo
fectionist. Before working for me, she h
tal. Therefore, she was familiar with me
testing in both inpatient and outpatie
asked me to clarify her job description.
take care of the patients and her job w
this job description with enthusiasm a
tained her enthusiasm and evolved into

The job description of the office mar
not only in its length but also in the ne
all of its components. The difficulty o
constant busyness of an oncology office
the patients are often angry and confuse
have cared deteriorate and die on a regu

In a group practice, any one of th
office manager is responsible may be a f

1. Maintain patient accounts, send
review all reimbursements and adjust
third-party payors.

2. Identify office equipment and
appropriate products and services, and
ment working properly and supplies sto

3. Hire, train, schedule, and super

4. Review office expenses, write ou
and maintain the office checkbook.

5. Keep the office clean, welcoming

6. Maintain patient medical record

7. Open and distribute office mail.

8. Take, deliver, and file phone me

9. Interact with hospital, health pl
tient care.

10. Interact with hospital, health pl
policies and procedures.

11. Screen and schedule new patien
before the first visit.

12. Maintain and revise appointmen
conflicts and adequate time between ap

13. Schedule patients for admission
and office appointments.

my patients have rarely suffered financially or medically because of the limits of managed care.

BE AVAILABLE AND ACCESSIBLE

Availability and accessibility are reliable practice builders and obviously improve quality of care. I arrange to be available to my patients for routine follow-up by scheduling the next visit before the patient leaves the office. I rarely rely on a patient to contact me to make a routine follow-up appointment. I take calls for my practice seven days a week. I refer calls to another oncologist only when I leave town or for a special holiday or family event. My patients know that if they call me, they get me. They know that I am available by beeper within 10–30 minutes at all times. I carry a beeper with me nights and weekends, and I carry a phone on my person. I also have a phone in my car if I am away from my home or office. This often makes me more accessible than the patient's primary care physician. Frequently, primary care physicians practice in groups, and the person on call may not be the patient's primary physician. For this reason, patients often feel that they would rather contact me than the primary care doctor on call. Consequently, I am often the first doctor who is called when there is a problem, even if it is not related to oncology. This kind of availability and accessibility also helps in receiving referrals.

Although a diagnosis of cancer is rarely a medical emergency, it is frequently a psychological one. If requested by the patient or the referring doctor, I am usually able to see new patients within 24 hours. If this is not possible, I offer the patient the option of seeing another oncologist. I may lose a few patients, but the patient and the referring doctor are better served.

Although this kind of availability can interfere with family activities and personal life, I believe that my practice style allows me more freedom to accommodate my family's needs and expectations. I finish my office schedule each day at 3:30 PM to attend after school athletic events and to cook dinner most evenings. I routinely carve out time during the day to take my children to the orthodontist or to attend mother-child time at preschool. When my youngest child was an infant, I brought him to the office for six weeks to nurse him between blocks of scheduled office visits. Group practice usually cannot permit such flexibility and opportunity. This flexible practice style has positively affected my relationships with my family. I have been married for 27 years and have had the pleasure of raising four sons, who now range in age from 9 to 21.

BE PERSONABLE AND PROVIDE PERSONALIZED CARE

Personalized care is always a top priority. My patients appreciate that I know them personally. I know their medical diagnoses, the course of each patient's

disease, and what their recent treatmen
medical record the specifics of drug al
remember the significant aspects of m
to make each patient feel that I am inte
rather than as a diseased person. My fat
try to discuss something personal wit
may relate to family experiences, travel
the patient's chart, and the next time t
the daughter's wedding. I believe that
tients' lives provides an extra measure o

In addition to asking my patients a
verse with them about events in my ow
experiences on their baseball or basket
lege applications. Such conversations n
not previously available. Furthermore,
also with some of the same vulnerabilit
their confrontation with cancer.

BE COST-EFFECTIVE

As a solo practitioner, I can provide b
cost-effectiveness. Because I make dail
tients, they receive continuity of care
tween the hospital and outpatient car
history, and this knowledge helps in t
identifying tests that have already been
tion to testing that has not been done
This approach promotes cost-effectiven
possible if I were less familiar with my

MANAGING THE BUSINESS

Many physicians choose to avoid the b
going into group practice. One of the st
physicians can concentrate on medical
side of medicine. However, when group
tors demand more productivity and co
but be aware of the business side of m
medicine is the fun part, the adventure
and error. I have no business training, a
medicine rather naively. Fortunately, I h
port people who have the expertise nece

14. Interact with other business consultants, such as the accountant, lawyer, and insurance agents.

My accountant also helps me manage the business side of my practice. Although I initially worked with a mid-size accounting firm, I quickly learned that it was too large to provide me with personalized service. My accountant is also solo and has had considerable experience with the business of medicine in the Twin Cities. Besides her expertise in the realities of the medical marketplace and medical reimbursement issues, she also demonstrates other qualities on which I rely, including her demand for meticulous recordkeeping and accurate and timely filing of all employment and tax forms and payments. She reviews my cash flow and bank statements for accuracy and completeness on a scheduled basis. She interacts with my employees about their benefit plan options and assets. She advises me about hiring and salary issues. Her attention to detail and expertise in issues of running a small corporation, taxation, and business practices give me confidence in knowing that I am complying with all regulatory requirements. As a solo accountant, she is accessible to me in the day and in the evening and provides continuity of service.

The roster of my support staff also includes two or three part-time receptionists and bookkeepers. I have found that part-time employees make a lot of sense in a small office. We can increase or decrease hours as demanded by the patient schedule. In addition, we can reorganize the schedule to allow for vacations, illnesses, and school holidays. Many of my part-time employees are mothers with school-age children who appreciate a 9 to 3 schedule 3 or 4 days per week. This schedule allows them to get their children off to school and be at home upon their return. Furthermore, to keep my office running smoothly, I encourage my employees to bring their children with minor illnesses to the office. We can usually find a place for them to read, color, or play away from patients. Consequently, an employee can come to work and still be available to her child. This approach improves efficiency in the office and is a benefit that increases employee loyalty.

PAY ATTENTION TO NUMBERS AND DETAILS

Despite my reliance on the honest efficiency and common sense of my office manager, the meticulousness of my accountant, and the loyalty of all my employees, I am not excused from the continuous and detailed monitoring of the business of my practice. I review selected explanation of benefit forms and try to stay current with various payor reimbursement issues. I analyze patient billings, receipts, and adjustments on a monthly basis. I am solely responsible for signing checks. I am constantly challenging my office manager to keep expenses down and the cash flow accurate and timely. We have been successful in that our accounts receivable are often less than 45 days and our expenses over the past five years have averaged 48% of receipts (excluding my personal salary and benefits). Few large groups or integrated health care networks can duplicate these numbers. In addition, average billings have increased 65% over the past five years, although fees have increased by only 17%.

MAKE GOOD DECISIONS BASED ON QUALITY AND COST

When I opened my practice, I made an economic decision not to give chemotherapy in my office. I did not want to spend the money required to develop a state-of-the-art facility and to keep cash tied up in inventory. Furthermore, I did not want to be responsible for paying a full-time oncology nurse when I am in the office only half of the work week. Because chemotherapy should be given only with a physician in the office, a full-time nurse would be underutilized. Finally, even in 1982, reimbursement for drugs and chemotherapy administration expenses in the Twin Cities managed care marketplace was not adequate to justify the investment in a nurse, treatment facility, drugs, and supplies. However, as the number of my patients increased, more time was required to discuss the nature of their illness, adjustment to its debilities, and treatment options. I recognized that a warm, caring, and approachable nurse would increase access to care and improve personalization. Therefore, I hired a nurse in 1991. Although she performs a few nursing tasks in the office, such as Port-o-cath flushes, laboratory draws, and selected injections, most of her time is unscheduled. She returns phone calls and spends her time in the office answering questions and reviewing treatment options and medication schedules. Patients often relate concerns to her that they believe are not important enough for the doctor's attention. Thus, my nurse increases communication and improves the personalized care that my patients receive.

As the need for oncology services grows, I expect that my nurse will help me to see more patients. She is currently enrolled in a program to become a nurse practitioner. After completion and licensure, she will be able to see patients independently, thereby increasing my ability to care for more patients.

All employees who have worked for me the requisite time get benefits, such as pension, profit sharing, and medical expense reimbursement, commensurate with their hours of employment. Although in the short term such benefits increase my overhead, in the long term they help me to keep the loyalty and expertise of my employees. Ultimately, the low turnover of employees in my office and good employee morale make my office a desirable place to work.

Other resources for business advice and products are lawyers and insurance agents. My lawyers are extremely useful and savvy when it comes to the business of running my practice. The one exception is that I have not asked my lawyers to review health plan documents (which are generic for all doctors in my marketplace). Because large multispecialty and single-specialty groups have been unsuccessful in getting changes in their contracts, it makes no sense for me to spend money on legal fees with little chance for improved access, market-share, or reimbursement.

Insurance agents are also knowledgeable and helpful when I confront myriad insurance issues. When getting a quotation for business insurance, I usually contact at least two agencies. Sometimes I have asked each agent to critique the opposing offer. This approach helps to identify subtle differences in service and cost that otherwise I may miss. As in the case of my accountant, I usually favor solo attorneys and insurance agents from small offices, who usually provide better access and more personalized service.

MARKETING FOR GROWTH

Providing the best quality of care and organizing a well-run business do not guarantee success without efforts to gain access to the market and to promote growth of business. Every activity that I perform is a marketing activity. To practice medicine, one must have access to patients. Solo specialists should enroll in all available health plans and payor networks. I am fortunate to provide a needed set of services in my marketplace. As the population ages and more cancers are diagnosed, the need for oncology care rises. Many primary care physicians do not have the expertise or willingness to provide ongoing care to oncology patients. Thus, my niche in the marketplace will continue to grow. With appropriate credentials and a track record of high-quality, cost-effective service, specialists in the Twin Cities marketplace have not been excluded from health plan networks. In fact, as physicians group themselves into care systems that contract directly with employers, physicians with established referral bases and hospital associations will be able to participate across a broader range of care plans.

Because every activity is a marketing activity, all interactions with patients, families, other doctors, and health plan administrators should be considered an opportunity to prove oneself a competent, caring, and compulsive provider of health care. Looking the part has much to do with playing the role. Therefore, I wear clothes that add brightness and color to my patients' days and reinforce a businesslike approach to the complexity and seriousness of their condition. I market myself to my referring physicians with frequent and timely verbal and written communications. My accessibility and availability make it easy for primary care doctors, emergency physicians, and other specialists to curbside me with a concern or a question in the hospital corridor or by phone in the evening or on weekends. If they decide that a particular patient problem does not require my services, they may remember me the next time one of their patients needs oncology care.

INTEGRATING WITH THE MEDICAL MARKETPLACE

Integrating with the medical marketplace can be used by the solo practitioner to improve the quality of care provided and to guarantee access to the market.

Despite being independent, solo practitioners must use various strategies to integrate their practice patterns with other practices and with health plans, hospitals, and other medical organizations. Solo practitioners can easily become isolated from colleagues in the same specialty as the practice of medicine becomes more outpatient- and office-based. I guard against this by presenting interesting and more difficult cases at local hospital cancer conferences and by attending national meetings. I discuss case management with other providers participating in patient care, and I enter patients in protocol studies.

To gain access to patients, I have enrolled in all available provider panels for health plans, HMOs, PPOs, and care systems. I have made it a policy to sign on to all available third-party payor programs, regardless of the reimbursement. I do not want a referring physician to have to think twice about which insurances I take. Once the patient is in my practice and we have developed a rapport, he or she generally continues to select a health plan for which I am listed as a provider.

Although most health plans continue either to cut reimbursement or to reduce the rate of inflation on fees, growth of one's expertise, reputation, and bottom line depends on accessing more patients. Because most of my expenses are already fixed, adding patients generally does not affect my overhead significantly. As long as I can take good care of the patients already in my practice, I continue to take new patients from all available third-party payors. Because I do not give chemotherapy in the office the overhead of seeing a patient is related to rent and employee salaries. Any open space in my schedule should be filled with patient visits because the reimbursement only adds to the bottom line once my overhead has been paid.

Integration with the health care delivery system also means participation in the governance of relevant organizations. Involvement on committees gives me first-hand information about issues that may affect my practice and a voice in policy development, despite the fact that my voice may be overshadowed by more powerful constituencies. Finally, my presence reminds health plan administrators, community board members, and other physicians that solo independent physicians can integrate with care delivery systems, take good care of patients, and develop thriving practices despite managed care, consolidation, and integration.

Over the past 10 years, I have served on various hospital committees and have been an active member on two foundation boards of directors (the Methodist Hospital Foundation and the Minnesota Medical Foundation), a health plan board (Medica), a health system board (HealthSystem Minnesota), and a medical malpractice insurance company board (Midwest Medical Insurance Company). These experiences have enabled me to develop a sophisticated and comprehensive view of how the various aspects of the business of medicine affect the way in which I practice oncology and run my business. As the chief executive officer of my corporation, I am reminded that the only real

of the financing of health care through large managed care contracts, and the relative stability offered by larger organizations. Like the larger single-specialty groups, some multispecialty groups have been acquired by for-profit, publicly traded PPMCs. Some groups also have affiliated with nonprofit health care organizations. Most multispecialty groups are organized as professional corporations or partnerships.

PHYSICIAN–HOSPITAL ORGANIZATION

Physician–hospital organizations (PHOs) are corporations structured to include physicians and hospitals as members. PHOs are usually structured as professional corporations separate and distinct from the related organizations of the hospital and physician members. The organization is designed to represent both parties in key insurance company negotiations and contracts. Governance of the PHO usually includes representation from both entities and is often structured so that each has equal board representation. Hospitals have been especially interested in the development of PHOs as a mechanism to link physicians to their organizations. Some physicians view PHOs as a mechanism to access contracts and capital as well as to align their interests with those of hospitals in their marketplace. PHOs have grown rapidly throughout the United States, given the increased complexity of the marketplace and subsequent need to gain leverage with third-party payor negotiations. With their growth have come a few significant challenges, including the difficulty of aligning incentives for hospitals and physicians, which usually manifests itself in the distribution of funds from capitated contracts. The distribution of "capitated" funds among organizational entities may be complex and highly charged as participating members divide a fixed pool of dollars.

MANAGEMENT SERVICE ORGANIZATIONS

Management service organizations (MSOs) are relatively new structures developed to support practicing physicians. An MSO is generally not an organization that requires physician membership. MSOs are best described as service organizations that are compensated for the provision of management expertise. Some MSO models, however, offer physicians equity or "ownership" of the company. Usually operated by hospitals or large corporations, an MSO offers management services targeted in two areas—general practice operations and managed care. A physician may contract with an MSO to oversee day-to-day operations. In such cases, the MSO usually hires all of the practice staff, provides billing services, and supports contracted physicians with the transition from fee-for-service operations to managed care. MSOs have propagated rapidly but are in too early a stage of development to prove their full value. Their legal constitution is variable and usually depends on the founding organization's legal structure.

NETWORKS AND INTEGRATED DELIVERY SYSTEMS

Increased competition and the growth of managed care have combined to create fertile ground for the development of physician networks. Also relatively new to the market, networks take advantage of consolidation and leverage to drive competitive payor contract terms. Networks may include members representing a number of organizational models, linked together by exclusive contracting agreements. In some cases, networks are linked to hospital systems to create an integrated delivery system (IDS). As with other new organizational models, it is too soon to comment on the effectiveness of provider networks and integrated systems.

EMPLOYMENT

The final practice option is the employment model. Hospitals and corporations may employ physicians if they are not limited by laws governing the corporate practice of medicine. The presence of such legislation is unique to each state and will dictate whether this option is available in a given geographical region.

As an employee, the physician is generally salaried and receives compensation from the corporation. Although considered restrictive by some, the employment model may be less risky than other models and provide a modicum of protection from a dynamic marketplace. Employment usually includes established working hours and defined productivity expectations. Physicians are legally employees of the corporation and cannot access the potential benefits of incorporation or partnership.

EVALUATION OF ORGANIZATIONAL MODELS

Comprehensive evaluation of the organizational models available to physicians is a critical step in the decision-making process. Several key factors are recommended for review in considering options. Although these factors vary in importance among individuals, a review at least should include an understanding of compensation principles, ownership options, exposure to risk, culture, lifestyle, productivity requirements, and participation expectations, such as exclusivity, degree of autonomy, and ease of exit. Although this list is far from exhaustive, it gives the reader a sense of the variability of the models. Figure 1 demonstrates the level of variability of the models.

LEGAL CONSIDERATIONS

With the many choices of organizational models come various legal issues and considerations. Solo practitioners must decide whether they should incorporate

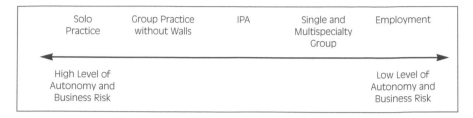

FIGURE 1. The relationship of organizational models to the potential for member autonomy and exposure to business risk.

or maintain their sole proprietor status. Group practices may take the form of partnerships or professional corporations, each with its own set of benefits and limitations. The legal options available to a practicing physician mirror the growth and complexity of the many organizational options discussed herein. Clearly, legal structure affects many key areas (e.g., taxation, protection from liability exposure, pension options, shareholder equity). New and currently practicing physicians must take time to understand the implications of these important options. In most cases, understanding is best accomplished with the help of retained legal counsel. Table 2 outlines some of the key characteristics of the models reviewed, including exclusivity requirements, potential for equity sharing, and customary degrees of business integration.

RECOMMENDATIONS

The decision to launch a new practice or join an existing group or health care delivery organization is a significant step for most physicians. As with other

TABLE 2.   Key Attributes of Various Models

Model	Required Exclusivity	Potential to Hold Equity	Business Integration
Solo practice		X	
Group practice without walls		X	X
Independent practice association	X*	X	
Single specialty group	X	X	X
Multispecialty group	X	X	X
Physician–hospital organization	X*		
Management service organization	X*	X*	X
Networks and integrated delivery systems	X		
Employment	X		X

* May be optional.

TABLE 3.   Key Evaluation Criteria

---

1. Complete a personal inventory of your interests and rank them in order. It is vitally important to understand where your professional life will sit in relation to other important factors such as family and other interests.

2. Talk with other physicians involved in various practice models. There is no substitute for hearing the benefits and drawbacks of the available models from those involved with them. It is usually best to talk to practitioners who are not involved with the organization that you are interested in joining. Objectivity is improved if there is no relation between the two.

3. If you plan to join an existing organization, request a copy of their bylaws, financial statements, and a sample contract. Each of these documents is important in the evaluation of the organization and the limitations imposed on new participants.

4. Check out the competition. If you are joining a group or entering solo practice, your ability to build a practice may depend on the level of competition.

5. Ask for the appropriate help from professionals. This is not the time to skimp on good counsel. A good accountant and attorney can assist with decision-making. Costs can be kept to a minimum if you set billing limits clearly.

---

critical decisions, the appropriate evaluation of individual desires, goals, and interests is an important first step. Furthermore, spending the time to do a comprehensive evaluation of the available options will result in a more informed decision and hopefully reduce the likelihood of dissatisfaction. Table 3 outlines some of the key evaluation criteria recommended to support a decision of such magnitude. A comprehensive and honest review of these and other important criteria will greatly improve the probability of a good match and long-term professional satisfaction.

REFERENCES

1. Boland P: The role of reengineering in health care delivery. Managed Care Q 4(4):1–11, 1996.
2. Cochrane J, Miller J: Integrated healthcare report. Health Care Megatrends, Dec 1996/Jan 1997:12–15, 1997.
3. Mehn J, Riefberg V, Russi E, Wanfried C: 1996 Health Care Annual Issues and Comparative Payor Performance Data. New York, McKinsey & Co., 1997.
4. Shenkin K: Models of managed care: The potential power of the IPA. Managed Care Q 4(4):68–74, 1996.

4

How to Find the Perfect Job
What You Need to Know before, during, and after the Interview

Looking for a job can be exciting and challenging. It can also be emotionally and financially draining. Television shows such as *ER* and *Chicago Hope* portray doctors working in glamorous settings with plenty of heroism, money, and time off to play. Real-life doctors know that the glamorous and heroic moments are few and far between, the financial rewards are decreasing, and time off to relax is often spent sleeping after long hours in the hospital or office. Despite these obstacles, the medical profession can still be economically and emotionally rewarding. The trick is finding a job that is right for you.

Most physicians find themselves looking for a job at a time when they are extraordinarily busy. Whether you are finishing a residency or are already in practice, the effort of searching for a new job coupled with ongoing personal and professional responsibilities can be overwhelming. This chapter describes five steps needed to complete a successful job search:

Step 1: Developing a strategic plan
Step 2: Starting the search
Step 3: Acing the interviews
Step 4: Closing the deal
Step 5: Preparing to start a new job

STEP 1: DEVELOPING A STRATEGIC PLAN

Successful businesses begin with a development of a cohesive and comprehensive strategic plan. Similarly, successful job searches begin with developing an individualized strategic plan. The type of position you are seeking will greatly influence what should be considered in the plan. The first consideration is matching your skills and interests with a potential job opportunity. There are multiple variables to consider in selecting opportunities that best suit your present and future career goals. Examples include geography, hobbies, cultural interests, location of family and friends, potential to grow professionally, and financial opportunities.

GEOGRAPHIC AND SALARY CONSIDERATIONS

Begin developing your strategic plan by narrowing your choices. Considering geographic location and salary expectations is a good place to start. Immediately eliminate geographic areas in which you would not consider living or practicing. Avoiding expenditures of unnecessary time and money on potential job opportunities that you are not likely to consider seriously allows you to focus on potential job opportunities that are more appealing. Keep in mind that spending an initial investment of time on a focused strategic plan will make it easier for you to maintain your current level of personal and professional obligations while looking for a new position.

Geographic considerations are frequently influenced by factors such as location of family members, weather, proximity to recreational areas, religious and cultural values, and educational opportunities for yourself or family members. Geographic choices are also influenced by the type of environment in which you wish to practice. Deciding whether you want to practice in an urban, rural, or suburban environment certainly will affect your geographic choices. You also may want to consider your area of medical expertise as it relates to the geographic area in which you choose to practice.

When you have narrowed your search geographically, next focus on salary and compensation issues. Salary considerations are critical in nearly every job search and generally depend on three factors: geographic location, medical specialty, and number of years in practice. Salary is also influenced by the type of practice setting and whether the responsibilities are strictly clinical or involve academics. Tables 1 and 2 reflect current tends for physician salaries.[16]

Typically, rural practice opportunities such as those located in federally designated Health Professional Shortage Areas (HPSAs) offer physicians loan forgiveness in an attempt to improve the distribution of physicians, particularly those practicing primary care. These opportunities may be attractive because of monetary incentives and the opportunity to be autonomous. Rural hospitals are often quite generous in offering recruitment incentives. A rural setting may be appealing for a physician with extensive loans, limited family ties to a specific geographic region, or those seeking sponsorship. Disadvantages to considering rural opportunities include possible professional isolation, limited support services, excessive work loads, lack of social or cultural activities, and limited back-up support from other physicians.

The 1990s' emphasis on cost containment strategies, telemedicine, and the reengineering of free-standing hospitals into health care systems have helped

TABLE 1. Physician Compensation by Years in Specialty

Specialty	1–2 yr		3–7 yr		8–17 yr		18 yr +	
	No.	Median	No.	Median	No.	Median	No.	Median
Allergy/immunology	5	*	43	152,332	36	183,891	46	189,904
Anesthesiology	47	175,000	307	213,128	423	249,500	208	238,200
Cardiology: invasive/ interventional	53	241,465	173	344,919	312	385,707	171	380,361
Cardiology: noninvasive	26	182,087	116	229,002	138	272,116	119	244,800
Critical care	2	*	10	174,395	14	201,539	11	146,496
Dentistry	2	*	3	*	8	*	8	*
Dermatology	22	150,119	68	171,432	88	194,385	86	196,754
Emergency medicine	41	160,440	161	180,000	175	180,000	88	187,986
Endocrinology/ metabolism	3	*	27	143,440	51	158,410	40	150,470
Family practice (with OB)	108	110,312	257	126,417	441	140,000	250	138,649
Family practice (without OB)	174	110,100	461	123,500	827	137,922	604	135,668
Gastroenterology	21	183,567	125	206,013	190	242,249	116	220,069
Geriatrics	1	*	2	*	6	*	6	*
Gynecology (only)	3	*	8	*	15	150,350	45	161,263
Hematology/oncology	22	150,000	71	179,600	133	200,00	111	202,408
Infectious disease	1	*	25	152,404	44	147,259	18	153,800
Internal medicine	277	118,647	722	134,030	1026	148,050	677	152,765
Maternal and fetal medicine	3	*	5	*	11	300,000	5	*
Neonatal medicine	*	*	11	181,229	25	195,000	14	210,369
Nephrology	12	132,149	41	179,019	73	212,158	79	196,500
Neurology	28	132,418	89	158,979	125	161,648	114	159,627
Nuclear medicine	1	*	5	*	5	*	10	194,261
Obstetrics/gynecology	110	171,602	322	209,468	441	231,000	282	232,630
Occupational medicine	10	132,597	20	144,000	42	144,784	17	142,134
Ophthalmology	29	128,350	157	195,314	179	221,420	171	215,766
Ophthalmology: pediatric	1	*	4	*	6	*	9	*
Ophthalmology: retinal	6	*	15	229,540	16	388,078	12	464,992
Otorhinolaryngology	33	162,913	80	202,139	141	235,502	115	239,870
Pathology: anatomic	6	*	16	157,461	38	183,459	40	226,826
Pathology: clinical	5	*	25	154,312	36	193,178	29	212,930
Pediatric cardiology	6	*	5	*	6	*	4	*
Pediatric critical care	0	*	4	*	4	*	2	*
Pediatric gastroenterology	1	*	8	*	5	*	6	*
Pediatric hematology/ oncology	1	*	1	*	4	*	4	*
Pediatric neurology	0	*	3	*	4	*	2	*
Pediatrics	108	104,383	365	126,532	479	142,900	437	148,625
Physical medicine	20	129,777	61	149,715	56	155,832	15	150,000
Podiatry	7	*	16	98,823	31	130,131	11	140,000
Psychiatry	46	123,069	104	140,562	102	149,842	53	150,000
Pulmonary disease	16	132,901	72	157,082	112	178,098	64	173,561
Radiation oncology	4	*	16	272,950	22	312,460	11	275,000

(Table continued on following page.)

TABLE 1. Physician Compensation by Years in Specialty *(Continued)*

Specialty	1–2 yr		3–7 yr		8–17 yr		18 yr +	
	No.	Median	No.	Median	No.	Median	No.	Median
Radiation: diagnostic (invasive/interventional)	14	213,750	63	240,000	101	275,000	51	275,066
Radiation: diagnostic (noninvasive)	18	175,527	99	232,000	154	269,236	174	274,100
Reproductive endocrinology	1	*	6	*	4	*	4	*
Rheumatology	9	*	33	140,929	64	144,739	40	156,149
Sports medicine	1	*	2	*	7	*	1	*
Sports medicine: surgical	3	*	4	*	9	*	4	*
Surgery: cardiovascular	8	*	39	366,609	55	606,052	38	580,177
Surgery: colon & rectal	1	*	4	*	13	274,741	9	*
Surgery: general	42	178,824	171	199,293	277	238,370	273	222,116
Surgery: hand	1	*	12	263,000	20	253,263	14	289,067
Surgery: neurologic	20	288,334	42	385,399	58	361,919	69	394,473
Surgery: oral	1	*	3	*	4	*	5	*
Surgery: orthopedic	77	206,682	262	297,756	409	349,399	367	300,000
Surgery: orthopedic (foot & ankle)	0	*	5	*	3	*	2	*
Surgery: orthopedic (joint replacement)	2	*	10	454,242	9	*	8	*
Surgery: orthopedic (spine)	6	*	27	409,693	17	449,641	5	*
Surgery: pediatric	2	*	4	*	4	*	3	*
Surgery: plastic	8	*	34	219,802	26	229,497	21	300,000
Surgery: vascular/thoracic	13	217,709	38	289,506	80	338,224	55	353,631
Urology	24	157,460	99	204,447	143	224,658	175	227,580

Notes: Compensation, based on 1996 data, is reported by the number of years in specialty. The count for years in specialty begins at the time the provider completes the latter of residency or fellowship. No. indicates number of providers; median salary in dollars. An asterisk indicates that data are suppressed when the number of provider responses is less than 10 or the number of medical practice responses is less than 3. Data for academic faculty are excluded. (Reprinted with permission from the Medical Group Management Association, Englewood, CO, 1997.)

to facilitate relationships between rural hospitals and physicians who are seeking ties with colleagues, networks, and other hospitals. Such developments make rural practice more palatable.

Regardless of where you choose to practice, spending some time initially to narrow your choices will enable you to concentrate on specific job opportunities that are most appealing to you professionally and personally.

SELECTING THE IDEAL PRACTICE SETTING

Deciding which setting suits your personality and professional aspirations will also help to narrow the job search process. You need to consider whether you want to be a clinician, administrator, or academician. Some opportunities will include a combination of these activities. Next, consider whether you want to

TABLE 2. Physician Compensation by Geographic Section

Specialty	Eastern No.	Eastern Median	Midwest No.	Midwest Median	Southern No.	Southern Median	Western No.	Western Median
Allergy/immunology	25	195,000	44	162,995	37	184,518	60	155,841
Anesthesiology	237	228,500	242	282,730	399	273,850	469	217,245
Cardiology: invasive/ interventional	123	277,000	359	378,000	263	404,486	170	288,224
Cardiology: noninvasive	112	244,014	98	279,258	166	281,759	102	191,798
Critical care	4	*	11	142,000	5	*	24	182,517
Dentistry	16	91,275	1	*	6	*	1	*
Dermatology	39	196,029	90	180,190	66	200,807	135	175,786
Emergency medicine	98	153,783	147	172,091	98	200,000	239	182,947
Endocrinology/ metabolism	30	145,250	38	154,137	57	167,784	41	149,166
Family practice (with OD)	98	121,571	836	136,014	135	156,067	279	126,824
Family practice (without OB)	429	120,319	829	127,330	672	148,883	788	132,297
Gastroenterology	99	200,660	178	246,326	131	260,080	182	204,658
Geriatrics	2	*	16	121,469	1	*	8	*
Gynecology (only)	17	197,000	19	138,099	30	194,175	28	151,227
Hematology/oncology	80	179,119	105	192,300	90	243,413	133	178,662
Infectious disease	17	140,600	44	155,675	29	146,585	27	152,420
Internal medicine	560	138,894	1035	137,237	727	145,370	1163	137,867
Maternal and fetal medicine	*	*	7	*	8	*	21	285,002
Neonatal medicine	4	*	31	190,750	9	*	28	209,976
Nephrology	44	237,042	82	196,500	62	237,680	49	173,000
Neurology	71	156,000	157	160,000	101	170,000	89	157,616
Nuclear medicine	1	*	1	*	9	*	14	185,895
Obstetrics/gynecology	218	210,307	439	223,255	275	251,054	444	204,355
Occupational medicine	9	*	39	138,718	15	165,645	39	144,000
Ophthalmology	109	231,892	164	248,376	175	206,000	161	190,021
Ophthalmology: pediatric	4	*	2	*	15	252,640	*	*
Ophthalmology: retinal	11	262,000	13	423,000	18	416,981	7	*
Otorhinolaryngology	72	241,226	146	250,000	111	240,000	113	195,000
Pathology: anatomic	37	173,466	15	175,006	8	*	46	240,200
Pathology: clinical	9	*	34	197,583	30	201,500	43	163,398
Pediatric cardiology	3	*	8	*	8	*	8	*
Pediatric critical care	4	*	2	*	5	*	4	*
Pediatric gastroenterology	5	*	3	*	3	*	12	174,664
Pediatric hematology/ oncology	4	*	4	*	3	*	2	*
Pediatric neurology	3	*	9	*	3	*	1	*
Pediatrics	259	128,177	490	133,623	356	133,600	704	132,000
Physical medicine	20	149,684	40	168,387	15	176,938	101	144,004
Podiatry	9	*	41	107,117	20	118,442	18	127,750
Psychiatry	41	127,500	115	135,000	51	134,000	130	144,647
Pulmonary disease	58	152,750	86	173,322	107	188,600	108	160,962
Radiation oncology	17	231,628	35	292,164	18	433,699	10	300,000

(Table continued on following page.)

TABLE 2. Physician Compensation by Geographic Section *(Continued)*

Specialty	Eastern No.	Eastern Median	Midwest No.	Midwest Median	Southern No.	Southern Median	Western No.	Western Median
Radiation: diagnostic (in-vasive/interventional)	39	252,196	92	291,504	68	255,424	88	232,250
Radiation: diagnostic (noninvasive)	86	256,250	167	310,708	99	274,800	192	233,286
Reproductive endocrinology	8	*	2	*	2	*	5	*
Rheumatology	29	130,000	50	147,942	55	155,600	66	131,143
Sports medicine	*	*	8	*	2	*	4	*
Sports medicine: surgical	6	*	8	*	6	*	3	*
Surgery: cardiovascular	48	607,502	48	501,883	58	618,517	26	385,680
Surgery: colon & rectal	8	*	6	*	10	237,650	10	192,486
Surgery: general	164	215,396	302	221,756	247	263,604	205	197,089
Surgery: hand	7	*	20	290,882	18	561,320	20	224,548
Surgery: neurologic	35	371,613	77	357,430	50	408,500	41	318,904
Surgery: oral	7	*	3	*	6	*	2	*
Surgery: orthopedic	330	315,582	355	334,534	290	316,000	345	279,027
Surgery: orthopedic (foot & ankle)	7	*	4	*	*	*	3	*
Surgery: orthopedic (joint replacement)	15	394,848	11	670,289	6	*	6	*
Surgery: orthopedic (spine)	27	371,634	24	556,168	13	310,600	4	*
Surgery: pediatric	6	*	5	*	5	*	4	*
Surgery: plastic	13	232,881	20	250,403	39	262,759	31	216,962
Surgery: vascular/thoracic	65	367,286	39	294,556	62	373,509	38	237,525
Urology	84	221,342	168	235,377	143	254,163	139	197,340

Notes: No. indicates number of providers; median salary in dollars. An asterisk indicates that data are suppressed when the number of provider responses is less than 10 or the number of medical practice responses is less than 3. Data for academic faculty are excluded. *Eastern Section*: CT, DC, DE, MA, MD, ME, NC, NH, NJ, NY, PA, RI, VA, VT, and WV. *Midwest Section:* IA, IL, IN, MI, MN, ND, NE, OH, SD, and WI. *Southern Section:* AL, AR, FL, GA, KS, KY, LA, MO, MS, OK, SC, TN, and TX. *Western Section:* AK, AZ, CA, CO, HI, ID, MT, NM, NV, OR, UT, WA, and WY. (Reprinted with permission from the Medical Group Management Association, Englewood, CO, 1997.)

be a solo practitioner, join a group practice, become an employee of a hospital, join a physician's organization, or pursue some other option.

If you want to combine clinical excellence with academics, identify centers highly rated in your field of expertise by peer organizations or professional journals. Centers that have attained the designation of "center of excellence" are identified by reports such as the entire issue of *U.S. News & World Report* [25] devoted to ranking the leading hospital departments across the country by specialty area. Other resources for this information include the American Medical Association, the American Hospital Association, the Joint Commission for Hospital Accreditation, and residency/fellowship training programs. Positions at centers that are nationally recognized for their excellence are generally highly competitive. However, they often afford excellent career opportunities and should be considered if this type of practice setting appeals to you.

Academic positions generally include components of teaching and research. Often such positions can be combined with clinical responsibilities. Some academic programs place limits on direct and indirect compensation to ensure that physicians maintain a focus on teaching and research. Miller et al. surveyed program directors about the career status of residents who completed graduate education training programs in selected specialties and subspecialties during the 1993–1994 academic year.[18] This study reported wide variation among specialties in the percentage of graduates pursuing academic versus clinical positions; however, a higher percentage of residents in all of the internal medicine subspecialties, emergency medicine, pathology, psychiatry, and plastic surgery pursued academic careers (Tables 3 and 4).

TABLE 3. Distribution of Career Status of Residents Potentially Seeking a Professional Position

Specialty and Subspecialty*	% Full-time Clinical Positions (% Difficulty)[†]	% Academic Positions
Core specialties		
Family practice (n = 1598)	79.6 (1.2)	6.4
Internal medicine (n = 1595)	63.6 (3.2)	14.4
Pediatrics (n = 944)	68.2 (2.0)	12.1
Obstetrics and gynecology (n = 765)	84.1 (1.9)	10.2
Surgery—general (n = 318)	71.1 (4.9)	17.9
Psychiatry (n = 449)	50.3 (2.2)	27.2
Hospital-based specialties		
Anesthesiology (n = 908)	73.8 (25.5)	17.5
Radiology—diagnostic (n = 192)	69.3 (8.3)	18.2
Pathology (n = 231)	55.0 (8.7)	29.9
Emergency medicine (n = 509)	68.2 (2.9)	25.5
Surgical subspecialties		
Ophthalmology (n = 169)	85.8 (12.4)	5.9
Orthopedic surgery (n =135)	88.9 (5.0)	5.9
Otolaryngology (n = 133)	77.4 (3.9)	15.8
Plastic surgery (n = 101)	71.3 (20.8)	22.8
Urology (n = 138)	87.0 (6.7)	12.3
Internal medicine subspecialties		
Cardiovascular disease (n = 391)	70.1 (12.4)	24.0
Critical care medicine (n = 165)	58.2 (11.5)	36.4
Endocrinology, diabetes, metabolism (n = 97)	56.7 (16.4)	35.1
Gastroenterology (n = 300)	72.7 (21.1)	22.3
Hematology (n = 120)	60.8 (6.8)	30.8
Infectious disease (n = 185)	41.6 (14.3)	45.4
Oncology (n = 157)	40.8 (7.8)	47.1
Nephrology (n = 152)	61.8 (3.2)	25.7
Pulmonary disease (n = 178)	56.7 (6.9)	36.5
Rheumatology (n = 109)	69.7 (13.2)	22.9
Geriatric medicine (n = 65)	36.9 (8.3)	53.8
Total (n = 10,104)	69.4 (6.9)	17.1

* Number of residents seeking professional positions.
[†] Percentage having difficulty finding their full-time practice position.
From Miller et al: Initial employment status of physicians. JAMA 275:708–712, 1996, with permission.

concentrated on the regional (40.3%), national (32.6%), or local (22.5%) levels.[8] Networks are poised to service a large number of patients and to obtain managed care, indemnity, and capitation contracts. Such resources can greatly enhance your ability to practice in a given setting.

Regardless of whether you are considering an opportunity that is part of a larger network, you will likely need access to other medical services such as laboratory, radiology, physical therapy, surgical suite, and pharmacy. Try and assess how easy it will be for you to access support services and to provide a continuum of care for your patients. If these services are not readily available, this will probably affect your ability to obtain referrals and build your practice.

HOW MEDICAL TRAINING AND RESIDENCY PROGRAMS INFLUENCE AVAILABLE POSITIONS

Both the geographic location and the practice setting you choose may reflect the type of medical training you pursued in the past. Medical training programs respond to changing characteristics of physician supply and demand, which are influenced by factors such as managed care and health care reform initiatives.

Accreditation Alert, a publication targeted for residency training programs, studied the changes in resident complements within 26 graduate medical education specialties between 1992 and 1995.[1] This study suggested that a significant decrease in the number of residency training slots is a response to an anticipated decrease in physician demand within the marketplace. Marked decreases were noted in non-primary care specialties, including neurology, dermatology, nuclear medicine, allergy and immunology, anesthesiology, colon and rectal surgery, radiation oncology, and orthopedic surgery. Other surveys, such as the Medical Group Management Association (MGMA) survey in 1997, reported salary decreases in anesthesiology, neurology, ophthalmology, psychiatry, and pulmonary disease that correspond with an oversupply of these specialists.[16]

If you trained in a medical specialty that is currently in oversupply and have been unsuccessful in acquiring the type of practice setting and location you desire, consider options such as expanding your geographic scope, accepting a position that includes your specialty and primary care responsibilities, seeking additional training, and accepting a locum tenens position or a temporary position until you find a more appealing opportunity.

Within the specialties studied by *Accreditation Alert*, primary care specialties (including obstetrics and gynecology and pediatrics) experienced no significant change in the number of residents trained. This finding goes along with a national trend to achieve an improved balance between primary care physicians and specialists.

Conversely, an increase in residency training slots corresponds with an increase in demand in the marketplace. According to the *Accreditation Alert* study, an increase in the number of residency training slots was noted in emergency medicine, family practice, neurosurgery, physical medicine and rehabilitation, internal medicine, otolaryngology, pathology, and thoracic surgery.[1] Cejka & Company also reported a continued emphasis in hospital positions for internal medicine, family practice, pediatrics, obstetrics and gynecology, psychiatry, orthopedics, and emergency medicine.[8] Recent MGMA annual surveys noted that specialties with continued growth in median compensation include primary care, gastroenterology, psychiatry, and urology. Training in a specialty that is currently in high demand allows greater opportunity to choose a practice setting and location.

Changes in legislation can affect the income of physicians. The recent enactment of the Balanced Budget Act of 1997 (Public Law 105-33) provides a mechanism for a balanced federal budget for the first time in 28 years. The act will decrease the amount of federal dollars spent on Medicare and Medicaid beneficiaries and graduate medical education. The reduction in spending negatively affects the income of physicians, hospitals, and other health care providers. The projected cuts over a five-year period will result in a decrease in income by a total of $5.3 billion for physicians and $48 billion for hospitals. The income decrease for hospitals will limit the support and collaborative efforts with physicians in the development and implementation of patient care services. The Federal Register suggests greater impact on the surgical specialties and lesser impact on primary care specialties.[11]

THE APPLICATION PROCESS

Once you have decided on a practice setting and location, you need to prepare your curriculum vitae and cover letter. This is a critical part of the process and may be your first and only introduction to a potential employer. The old adage, "Make the first impression count," is meaningful advice because you are likely to be one of many candidates applying for any given position.

Developing your cover letters early is essential if you are to respond quickly to an advertised job opening. Ideally, you should prepare several different cover letters that reflect differences in practice setting (i.e., hospital vs. private practice or academic vs. clinical position) and geographic location. Keep in mind that the goal of the cover letter is to introduce the reader to you. This is your first attempt to create a positive impression. Include in the first paragraph how you found out about the job opening (e.g., journal, conference, job posting, Internet). If you were referred by someone in particular, it may be helpful to mention his or her support in the opening paragraph. Because employers receive multiple applications for the same position, the name of a familiar colleague may differentiate you from other candidates.

The subsequent paragraph(s) in the cover letter should describe succinctly your qualifications and your interest in the position. Summarize similar clinical and academic experiences during your training or other employment. Think of who matches a specific criterion, it does not obligate the employer to hire a physician presented by the PRF.

In a retained search, a firm is working with an employer on an exclusive basis to fill a position. The retained search involves a formal contract between the employer and search firm. The firm continues to work with the employer until the search is completed. Recruitment firms are committed to fulfilling such agreements and offer dedicated resources, including direct telemarketing, mailing list, and attendance at job fairs. Generally, fees are paid to the PRF to initiate the search and at the closure of a search when a contract between the physician and employer is executed.

The cost to an employer to hire a recruitment firm is often substantial. It may range between 20 and 30% of the physician's salary for the first year. The obligatory payment to the recruitment firm may create a disincentive for an employer to hire a candidate presented by a firm in a contingency search if the employer has generated other candidates. PRFs are often used in rural areas where positions may remain open for long periods. They also may be used in competitive areas or when a job opening needs to be filled in a short time. Employers may hire a PRF because they do not have the resources or experience to complete a search independently.

Physician couples have the added challenge of locating two jobs in a geographically narrow region. PRFs may be helpful in areas that are known to be competitive because of a limited number of positions or may be able to assist the second person in relocating to an adjacent community. Recruiters may provide assistance to nonmedical professionals. Finding a PRF is generally fairly easy since recruiters often maintain contact with physicians and are in contact with training programs. Table 5 provides a partial list of recruitment firms.

Many employers, such as hospitals and large group practices, employ someone specifically to conduct physician recruitment searches. Other options for employers include contacts to physicians directly by phone or mail. Nationally based mailing companies may be hired by the employer to develop a list of potential candidates for a particular job. The criteria may be as inclusive as all physicians licensed in the state of Maine or more specific, such as physicians who have trained in hematology in New York during the past two years. Many professional societies also coordinate mailings to assist members in locating job opportunities.

If you are still in training, consider doing an elective rotation at a site that mirrors your area of interest, practice type, or geographic region. You will gain exposure to people who may be helpful in the search process.

Consistent review of advertisements in medical journals and the Internet provides a resource for leads. Formal advertisements include information such as location, salary, and features of the job. Numerous journals and organizations offer free on-line access. Some addresses allow you to make your initial inquiry via the Internet.

TABLE 5. Physician Recruitment Firms (PRFs)

Name	Address	Telephone
Locum Medical Group	3690 Orange Place Cleveland, Ohio 44122	1-800-752-5515
Fogarty and Associates	5200 West 73rd Street Edina, Minnesota 55439	(612) 831-2828
Weatherby Health Care	25 Van Zant Street Norwalk, Connecticut 06855-1786	1-800-365-8900
Physician Net	Suite 250, Browenton Place 2000 Warrington Way Louisville, Kentucky 40222	1-800-626-1857
Truesdale Associates		1-800-297-1979
Gilbert Tweed Associates, Inc.	3411 Silverside Road 100 Hagley Building Wilmington, Delaware 19810	(302) 479-5144
Phyllis Hawkins & Associates	3550 North Central, Suite 1400 Phoenix, Arizona 85012	1-800-736-3932
Inter-Face	222 South Central, Suite 400 St. Louis, Missouri 63105	1-800-210-7273
MSI Physician Recruiters	Place St. Charles Building, Suite 2205 201 St. Charles Avenue New Orleans, Louisiana 70170	(504) 522-6700
National Physician Register	P.O. Box 894 Brunswick, Maine 04011-9942	
Daniel Stern & Associates	The Medical Center East 211 North Whitfield Street Pittsburgh, Pennsylvania 15206	1-800-438-2476
Medsource	357 East Kellog Boulevard St. Paul, Minnesota 55101-9062	1-800-468-9362
Medical Recruiting Specialists	3383 Vineville Avenue Macon, Georgia 31204	1-800-888-1112
Healthcare Professional Placement	2505 Amin Street, Suite 209A Stratford, Connecticut 06497	1-800-610-4678
Physicians Professional Development Reception and Review	470 Boston Post Road Weston, Massachusetts 02193	1-800-869-2700
Alternative Solutions Inc.	396 Commonwealth Avenue P.O. Box 740 Boston, Massachusetts 02117-0740	(617) 262-7326
MedSearch America	10407 NE 32nd Place, Suite B-106 Bellevue, Washington 98004-1901	(206) 827-4676
Medical Link	P.O. Box 205 Newton, Massachusetts 02168-0205	(617) 332-0908
Eggers Consulting Co., Inc.	Eggers Plaza 11272 Elm Street Omaha, Nebraska 68144	(402) 333-9759
Mason & Associates	P.O. Box 12558 Ft. Wayne, Indiana 46863-2558	(219) 484-2007
H&F Medical	Pines Office Center One Pines Court St. Louis, Missouri 63141-6076	(314) 453-0800

(Table continued on following page.)

TABLE 5. Physician Recruitment Firms (PRFs) *(Continued)*

Name	Address	Telephone
International Medical Placement, Ltd.	University Corporate Centre 100 Corporate Parkway, Suite 314 Amherst, New York 14226	(716) 835-4000
Jackson & Coker	1150 Hammond Drive, Suite A-1200 Atlanta, Georgia 30328	(770) 552-1890
Comphealth/Kron	4021 South 700 East, Suite 300 Salt Lake City, Utah 84107-2184	1-800-453-3030
Olesky Associates	13 Eaton Court Wellesley, Massachusetts 02181	(617) 235-4330
Merritt, Hawkins & Associates	100 Ashford Center North, Suite 470 Atlanta, Georgia 30338	1-800-306-1330
Physician International	4 Vermont Street Buffalo, New York 14213-2498	1-800-846-0220
Bradford Barnes	100 Franklin Street Boston, Massachusetts 02110	(617) 451-1100
Cejka & Associates	222 South Central, Suite 400 St. Louis, Missouri 63105	1-800-678-7858

Some practice opportunities provide a written job description, and others may not. Request a copy of the description and literature describing the practice, clinic, hospital, or group. Maintain a log to which you may refer at a later date. The log should contain details such as requests for written information, description of clinical/academic duties, vacancies, contact persons, time frame for making a decision, and salary range.

Successfully completing step 2—the search—involves pursuing all potential leads that may be of interest of you. Developing systems for keeping track of potential job opportunities and staying organized is critical.

STEP 3: ACING THE INTERVIEWS

TRAVEL AND DRESS

When you are invited for an interview, confirm whether you are responsible for your own travel plans. Request an itinerary for travel arrangements and the interview schedule. Assume that there may be some schedule changes and plan accordingly. In addition, clarify whether your significant other is invited and whether both of you will be reimbursed for the trip. Employers who consider family members and significant others in the relocation process demonstrate a level of support. Because of budgetary constraints an employer may not be able to include your significant other. Unexpected guests pose an awkward situation for both you and the employer; clarify the arrangements before the interview.

During an interview, an employer's first impression of a candidate will focus on his or her physical appearance. Dressing for success means wearing fashionable, tailored clothing that is clean and pressed. Avoid overly casual or trendy clothing. Men and women should wear professional business attire. You may want to include a change of clothing for a less formal dinner in the event the opportunity arises. In your briefcase, pack additional copies of your curriculum vitae, list of references, and a notebook to maintain your log.

THE COMPOSITION OF THE INTERVIEW

The interviewing process is arduous for both you and the employer. Both of you spend a significant amount of time and energy exploring the possibility of a mutual relationship. If you will be reimbursed for the trip, maintain the original receipts and itemize your expenses. Try to keep your spending moderate.

During the interview, be courteous to everyone you meet. Do not underestimate the input of secretaries, office managers, or administrators. Strong interpersonal skills will work in your favor if the employer is trying to differentiate between you and another candidate with similar qualifications and experiences. Your goal during the interview is to be sincere and confident without being arrogant. Avoid discussing personal business such as school loans, tuition bills for your children, or sick family members. When discussing current and previous work experiences, focus on the positive aspects of your affiliations, training, and professional activities.

The interview is the time to inquire about the details of the job. Appropriate questions include the following:

- What will be my commitment to provide on-call services?
- What are the back-up support systems?
- Who will cover my patients when I am on vacation?
- Am I taking call with the same frequency as other members of the group?
- What will be my administrative responsibilities?
- Will I be involved with supervising medical students, residents, or fellows?

Ask about the past, present, and future of the practice. You may learn about the stability of the practice by asking about staff turnover, level of available supervision, competition for services within the marketplace, size of the marketplace, anticipated demand for services, fee schedules, and projected insurance case mixes. Developing a list of questions before the interview affords the opportunity to define your role while learning about essential aspects that will influence your success in the position.

Whether the position is an ownership or employee relationship, it is important to measure the fiscal viability of the practice. Often fiscal viability can be assessed by asking questions about the billing and collection history of the practice. Learn about the collection rate for the group and the anticipated collections for the first and second year of your practice.

TABLE 6.   Checklist for Evaluating a Practice Opportunity

Contact Information	Notes		
Location			
Address			
City, state, zip			
Contact(s)			
Date of visit			

Criterion	High	Medium	Low
Geography—proximity to family members, weather, educational opportunities			
Environment—urban, suburban, rural, population density, convenience to shopping, convenience of services for patients			
Economy—cost of living, tax rate, affordability of housing, per capita income, proximity to practice location			
Family interests—availability of work for spouse/ significant other, social opportunities, leisure interests, consideration by employer, proximity to family			
Children—school system, public vs. private school, special needs, peer group, recreational activities, day care options, affordability of day care			
Social interests—proximity to friends, restaurants, theater, etc.			
Religion—access to denomination, social opportunities, cultural diversity, and events			
Recreation—sports and hobbies			
Viability of practice—size, stability/turnover, demand for service, marketing support, secretarial support, office space, availability of colleagues, paperwork, administrative work, level of supervision			
Research—seed money available, protected research time, access to clinical lab, availability of colleagues for collaboration, track record in obtaining grants, administrative assistance/ support, laboratory setting, space, access to patients, equipment, credentialing, availability of state-of-the-art information systems			
Teaching—resident, fellows, medical students, academic appointment, tenure, career advancement, faculty practice plan, mentoring			
Fiscal viability—growth potential, demand for service, payer mix, number of visits per week, referral base, billing/collections, affiliation with other practitioners, anticipated market changes, competition, physician extenders			

(Table continued on following page.)

TABLE 6. Checklist for Evaluating a Practice Opportunity *(Continued)*

Criterion	High	Medium	Low
Practice management supports—billing, coding, marketing, record keeping, level of automation, managed care contracting, administrative support, patient flow, indirect benefits of participation			
Fringe benefits—health, dental, parking, secretarial support, disability, moving allowances, sign-on bonus, income guarantee, other			
Salary—clinical and administrative opportunities, salary vs. fee for service, salary range, bonus potential, overhead costs			

Notes:

conversation to eliminate positions that are below your target range or waiting to establish a relationship with a potential employer to gain support and interest before discussing salary. Remember that discussions about compensation are not official or binding until you have been given a genuine offer confirmed in a contract or "letter of understanding."

FRINGE BENEFITS AND EMPLOYMENT INCENTIVES

Fringe benefits greatly affect your level of compensation. They may be worth 15–35% above your annual salary. Factoring in the menu of benefits may cause a position with a lower salary to be worth more than anticipated. Other than the obvious fringe benefits such as health insurance, the package may contain benefits such as reimbursement for continuing medical education credits, travel expenses for conferences, reimbursement of professional fees, and reimbursement for journals. Also consider whether you are given a moving allowance, income guarantee, incentive programs, malpractice insurance, sign-on bonus, practice management services, pension, or other benefits.

Many employers make the compensation package more palatable by offering incentives. The 1996 study by Cejka and Company, reported in *Modern Healthcare*, revealed that the most popular incentives include moving expenses, compensation guarantees, paid malpractice insurance premiums, free office space, loan forgiveness, support staff, and sign-on bonuses. The survey also suggested that hospital executives were using new tactics such as recruiting residents earlier in their training, hiring physician extenders and mid-level practitioners, and contacting medical schools. Recruitment incentives are guided by antikickback provisions, Stark Laws I and II, Safe Harbor Regulations, and IRS/Herman Hospital Settlement.

Currently there is an increasing trend toward salaried positions. This trend is a change from previous years when the usual arrangement was fee for service. Merritt, Hawkins & Associates, a professional recruitment firm, reported that 67.5% of their placements included a one-year income guarantee and 27.2% included a two-year income guarantee.[17]

Another evolving trend is for employers to provide incentive arrangements to physicians. These arrangements reward a physician for productivity above an expected standard. Incentive arrangements should be outlined clearly in the contract. The contract should include a summary of when and how the payment will be made, the threshold for payment, the method of determining the amount of payment, and the type of report a physician can expect about accumulated earnings. The MGMA and other professional organizations provide data about physician productivity by specialty and region. This information can assist you in determining whether the standard set in the contract is attainable.

Many physicians hire an independent attorney to ensure that the contract is equitable for both parties. To expedite the process, you may want to select an attorney in advance of the negotiation stage. Be sure to choose an attorney with experience in negotiating contracts for physicians.

After completing step four—closing the deal—you should have a contract in hand. Now you are ready to move on to step five—preparing to start a new job.

STEP 5: PREPARING TO START A NEW JOB

Once you have accepted a new position and signed the contract, you need to begin preparing for your first day of work. Preparing in advance of your arrival will ensure that you have patients scheduled at the onset of your employment and that you get reimbursed for treating these patients. You may consider sending announcement cards, promotional brochures, informational mailings, fact sheets, and newsletters. Planning an open house will allow other physicians and potential referral sources to meet you. Newspaper articles or announcements and public service announcements on the radio are excellent ways to publicize your arrival. If you are affiliated with a particular hospital, the hospital may have a newsletter that features information about new physicians. Most hospitals have a media relations director who can assist with promoting your arrival. Web pages and hospital referral lines are also good vehicles to announce your arrival and help in facilitating patient referrals.

Six months before your arrival, obtain an application to join the staff of the local hospital in your community. Also obtain applications for all insurance

---

TABLE 7. Timeline of Events

Step 1: Developing a personalized strategic plan (1–2 years before start date)
- ☐ Discuss with family members and significant others to determine the geographic range of the search.
- ☐ Evaluate factors that affect the selection of a practice location, including geography; demographic environment; practice setting; academic, clinical, and administrative duties; research activities.
- ☐ Develop a curriculum vitae and sample cover letters.
- ☐ Survey marketplace demands by specialty and salary statistics.
- ☐ Select an attorney for contract review (optional).

Step 2: The search (ongoing until a contract is executed; 1–1½ years before start date)
- ☐ Review medical and professional journals.
- ☐ Network with peers, colleagues, and other professionals.
- ☐ Contact professional physician recruitment agencies.
- ☐ Review advertisements on the World Wide Web.
- ☐ Attend medical conventions or specialty meetings if possible.
- ☐ Prepare and rehearse questions and answers for telephone interviews and site visits.

Step 3: The interview (1 year to 6 months before start date)
- ☐ Select clothing that illustrates your professional persona.
- ☐ Travel to potential job opportunities (clarify who is responsible for expenses of self and/or guest).
- ☐ Meet with a realtor to locate a community for resettlement.
- ☐ Seek answers to questions on your list to gain information about the past, present, and future of the potential position.
- ☐ Send thank-you notes.

Step 4: Closing the deal (1 year to 6 months before start date)
- ☐ Review information from salary surveys and fringe benefit packages.
- ☐ Negotiate salary and fringe benefit package and compare with industry guidelines.
- ☐ Request written information about incentive packages, including a summary of when and how the incentive will be paid, the threshold for payment, method of determining the amount of payment, type of report to expect, and whether all income is pension-eligible.
- ☐ Send written contract with above information to attorney and/or review information carefully. Compare compensation and incentives to legal guidelines and industry standards.
- ☐ Ask questions about the contract and negotiate any changes.
- ☐ Sign the contract.

Step 5: The transition (6 months before start date)
- ☐ Contact the State Board of Medicine for an application for a medical license. Complete the application and mail with a check promptly. Call to confirm receipt of application. Call every 2–3 weeks to confirm the status.
- ☐ Obtain a federal and state Drug Enforcement Agency certificate to avoid delays in reimbursement.
- ☐ Obtain Medicaid and Blue Shield numbers for the state in which you will practice. Obtain a Medicare and UPIN number. Call agencies every 2–3 weeks about the status of the numbers.
- ☐ Apply to managed care entities that are dominant in the geographic region. The credentialing process may take between one month and one year, depending on the insurer.
- ☐ Forward copies of all credentialing materials to your employer as soon as you receive them, including the above items as well as diplomas, certificates, and letters that confirm examination or board results.
- ☐ Collaborate with your employer and/or the media relations director of the hospital with which you are affiliated about the development of announcements, promotional brochures, press releases, newspaper articles, or other mailings.
- ☐ Obtain malpractice insurance before your start date if possible. This will allow you to apply to managed care plans before your start date.
- ☐ Apply for hospital privileges. If you will be in town, plan to meet the chief of staff before your relocation.

---

providers with which your practice has affiliations. The application process may be lengthy, so begin early. Information that you are likely to need for the application process includes a copy of your wallet-size state medical license; a copy of the application for the state license; federal and state Drug Enforcement Agency Certificate; training certificates, including residency, fellowship, and internship; copy of medical school diploma; written explanations of any past or current malpractice claims; malpractice insurance fact sheet; Unique Physician Individual Number (UPIN); Medicaid, Blue Shield, and Medicare numbers; and updated copy of CPR certificates. Maintain photocopies of all applications.

Successfully completing your job search includes many complex decisions. An organized strategic approach is essential to match your goals and skills with potential job opportunities. Proper sequencing and organization of the events are essential. Table 7 provides a checklist of items to maximize your efforts and resources. Following the five steps as outlined above will set the stage for finding a job that is right for you.

BIBLIOGRAPHY

1. Accreditation Alert: Resident and Program Statistics by Specialty: Projected vs. Actual. vol. 3, nos. 3 &4, Fall/Winter, 1996.
2. Altieri R: Recruitment and compensation: The private sector. Phys Med Rehabil State Art Rev 7:291–298, 1993.
3. Angel JL: The Complete Resume Book: Do's and Don'ts for the Interview. New York, Simon & Schuster, 1990, pp 372–373.
4. Baker LC: Differences in earnings between male and female physicians. N Engl J Med April 11, 1996.
5. Burda D: Doc recruitment aggressive again. Modern Healthcare, October 21, 1996.
6. Burda D: How much depends on who asks. Modern Healthcare, July 10, 1995.
7. CCH Incorporated: Med-Manual, Med Guide 8106. Conditions for Costs of Physician's Services to Providers (Provider Reimbursement Manual, Part1, 2182.6).
8. Cejka & Company: 1996 Annual Physician Recruitment Practices Survey. Modern Healthcare, 1997.
9. Elsman M: How to Get Your First Job. New York, Crown Publishers, 1985.
10. Ernst & Young LLP: 1996 Physician Compensation Survey.
11. Federal Register, October 31, 1997.
12. Gilbert Tweed: 1992 Salary survey. AAP Newsletter, Winter, 1992.
13. Guertin RA: Recruitment, retention, and compensation: Academic departments. Phys Med Rehabil State Art Rev 7:275–289, 1993.
14. Hospitals & Health Networks, American Hospital Association Company, Chicago.
15. Medical Economics, Montvale, NJ.
16. Medical Group Management Association: Physician Compensation and Production Survey: 1997 Report (based on 1996 data).
17. Merritt J (Merritt, Hawkins, & Associates): Physician recruitment: The elements of a successful search. Medical Staff Counselor Vol. 6, No. 3, 1996/97.

18. Miller et al: Initial employment status of physicians. JAMA 275:708–712, 1996.
19. Modern Healthcare Weekly Business News. Crain Communications, Chicago.
20. National Association of Long Term Hospital: Medicare raises reasonable compensation limits for physician services to providers. Member Advisory, May 19, 1997.
21. National Institute on Physician Recruitment and Retention Conference, Atlanta, January 30–31, 1995.
22. National Rural Health Association Newsletter (NRHA): Kansas City, MO.
23. Physician Services of America: Annual Compensation Study, 1995–1996.
24. Roane S: How to Work a Room—Learning the Strategies of Savvy Socializing for Business and Personal Success. Shapolksy Publishers, 1988.
25. U.S. News and World Report, Washington, DC.
26. U.S. Public Health Services, Recruitment Programs, McLean, VA.
27. William SJ, Torrens PR: Introduction to Health Services, 4th ed. Delmar Publishers, 1993.

The following organizations and health care consulting firms monitor physician compensation and other health care issues. A fee may be charged for reprint of information:

American Group Practice Association, 1422 Duke Street, Alexandria, VA 22314, (703) 838-0033.

American Hospital Association, 840 North Lake Shore Drive, Chicago, IL 60611-2431, (800) AHA-2626. Publications include AHA Guide to Health Care Field, AHA Directory of Health Care Professionals.

American Medical Association, 535 North Dearborn Street, Chicago, IL 60610, (312) 464-5000 or 1-800-AMA-2260. Available books and pamphlets include The Environment of Medicine, Physician Characteristics and Distribution in the USA, The Directory of Graduate Medical Education Programs, http://www.AMA.2260.

Health Care Finance Management Association, Two Westbrook Corporate Center, Suite 700, Westchester, IL 60154-5700, (708) 531-9600.

Medical Group Management Association, 104 Inverness Terrace East, Englewood, CO 80122-5306, (303) 799-1111, http://www.mgma.com. 1997 Publications include Cost Survey, Management Compensation Survey, Academic Practice Faculty Compensation Survey & Production Survey, Academic Practice Management Compensation Survey.

National Health Care Consulting Firms:
Ernst & Young—(212) 773-2154
Hay Group—(510) 945-8220
Hospital & Healthcare Compensation Service—(201) 616-5722
National Association of Health Care Consultants—(800) 313-6242
Sullivan, Cotter, & Associates (313) 872-1760
Towers & Perrin—(201) 331-3546
William Mercer—(313) 877-7303

CHARLES M. KEY, BA, JD

WALTER E. SCHULER, BBA, JD

5

Signing the Contract

American business in general and the health care industry in particular function largely through contractual relationships. This chapter provides the physician with an introduction to the nature and substance of contracts in general and to the elements of contracts often encountered by physicians in professional practice. This chapter is not intended as a substitute for legal or other professional advice but should assist the physician in understanding the contracting process and identifying significant contract issues.

THE NATURE AND PURPOSES OF CONTRACTS

WHAT IS A CONTRACT?

According to a common dictionary definition, a contract is (1) "a *binding agreement* between two or more persons or parties," or (2) "a *document* describing the terms of a contract" (*Merriam-Webster's Collegiate Dictionary*, 1992 [emphasis added]). The first part of the definition explains the meaning of "contract" as a concept, whereas the second explains the meaning of "contract" as a tangible thing. An awareness of both meanings is essential to the following discussion.

LEGAL ENFORCEABILITY

Numerous attempts have been made to define the concept of a contract, yet no definition is entirely satisfactory. To refer to something as a "contract" is to draw a legal conclusion, as shown by the often-repeated tautology, "A contract is an agreement that the law will enforce." A contract is a promise given for a promise, a bargained-for exchange, or an offer and acceptance of sufficient specificity, supported by adequate consideration, such that the courts will recognize that the parties are legally bound to their obligations. This is what it means to say that an agreement is "binding."

It is not necessary for present purposes to go into when and under what circumstances the law will enforce an agreement (that is the subject of a full-year law school course and countless treatises). The important points to recognize are (1) that legal enforceability is one of the principal features—in fact, often one of the basic purposes—of a contract and (2) that a contract is fundamentally an agreement. The word "agreement" is in fact often used, in this chapter and elsewhere, as a synonym for "contract."

OTHER PURPOSES SERVED BY WRITTEN AGREEMENTS

Oral vs. Written Agreements. A contract may be consummated without the necessity of a written instrument. A contract may be established through oral communications or by the conduct of the parties evidencing their agreement. Although such an agreement is often difficult to prove, once proven, it may be legally enforceable. Reduction of an agreement to writing not only makes it easier to prove the agreement's terms but also serves other valuable purposes.

Communication. The principal purpose served by a written agreement is to communicate effectively the substance of the agreement between the parties. An agreement that seems clear after initial discussions between the parties is often shown to be less clear when the parties attempt to reduce the agreement to writing—in part because people are more precise when writing than when speaking and in part because most of us read better than we listen. While hammering out the language of the written agreement, the parties naturally narrow, refine, and focus the substance of the agreement. Thus, the act of reducing the agreement to writing improves communication.

Completeness. Another purpose served by reducing the agreement to writing is to help ensure the completeness of the agreement. Often the terms that were *not* discussed and agreed on result in a dispute between the parties. Taking time to put the agreement in writing, together with a careful review of the draft, often helps to identify gaps in the agreement that can best be resolved in advance.

Permanence. Written words on a page are more permanent than the memories of individuals. Memories fade, individuals come and go, but signed agreements in the file are available for review whenever there is a question about the substance of an agreement. It is important, therefore, not to overlook ambiguities or misleading statements in written agreements or to rely on oral representations about what the language of the agreement means. In the event of a dispute, the courts normally look to the language of the contract itself (within its "four corners") and will not consider extrinsic evidence of the intent of the contracting parties. The clear communication of the complete agreement of the parties, preserved in permanent form, helps to ensure a good working relationship between the parties, helps to avoid disputes, and, when disputes arise, facilitates their resolution.

THE ANATOMY OF THE CONTRACT

TYPES OF AGREEMENTS

Whether starting out in practice, changing from one practice group to another, or considering an employment offer from a health care system, most physicians at some point in their careers will be presented with an employment agreement or some other type of professional services agreement. Often, a supporting organization such as a hospital will offer recruitment incentives to encourage the physician to accept a position. These recruitment incentives are normally set forth in a separate form of agreement, referred to as a *recruitment agreement*.

Employment and independent contractor agreements as well as recruitment agreements and incentives are covered in separate sections. Many other types of contracts may be encountered in a physician's practice, such as partnership, stockholder buy-sell, operating, managed care, and practice management agreements. Space does not permit a full discussion of each type of agreement, but many of the principles and elements discussed in this chapter may be applied to many different types of contracts.

COMMON ELEMENTS

A contract need not be in any particular format or style. Many are written in plain language, whereas others are in arcane eighteenth-century prose. Regardless of form or style, however, a number of common elements may be identified. Most contracts consist of at least ten basic segments: (1) the preamble; (2) the recitals; (3) the definitions; (4) the primary obligations of the physician; (5) the primary obligations of the other party; (6) mutual obligations; (7) the term and termination provisions; (8) general terms and conditions; (9) the signature page; and (10) the exhibits. The individual contractual provisions contained in these segments vary significantly, depending on the type of contract and the nature of the relationship between the parties.

A discussion of some of the most common provisions in a professional services agreement follows. Specific examples are provided whenever their inclusion will significantly enhance the physician's understanding of the provision. Because some of these provisions are common only in certain types of professional services agreements, the following abbreviations are included next to the name of the provision to help identify in which type of agreement it is commonly found: IC = independent contractor, E = employment, MC = managed care, R = recruitment, and ALL = all professional services agreements. It must be stressed, however, that the contract provisions described below are included for illustrative purposes only and are not to be considered exhaustive.

Preamble [ALL]

The preamble generally consists of the identity of the parties, including their formal names, states of origin or residence, licensed status, and corporate or other organizational status. This segment also typically includes the execution date, which is the date that the agreement was signed by both parties or the date that the parties intend for the agreement to be effective.

Example: THIS AGREEMENT is entered into as of December 18, 20xx by and between AB, a Florida professional corporation (hereinafter referred to as "Employer") and CD, an individual duly licensed to practice medicine in the State of Florida (hereinafter referred to as "Employee").

Recitals [ALL]

The recitals generally provide an explanation of the roles of the parties in the agreement and the purposes of the agreement. The recitals also may include additional information about the parties, including the physician's qualifications, licensed status, and specialty area as well as the health care entity's organizational structure, licensed status, and physical location. This segment also may state whether the parties tend to create an employment or independent contractor relationship. The recitals are not terms and conditions but merely recitations of background information.

Example: WHEREAS, Employer is a group medical practice comprised of physicians duly licensed to practice medicine in the State of Florida;

WHEREAS, Employee is a physician duly licensed to practice medicine in the State of Florida; and

WHEREAS, Employer and Employee wish to enter into an employment relationship in which Employee will practice medicine for and on behalf of Employer.

The traditional (formal) contract form uses clauses beginning with *WHEREAS*, but this is simply a matter of form. A modern form of agreement may cover the same material in numbered paragraphs.

Definitions [ALL]

The definition segment is a glossary of terms used throughout the agreement. In the event that a dispute arises between the parties about a particular term, the meaning of a term as it is defined in the agreement should take precedence over common usage. Once defined, terms are usually capitalized when used elsewhere in the agreement to alert the reader that the term has a specialized meaning in the agreement. Some agreements have only a few defined terms, and definitions are included in the text of the relevant provision rather than in a separate definitions segment. Definitions are often used to improve readability and reduce ambiguity in the contract.

Parties frequently overlook the importance of the definitions and sometimes dismiss them as background information similar to the recitals. However, unlike the recitals, definitions may contain material terms and conditions of the agreement, because the way in which a particular term is defined can have a critical impact on the obligations of one or both parties. The example below is a broad definition of "Prohibited Outside Activities" under an employment agreement, which could be construed to prohibit any activity for which the Employee receives compensation, including, for example, hobbies, writing projects, and speaking engagements. Such a broad definition may or may not be within the contemplation of the parties. Defined terms must be carefully scrutinized and negotiated if necessary.

Example: "Prohibited Outside Activities" shall mean any activity for which Employee receives any compensation, other than those performed by Employee for and on behalf of Employer.

Primary Obligations of the Physician [ALL]

The primary obligations of the physician under a professional services agreement generally require the physician to obtain and/or maintain, at a minimum, the following:

- An unrestricted license to practice medicine within a particular state
- Valid registration with the United States Drug Enforcement Administration (DEA) to prescribe and dispense controlled substances
- Eligibility to participate in the Medicare, Medicaid (or substitute state/federal program), and CHAMPUS programs
- Active staff privileges at a particular hospital or hospitals
- Professional liability insurance coverage in specific amounts
- Board certification in his or her specialty within a certain time frame

Other requirements include:

- Notice to the other party of any medical malpractice or tort claims or other actions that may place the physician's professional credentials in jeopardy
- Confidentiality of proprietary information, patient information, and records
- Service on credentialing or other peer review committees
- Participation in utilization management and quality improvement programs adopted by the other party

Depending on the type of agreement and nature of the relationship between the parties, the physician also may be obligated in other ways:

Schedule [R, E, IC].   The physician may be required to perform services in accordance with a schedule established by the other party, which provides for a minimum number of patient contact hours, on-call hours, and attendance at medical staff meetings.

Relocation [R, E, IC]. The physician may be required to relocate to a particular community, establish residence, and actively practice his or her medical specialty within that community (rather than for a particular health care provider) for a certain time. A physician, of course, may have to relocate out of necessity when entering into any professional services agreement; however, unless the physician is recruited to a particular community for a certain time, there usually is no contract term requiring relocation.

Location of Residence [E, IC]. In a professional services agreement with a hospital, it is common for the physician to be obligated to maintain his or her residence within a certain distance of the hospital in order to be available "on call" with short notice.

Noncompetition Covenant [E]. Employment contracts sometimes require the physician to agree not to compete with the other party during the term of the agreement and for a period after termination of the agreement. Noncompetition covenants are generally disfavored in the law but are enforceable in most states as part of an employment contract if reasonable in geographic scope and duration, necessary to protect the legitimate business interests of the employer, and not against the public interest. Noncompetition covenants also may be enforceable in the context of the sale of a business but are generally not found, and may not be enforceable, in the independent contract context.

Noncompetition covenants frequently include "liquidated damages" clauses, which provide that if the physician breaches the noncompetition covenant, the physician must pay the employer a predetermined amount of money that the parties agree represents a fair and reasonable estimate of the employer's damages associated with the physician's breach. If a noncompetition covenant includes an unreasonably large liquidated damages figure, the liquidated damages clause may be deemed to be a "penalty" and rendered unenforceable. Contract terms that operate as a penalty against a party for breach of contract are generally void and unenforceable. Similarly, "punitive damages" are generally not available for a breach of contract alone. However, the employer still may be entitled to a lesser, more reasonable amount of monetary damages under the noncompetition covenant.

Noncompetition covenants sometimes include a "buyout" clause that provides the physician with an option either (1) to abide by the terms of the noncompetition covenant or (2) to pay the employer a previously agreed upon sum of money. Buyout clauses are similar to liquidated damages clauses, except that the physician does not necessarily breach the noncompetition covenant by exercising his or her option under a buyout clause. Instead, by exercising the buyout option, the physician pays for the employer's consent to the physician's ability to compete directly with the employer and for the employer's waiver of any right to enforce the noncompetition covenant against the physician. Thus, the physician *buys* his or her way *out* of the effect of the noncompetition covenant.

Like the liquidated damages clause, the buyout clause also should represent a fair and reasonable estimate of the employer's loss of revenue associated with the physician's direct postemployment competition with the employer. However, if a physician voluntarily pays a previous employer an unreasonably large sum of money under a buyout clause without challenging its reasonableness, the unenforceability of the the buyout clause as a penalty is not an issue.

Both the geographic scope and the duration of the noncompetition covenant must be reasonable for the noncompetition covenant to be enforceable. There is no hard and fast rule about the reasonableness of the restrictions. The reasonableness of the geographic scope of a noncompetition covenant depends on all of the facts and circumstances. For example, a clause in a noncompetition covenant that prohibits the physician from practicing medicine within a 150-mile radius of the employer may be reasonable for an urban ophthalmology practice with a large referral area but unreasonable for a family practitioner in a small town adjacent to a large city.

The reasonableness of the duration of the noncompetition covenant also may depend on the applicable health care market. A noncompetition covenant with a duration of one or two years after termination of a five-year employment contract probably will be reasonable in most cases, provided that all other aspects of the noncompetition covenant are reasonable. Again, the question is what is reasonably necessary to protect the legitimate business interests of the employer.

Noncompetition covenants frequently take effect regardless of the reason for termination of the agreement; in other words, they "survive" termination of the agreement for any reason. The effect of a noncompetition covenant on the employed physician may be reduced by providing for circumstances in which the noncompetition covenant would not apply. For example, the agreement may provide that the noncompetition covenant does not apply if the agreement is terminated (1) by the employer without cause or (2) by the physician for cause.

Nonsolicitation Covenant [E, IC].   A nonsolicitation covenant is similar to a noncompetition covenant in that it is designed to protect the legitimate business interests of the employer by limiting the activities of the employee after termination of the agreement. Employers often invest significant time and resources in the training and development of their employees and in building a practice; thus, they have a legitimate business interest in protecting both. A nonsolicitation covenant prevents a departing employee from unfairly taking other employees and patients away from the employer. Such a covenant is generally applicable during the term of the agreement and for a reasonable amount of time after termination of the agreement. (See discussion of reasonableness under "Noncompetition covenant" above.)

Nondiscrimination [IC, MC]. This provision typically requires that the physician agree not to discriminate against patients on the basis of race, color, sex, age, religion, national origin, disability, health status, veteran's status, or status as a beneficiary of a managed care plan. Nondiscrimination provisions also should specify that the physician is not required to accept any particular individual as a patient, at least when there is a legitimate, clinical reason for refusing to accept a patient or continue a physician–patient relationship.

Assignment, Reassignment, and Billing [E, IC]. This term usually provides that, in exchange for a compensation package set forth in the agreement, the physician will assign his or her rights to all payments for services rendered by the physician to the other party and that only the other party (not the physician) will be entitled to bill and collect all such payments. Because of stringent federal law governing the assignment and reassignment of Medicare benefits (discussed later in this chapter), the contract should make it abundantly clear that only one party has the right to bill for the physician's services. In an employment agreement, the employer usually has the sole right to bill and collect. In an independent contractor arrangement, either party may have the sole right to bill and collect. This is a fundamental distinction between an employment contract and an independent contract.

Billing Format [MC]. Under a managed care agreement in which the physician is compensated on a fee-for-service basis, the physician should specify that the physician (or his or her group) will bill the payor in a HCFA-1500 or compatible format so that the physician can maintain a standardized billing procedure consistent with Medicare program requirements. The contract should refer to a billing "format" as opposed to a billing "form" to allow for electronic billing.

Hold Harmless [MC]. A hold-harmless provision prohibits a physician from seeking reimbursement from a beneficiary for services rendered to the beneficiary under a managed care agreement in the event that the responsible third-party payor fails to pay the physician for any reason, including bankruptcy or insolvency. Such a provision is normally required by state law for prepaid health care services (those paid for on a capitated basis) but is normally *not* required when services are paid for on a fee-for-service basis. Physicians should resist overstated hold-harmless provisions.

Continuation of Services [MC]. The physician often has a common-law obligation to continue a patient's treatment, even if the patient cannot pay, until appropriate substitute care can be arranged. Similarly, managed care contracts often impose on the physician an obligation to continue to provide care to patients under the physician's care at the time of termination of the agreement until an appropriate transfer can be effected. Such a provision is helpful to the physician if it makes clear that the payor must continue to pay (on a fee-for-service basis) for services rendered after contract termination and if it sets a time limit for patient transfers to be accomplished (e.g., 90 days).

Indemnity Provisions [IC, MC]. Professional services agreements commonly include provisions requiring the physician to "indemnify" the other party for the physician's "acts or omissions" under the contract. (The contract also may use the words "hold harmless." This usage should not be confused with the beneficiary hold-harmless language discussed earlier.) The physician should understand that the effect of such a provision is to require the physician, in so many words, to *insure* the other party against the other party's risk of being named in a medical malpractice lawsuit that arises in whole or in part out of the physician's services under the agreement.

First, it is important for both parties to understand the nature of medical malpractice risk. The risk of being sued for medical malpractice is unavoidable. Even with the highest degree of care, mistakes will be made—and even when mistakes are not made, malpractice suits may be brought. Reasonable people recognize this risk as an unavoidable part of practicing medicine and purchase commercial insurance to cover the risk. Both the physician and the other party can purchase such insurance coverage for themselves. Often, however, the physician cannot purchase insurance to cover the other party's risk, especially when that risk is incurred by the physician under contract. *Contractually incurred obligations to indemnify are often expressly excluded from the physician's malpractice insurance coverage.*

Secondly, the patient's injury may be attributable, in whole or in part, to the other party's conduct. Although the law would normally hold the other party responsible to the extent of its fault, the indemnity agreement is designed to negate that responsibility and to require the physician to accept full responsibility, even for matters beyond his or her control.

Language requiring the physician to indemnify or "hold harmless" any other party with respect to liability for medical malpractice generally should be avoided. At a minimum, the physician should review such provisions carefully with his or her attorney and insurance broker.

Primary Obligations of the Other Party [ALL]

Compensation for Services [ALL]. The agreement should clearly set forth how the physician is to be compensated by the other party for services rendered. In many professional services agreements, the physician's compensation is set forth in detail in an exhibit.

In an employment agreement, the physician's compensation may consist of a base annual salary, plus a productivity bonus. Alternatively, the physician may be paid by the hour or other production unit. The employed physician's compensation may be subject to annual review by the employer; generally, however, there should be a minimum base amount that is not subject to reduction by an annual review. The agreement may include a clause that allows a tax-exempt hospital to reduce the physician's compensation if the hospital board of directors or trustees determines it to be excessive so that the hospital does not subject itself to intermediate sanctions or loss of tax-exempt status, as discussed later in this chapter.

Under a recruitment agreement, the physician may be provided with an income guarantee in which the other party pays the physician the amount by which the physician's monthly or quarterly practice income falls below a predetermined amount. The predetermined amount should represent a reasonable estimate of the physician's expected practice income. In many instances, the physician will be required to pay this amount back at some future point, or it may be forgiven if the physician agrees to continue practicing medicine within the patient community for an additional period.

In a managed care agreement, the physician may be compensated on either a fee-for-service basis, in which the physician is paid a specified dollar amount for each service performed, or on a capitation basis, in which the physician is paid a set dollar amount per member per month (PMPM), regardless of the number of services provided to the members under the managed care plan. Capitation payments normally should be made in advance, by a specified day in each month; just as importantly, the agreement should specify the full list of services that the physician is obligated to provide within the capitated rate. In a fee-for-service arrangement, the physician should make certain that the agreement obligates the other party to pay the physician's bills within a specified time.

Example: The applicable third-party payor shall, within thirty (30) days following submission of each claim by Participating Physician, either: (1) pay the claim; (2) request such additional information as shall be reasonably required to process the claim; or (3) deny the claim and issue a statement of its reasons for such denial to Participating Physician. Any resubmission of a claim by Participating Physician following a request for additional information shall be deemed a submission of a new claim for purposes of the foregoing thirty (30) day period.

Benefits [E]. In an employment agreement, the physician generally is provided with some form of benefits package, which may include various types of insurance for health, dental, disability, life, and professional liability (medical malpractice). The physician should consider whether the provided insurance is sufficient for the physician's needs, the circumstances in which the insurance will be paid, and the extent to which his or her family is covered. The benefits package also may include, for example, a deferred compensation plan; paid time off for sickness, disability, vacations, holidays, and continuing medical education (CME); and payment of expenses for relocation, CME, medical association dues, subscriptions to medical publications, cellular telephone, pager, or other business-related expenses. Some of these items are sometimes provided under other forms of professional services agreements, but in such agreements the items are better described as financial incentives or alternative forms of compensation. The term *benefits* generally implies an employment relationship.

Recruitment Incentives [R, E, IC].   As previously mentioned, professional service agreements sometimes contain financial incentives in addition to compensation and benefits to induce the physician to sign the agreement and to relocate to the patient community served by the other party, e.g., a signing bonus or educational loan forgiveness. Such recruitment incentives should be set forth clearly in the service agreement, either as part of the overall compensation and benefits provisions or under a separate recruitment agreement. The circumstances, if any, in which recruitment incentives are to be forgiven or repaid also should be stated clearly.

Buy-in to Practice [E].   An employment agreement may contain an option for the physician to become an equity member of a physician group practice at the end of the term of the agreement. This option generally will not contain a guaranteed right to buy an interest in the practice but may set the percentage of interest available, purchase price, and payment method in the event that the physician desires and is allowed to buy into the group.

Equipment and Working Facilities [E, IC].   The agreement should set forth which party is required to provide the equipment and working facilities necessary for the physician to complete his or her primary obligations under the agreement. The provision of office facilities, supplies, and the like by the other party is a strong indicator of the existence of an employment relationship, whereas an independent contractor normally provides his or her own facilities and materials. (See discussion below.) The contract should specify that facilities provided by the employer or other principal will be sufficient to permit the physician to perform his or her obligations under the agreement.

Promotion and Advertising [MC].   Managed care contracts typically authorize the managed care organization and/or third-party payor to list in its directory of providers the following information: physician's name, address, telephone number, and specialty and status of practice as either "open" or "closed" (i.e., whether the physician is accepting new patients). Physicians should *require* rather than merely *authorize* these listings—and should require that they be kept reasonably current. In addition, this provision should require the other party to promote and advertise the managed care plan actively and to provide a financial incentive for plan beneficiaries to select the physician as his or her provider. Each of these requirements describes a concept known as "steerage," which helps to ensure that in exchange for providing medical services to plan beneficiaries at a reduced rate of compensation or subject to utilization management protocols, the physician will be assured of a greater volume of patients.

Mutual Obligations [ALL]

Maintenance and Confidentiality of Medical Records [E, IC, MC].   This provision generally requires both parties to meet certain requirements in the maintenance of patients' medical records. The parties normally are required to maintain medical records for a specified number of years, which also may be prescribed by state law. Both parties may be required under this provision, upon proper request, to allow the United States Department of Health and Human Services, the Comptroller General of the United States, and their duly authorized representatives access to all books, documents, and records for the purpose of conducting an audit. Such a provision may be required by law to qualify for Medicare reimbursement. (See Section 952 of the Omnibus Budget Reconciliation Act of 1980, 42 U.S.C. §1395x(v)(1)(I).) The parties also are usually required, at all times, to maintain the confidentiality of all patient records and information and to agree not to disclose any such records or information without the express written consent of the patient in a form that complies with applicable federal and state law. This provision also should state which party is responsible for maintenance of medical records upon termination of the agreement and, in any event, should provide for reasonable access by the physician upon proper request. Any charges for copying medical records also should be included.

Professional Relationship [ALL].   The agreement should set forth the parties' contractual relationship as either an employment or an independent contractor relationship. Such a declaration most likely will not be determinative of the *actual* relationship between the parties but will be a strong indication of the *intended* relationship.

Utilization Management and Quality Improvement [IC, MC].   This provision describes the managed care organization's or third-party payor's utilization management and quality improvement programs. It usually refers to procedures more particularly described outside the contract and requires that the physician comply with such programs and procedures. The physician should require that the other party provide advance notice of any changes in these programs and procedures. Typically, this provision requires first that the physician agree to verify the patient's eligibility under the managed care plan for certain procedures or services—i.e., to contact plan administrators to verify that the patient is covered under the plan—before the plan will accept responsibility for payment. Second, the physician is typically required to obtain precertification from the plan for certain procedures—i.e., to contact plan administrators to ensure that the services prescribed by the physician are covered under the plan—before the plan will accept responsibility for payment. There is usually an exception to the precertification and verification of eligibility requirements for emergency situations. The contract should not allow the managed care organization or third-party payor to deny payment retroactively for services rendered when the physician has complied with the plan's verification of eligibility and precertification procedures. This provision also may describe any appeal procedures for an adverse utilization review decision by the managed care plan.

Coordination of Benefits [MC].   A managed care contract usually provides that whenever a beneficiary is entitled to payment for health care services from more than one source, the payor will pay the physician only the difference between what the physician receives from the other source and the amount to which the physician is otherwise entitled under the contract. The coordination of benefits provision should not allow the managed care plan to deduct amounts "owed" to a physician by the primary payor or amounts that the physician is "obligated to bill" the primary payor, which may leave the physician without payment from either source.[1]

Compliance with Laws, Rules, and Regulations [ALL]   The agreement may specify that both parties will comply with applicable laws, rules, and regulations in carrying out their respective obligations under the agreement. Such a provision helps to ensure that neither party will be implicated in any illegal or inappropriate activity as a result of the other party's actions or inactions and that the agreement will not be rendered unenforceable as an illegal agreement.

Notices [ALL].   Formal written agreements often include specific time frames for certain things, such as notice of termination of the agreement. A precise method of giving notice should be specified to avoid unnecessary disputes about whether contractual time frames were met. The street address (as opposed to post office box), city, state, zip code, and contact person (or position title, e.g., administrator) for both parties should be set forth in the agreement and specified as the address to which notices should be sent. The means of delivery of notices should be specified (e.g., certified mail, overnight delivery), and the agreement should say when notice is effective (e.g., two business days after deposit in the United States Mail or on receipt by the other party). If the effective date of notice is not stated in the agreement, state law may prescribe a particular time frame in which notice becomes effective.

Term and Termination Provisions [ALL]

Term of Agreement [ALL].   The "term" of the agreement is the length of time that the agreement will remain in effect. The date that the agreement is signed by the parties or some other designated date (in the past or future) as of which the agreement becomes enforceable and binding on the parties is often referred to as the "effective date." In employment contracts and independent contracts for professional services, another date is often specified on which the physician is to begin performing his or her service obligations under the agreement (the "commencement date"). Some agreements provide for automatic renewal for additional months or years without requiring either party to do anything ("extended terms"). In such agreements the "term" of the agreement generally is referred to as the "initial term," indicating that extended terms are possible under the agreement. Also, when extended terms are possible, a party not wishing to enter into such an extended term generally must give the other party advance notice of termination before the end of the initial term.

Example: This Agreement shall become binding on the parties as of December 18, 20xx (the "Effective Date"). Physician's employment under this Agreement shall commence on January 1, 20xy (the "Commencement Date") and shall continue for a period of three (3) years until December 31, 20xz (the "Initial Term"). This Agreement shall be automatically extended upon the same terms and conditions for additional one (1) year terms (each an "Extended Term") unless sooner terminated by one of the parties by giving the other party ninety (90) days written notice of termination prior to the end of the Initial Term or any Extended Term.

Termination by Mutual Agreement [ALL]. Some agreements may include an express provision allowing termination by written consent of both parties. Even if not expressly stated, however, any contract may be terminated when both parties expressly consent to such termination in writing. Termination by mutual agreement may occur when one party experiences or anticipates difficulty in fulfilling its obligations under the agreement and requests the other party's permission to terminate the agreement. The other party may make consent to such termination conditional on payment of a certain amount of money to cover the costs associated with such termination. In other instances, both parties may find it convenient to terminate by mutual agreement without holding either party responsible to the other for costs associated with the termination.

Example: This Agreement may be terminated at any time with the express written consent of both parties.

Termination without Cause [ALL]. Many contracts include a provision that allows a party to terminate the agreement for any lawful reason or for no reason at all by giving the other party a certain amount of notice, usually somewhere between 60 and 120 days. This is often referred to as "voluntary" termination or "termination without cause." An unqualified termination-without-cause provision essentially overrides the stated "term" of the agreement and in effect creates a contract term of whatever number of days' notice is required to terminate without cause. A termination-without-cause provision can have significant ramifications for both parties.

Early termination of an employment agreement, for example, may be problematic for both the physician and the other party. If the physician terminates without cause, the physician may find that he or she is required, under other terms and conditions in the agreement, to pay back money advanced to the physician, such as signing bonuses, educational expense reimbursements, moving expenses, or any number of other financial incentives. The physician also may be required to pay for the cost of the other party's recruitment of another physician to replace him or her. In addition, if the contract contains a noncompetition covenant, which, as discussed above, often survives termination of the agreement for *any* reason, the physician may be prohibited from practicing medicine in the geographic area covered by the noncompetition covenant. The downside for the other party if the physician terminates without cause is that, even with notice, the other party may not be able to locate an adequate replacement before the physician leaves.

If the other party terminates without cause, it may find that it is required to forgive certain financial incentives advanced to the physician or that it must waive a noncompetition covenant, depending on the terms of the agreement. The downside for the physician if the other party terminates without cause is that the physician may have relocated to the area at substantial expense and may have passed up other promising career opportunities in reliance on a longer-term agreement.

A termination-without-cause provision must be carefully considered by both parties before it is included in a professional services agreement.

> **Example:** This Agreement may be terminated by either party at any time, with or without cause, upon ninety (90) days' prior written notice to the other party.

Termination for Failure to Cure [ALL]. A common contract provision called a "cure clause" allows a party who has failed to perform, or "breached" the contract, an opportunity to remedy the breach in lieu of termination. The cure clause requires the aggrieved party to provide the other party with an opportunity to correct or "cure" the breach by giving the other party written notice of the breach and a certain period (usually 30 days) to cure the breach. If the other party does not cure the breach to the reasonable satisfaction of the aggrieved party within the specified time, the aggrieved party may terminate the agreement.

If the contract requires the physician to provide the other party with an opportunity to cure a breach before the physician terminates the agreement, there should be a reciprocal provision requiring the other party to provide the physician with an opportunity to cure any breach before it terminates the agreement. Before terminating an agreement for cause, one must be certain that the other party is in breach of the agreement; otherwise, the terminating party may commit a breach by terminating the agreement without cause.

> **Example:** In the event that either party fails to substantially perform any of its material obligations under this Agreement, the nonbreaching party shall be entitled to terminate this Agreement upon thirty (30) days advance written notice to the breaching party specifying such breach. If the breaching party fails to cure the specified breach to the reasonable satisfaction of the nonbreaching party within such thirty (30) day period, the nonbreaching party may terminate this Agreement by providing an additional ten (10) days advance written notice of termination to the breaching party.

Termination for Cause [ALL]. This provision allows a party to terminate the agreement when the other party has failed to perform its obligations under the agreement. Allowable "cause" for termination should be clearly defined and notice requirements clearly specified.

Professional services agreements sometimes include a catch-all provision that allows the other party to terminate the agreement for a variety of loosely defined reasons, such as whenever the other party determines at its "sole and absolute discretion" that the physician has engaged in "unprofessional conduct." The physician should be aware that such catch-all provisions may give the other party the unbridled discretion to terminate the agreement for little or no reason, thus eroding the security otherwise gained by a contract for term. On the other hand, our experience has shown a legitimate need for a provision allowing the other party to terminate a physician whose aberrant behavior causes damaging embarrassment or places the health, safety, or well-being of patients in jeopardy. If such a catch-all provision is included, it should be stated objectively—i.e., not at the "sole discretion" of the other party but tied to some verifiable fact.

Example: Employer may terminate this Agreement immediately upon written notice to Employee upon the occurrence of any of the following events:

(1) The failure of Employee to correct any material breach of this Agreement to the reasonable satisfaction of Employer within thirty (30) days following written notice from Employer specifying such breach.

(2) The revocation, termination, restriction, or suspension of Employee's license to practice medicine in the State of Tennessee, Employee's DEA permit, or Employee's admitting privileges at any general medical-surgical hospital within twenty (20) miles of Employer's location, or the exclusion of Employee from participation in Medicare or Medicaid.

(3) The inability of Employer to obtain or maintain professional liability coverage for Employee at an annual premium of less than $———.

(4) Any unprofessional or illegal conduct by Employee which is injurious to the good name and reputation of Employer, including, but not limited to, the conviction of a felony.

Effect of Termination [ALL].   This provision can be helpful to both parties in understanding the extent of their obligations and in determining whether to terminate the agreement. A number of provisions of the agreement may survive the termination of the agreement for certain specified reasons or for any reason. An effect-of-termination provision can help both parties think about issues that otherwise may not have occurred to them and thus help reduce the possibility of a later dispute. For example, the effect-of-termination provision may detail the following:

- The circumstances under which the physician will be required to repay any financial incentives or other payments advanced to the physician and the terms and conditions of such repayment obligation [R, E, IC].
- The circumstances under which the physician will be subject to any noncompetition or nonsolicitation covenants [E].
- The obligation of the physician to continue to render medical services to patients who are under the care of the physician at the time of termination or to effect the appropriate transfer of patients as well as the other party's obligation to continue to compensate the physician for such continuing care [MC].

General Terms and Conditions [ALL]

This segment of the contract contains important terms and conditions that apply generally to the contractual relationship between the parties. The fact that they often consist of standard contract language ("boilerplate") should not lead to their being overlooked. These provisions (or the absence thereof) may have significant and even determinative effect on the parties' mutual obligations. Therefore, miscellaneous terms, conditions, and governing provisions must be carefully scrutinized and negotiated, if necessary. A brief explanation of the most common provisions found in this segment of a contract follows.

Benefit to and Binding Effect upon Others [ALL].   Any rights, privileges, or benefits of the parties to the agreement will be binding on and enforceable by the parties themselves and by the parties' lawful representatives, heirs, successors, or permitted assignees. For example, the contract can be enforced by (and against) the administrator of the physician's estate (if he or she dies during the term) or by (and against) a company that acquires the other party's stock or assets. To prevent persons outside the agreement (e.g., patients) from claiming a right to enforce any part(s) of the agreement, this provision often explicitly states that the parties to the agreement do not intend to create any rights or remedies in any third parties.

Titles, Captions, Headings [ALL].   The titles, captions, and headings of the provisions of the agreement are not to be construed to add to, detract from, or otherwise be used in the interpretation of the provisions or to explain the intentions of the parties; they are to be used only for reference purposes. Therefore, the physician should not rely on the paragraph headings in the agreement but should read the entire text to be sure that he or she understands the full agreement.

Governing Law [ALL].   This provision identifies which state's law will be used to interpret the terms and conditions of the agreement. This provision also may state the city or county and court in which any legal proceedings to enforce the agreement must be brought (known as *venue*). Contracts entered into between United States citizens on U.S. soil to be performed fully within the United States will normally be subject to federal law as well. Contracts that have no substantial effect on interstate commerce will be outside of federal jurisdiction in a number of areas, however, such as federal antitrust law. International service agreements are beyond the scope of this chapter.

Binding Arbitration [ALL].   This provision specifies an alternative and often exclusive means of resolving disputes between the parties arising out of the agreement. Such a provision may provide for mediation, a process in which the parties meet with a mutual third party (called a "mediator"), who will attempt to facilitate discussion and a mutually acceptable resolution. If mediation is unsuccessful, the agreement may require that the parties submit the dispute to an arbitrator who presides over the proceedings, acting as both fact finder and decision maker. The decision of the arbitrator is usually final and binding on both parties. Arbitration provisions may provide that arbitration is the exclusive method of dispute resolution (known as "mandatory arbitration") or that arbitration is an alternative method of dispute resolution to which both parties must agree at the time of the dispute. One of the purposes of arbitration and mediation (collectively referred to as "alternative dispute resolution") provisions is to reduce the likelihood that either party will be required to incur large litigation costs in resolving disputes that may arise as a result of the agreement. Because physicians typically do not have the financial resources to expend large sums of money to resolve a contract dispute, provisions for alternative dispute resolution often benefit physicians. However, in agreeing to arbitration, both parties may be giving up certain fundamental assurances of fairness that are otherwise guaranteed by the courts.

Invalid Provision [ALL].   This element states the parties' intent that if one provision of the agreement is determined to be invalid, the remaining provisions of the agreement will be unaffected by such determination and will remain in full force and effect (known as *severability*). An exception should be recognized if the effect of such severance is to deprive the physician of compensation for his or her services.

Subsequent Change in Law Governing Contract [ALL].   This provision requires that if any laws or regulations that govern the agreement change to the extent that a change in the terms and conditions of the agreement is necessary or appropriate, the parties will negotiate, in good faith, a modification that brings the agreement into accordance with the law. This provision also typically provides that if a subsequent change in the law makes the continued performance of the agreement (even with modification) unduly burdensome to either party, the contract is terminable by the burdened party or parties upon reasonable notice to the other party.

Patient Referrals [ALL].   The agreement should disclaim any intent to compensate for or induce patient referrals. As discussed later in this chapter, such conduct may be illegal. The physician should be free under the contract to establish staff privileges at and to refer patients to any entity of the physician's choosing.

Assignment [ALL].   This provision states whether the rights and obligations of either party under the agreement may be transferred by that party to another person or organization. A hospital or other health care organization may insist that it be allowed to assign the agreement to another organization that it controls (a subsidiary), is controlled by (a parent), is acquired by, or with which it is merged. Typically, however, the physician is not allowed to assign his or her rights and obligations under the agreement, because the physician's services are said to be personal in nature and involve the unique skills of the particular physician with which the other party has contracted. Nevertheless, the contact should permit the physician to assign the agreement to his or her employer or practice group.

Entire Agreement [ALL].   This provision clarifies that all of the terms and conditions of the agreement are contained in the written agreement, including any exhibits, attachments, appendices, schedules, amendments, or addenda, and that any previous or contemporaneous representations or promises, either oral or written, are superseded and of no force or effect.

Amendments [ALL].   The terms and conditions of the agreement should normally not be subject to change without the express written agreement of both parties. Agreements permitting amendment without the physician's advance written approval generally should be avoided. Such provisions may be necessary and appropriate in some managed care agreements between physicians in solo or small practices and managed care plans, but even then they should offer the physician a reasonable opportunity to avoid the effect of any amendment adopted unilaterally by the other party, e.g., by terminating the agreement.

Counterparts [ALL].   Multiple copies of the agreement may be signed, and each copy will be considered an original of the same agreement.

Waiver of Breach [ALL].   Either party's decision not to enforce a breach of one of the provisions of the agreement in one instance does not preclude that party from later enforcing a breach of the same provision or a different provision of the agreement. The need for this provision arises from an established legal principle that if a party is not diligent in pursuing its rights, it loses them (known as the doctrine of *laches* or *estoppel*).

Opportunity to Discuss with Legal Counsel [ALL].   Contracts sometimes recite that each party has had an opportunity to discuss the terms and conditions of the agreement with legal counsel and to bargain for and negotiate the terms and conditions of the agreement. The physician should be sure that any such representation is accurate. Such a provision is designed to help ensure that the agreement will be enforceable by the parties in the event of a dispute.

Trademarks and Trade Names [E, IC, MC].   Contracts often provide that neither party will have the right to use the name, symbols, trademarks, trade names, service marks, or copyrights of the other party or any third-party payor, and neither party will use any such items in advertising, promotional materials, or otherwise without the prior written consent of the other party. Any consent given should terminate no later than at termination of the agreement.

Signature Page [ALL]

The signature page evidences that the parties have entered into the agreement with the intention of being legally bound by its terms and conditions. Before signing the contract, the physician should be confident that he or she understands fully each of the terms and conditions. The physician also should ensure that all blank spaces throughout the contract, such as those for dates, initials, and addresses, have been completed. The physician should retain a signed original of the agreement that includes all exhibits, attachments, appendices, schedules, or addenda. The physician should make a copy of each of these documents for occasional reference and keep the originals in a secure location. The physician also may want to provide copies of the agreement to his or her attorney or business advisor. If the physician cannot access a complete, signed agreement when needed, any effort expended on review and negotiation may be wasted. This fundamental, practical point is too often overlooked.

Exhibits [ALL]

Many contracts include exhibits, attachments, appendices, schedules, or addenda, which consist of supplementary, explanatory, or more detailed information that has been referenced in one or more provisions of the agreement. Whether these items contain substantive compensation and benefits information or simply helpful reference information, they are a material part of the agreement and should be carefully reviewed and negotiated.

EMPLOYMENT AND INDEPENDENT CONTRACTOR AGREEMENTS

Professional services agreements usually can be classified as either employment agreements or independent contracts. The distinction between employee and independent contractor status is important, and both parties in a professional services arrangement should have a clear understanding of which type of relationship they are establishing.

A major difference between employment and independent contractor status is that the employer generally has control over the manner and means by which the employer performs his or her duties. The employer directs not only *what* the employee does but also *how* he or she does it. In an independent contractor relationship, by contrast, the principal has the authority to direct the outcome but not the manner and means by which the independent contractor performs his or her tasks.

To use a classic example, a person hired to build a barn is probably an employee if he or she is subject to the specific direction of the owner as to how to cut and assemble the material. An independent contractor, in the purest form, is left free to complete the construction by whatever means he or she sees fit as long as the end result is a barn of the description called for by the contract. The importance of the distinction in common law is that the employer is responsible for damage done by an employee within the scope of the employment, because the employer has the right to control the employee's actions. The same is generally not the case with an independent contractor, because the principal does not control the contractor's actions.

In the context of professional services, the lines are not so clearly drawn. No one has the authority to direct the manner and means by which a physician performs his or her professional services. The physician is personally responsible for the professional services that he or she provides and cannot delegate that responsibility, even to an employer. For this reason, more subtle rules have been developed to determine when a physician is an employee versus an independent contractor. Rather than focusing on the manner and means by which the physician performs his or her professional services, the analysis of the physician's status as an employee or independent contractor is more likely to focus on "the *independence* of the physician's *business operations* from those of the business operations of the organization for which or in which the physician performs his or her services"[3] [emphasis added].

Table 1 sets forth twenty characteristics that may be used to help determine whether a physician is an employee or an independent contractor. Although these characteristics were developed by the Internal Revenue Service (IRS) as a part of a test to help determine responsibility for the withholding and payment of federal income taxes, they are derived from traditional common law distinctions. The test is thus useful for distinguishing between employment and independent contractor relationships for both tax and nontax purposes. This area of law, however, is developing. Several recent legislative proposals have attempted to simplify the determination of employee versus independent contractor status.

RECRUITMENT AGREEMENTS AND INCENTIVES

A recruitment agreement is an agreement by a physician with a recruiter or another health care provider to perform medical services either (1) for or on behalf of the recruiter or other provider or (2) for a specific patient community at large. Recruitment agreements are often ancillary to employment or independent contractor agreements but also may be used to encourage a physician to establish an independent professional practice. For example, a hospital may recruit a physician to perform medical services for or on behalf of the hospital as an employee, or the hospital may recruit a physician to establish an independent practice to perform medical services for the community at large as a member of the hospital's medical staff.

TABLE 1.　Employee or Independent Contractor?

Characteristic	One is More Likely to Be an Employee If He or She:	One is More Likely to Be an Independent Contractor If He or She:
1. Instructions	Must comply with another's instructions as to how, when, and where services are rendered.	Determines how, when, and where services are rendered.
2. Training	Is required to work with another's employees, or attend meetings, or other training in order to perform services in a particular method or manner.	Comes to the relationship already trained.
3. Integration	Performs services on which the success or continuation of a business appreciably depends, or which are an integral part of the business operations.	Performs services which are not so integrated into the operations of a business so as to subject themselves to the direction and control of another.
4. Services rendered personally	Must perform services personally.	Is not required to personally perform services.
5. Hiring, supervising, and paying assistants	Is not allowed to hire, supervise, or pay his or her own assistants to complete work.	Is allowed to hire, supervise, and pay his or her own assistants in the completion of the work and is only responsible for the result.
6. Continuing relationship	Has a continuing relationship with the one for whom services are performed.	Does not necessarily have a continuing relationship with the one for whom services are performed.
7. Set hours of work	Is subject to a work schedule established by the one for whom services are performed.	Determines his or her own work schedule.
8. Full time required	Must devote substantially all of his or her working hours to the business of the one for whom services are performed, if required.	Is free to choose when and for whom he or she performs services.
9. Work on premises	Must perform services on the premises of the one for whom services are performed, or within other routes, territories, or places designated by the one for whom services are performed.	Is free to perform services at such location as he or she deems appropriate.
10. Order or sequence set	Must perform services in the order or sequence established by the one for whom services are performed, if required.	Determines the order and sequence in which services are performed.
11. Oral or written reports	Must submit regular or written reports to the one for whom services are performed, if required.	Is not subject to regular or written reporting requirements.
12. Payment by hour, week, or month	Is paid by the hour, week, or month, provided that this is not simply the most convenient way to pay a lump sum for the cost of a particular job.	Is paid by the job or on straight commission.
13. Payment of business/traveling expenses	Receives payment from the one for whom services are performed for business and/or traveling expenses.	Must pay his or her own business and/or traveling expenses.

(Table continued on following page.)

TABLE 1.   Employee or Independent Contractor? *(Continued)*

Characteristic	One is More Likely to Be an Employee If He or She:	One is More Likely to Be an Independent Contractor If He or She:
14. Furnishing of tools and materials	Is furnished with a significant amount of tools, materials, and other equipment necessary to perform services.	Must provide his or her own tools, materials, and equipment necessary to perform services.
15. Significant investment	Depends upon the one for whom services are performed for facilities in which to perform services.	Invests in the facilities in which the services are performed when such facilities are not typically maintained by employees.
16. Realization of profit or loss	Cannot realize a profit or suffer a loss as a result of the performance of services.	May realize a profit or suffer a loss due to significant investments or liability for expenses such as salary payments to others in conjunction with the performance of services.
17. Working for more than one firm	Does not perform more than an insignificant amount of services for more than one person or firm at a time unless each person or firm is part of the same service arrangement.	Performs more than an insignificant amount of services for multiple unrelated persons or firms at the same time.
18. Service available to general public	Does not make his or her services available to the general public on a regular and consistent basis.	Makes his or services available to the general public on a regular and consistent basis.
19. Right to discharge	May be discharged by the one for whom services are performed.	May not be discharged by the one for whom services are performed so long as he or she produces a result which is consistent with contract specifications.
20. Right to terminate	May end his or her relationship with the person for whom services are performed at any time without incurring liability.	May incur breach of contract liability for early termination of his or her relationship with the one for whom services are performed.

From Internal Revenue Service, Rev. Rul. 87-41, 1987-1 C.B. 296.

TYPES OF INCENTIVES

Financial incentives, such as student loan repayment options, signing bonuses, moving expenses, and others, are sometimes included in an employment or independent contractor agreement to persuade the physician to sign. However, recruitment agreements are more often separate and distinct documents from the employment or independent contractor agreement. Recruitment agreements typically require the physician to relocate to a particular community and to continue to provide medical services there for a specified period in exchange for certain financial incentives in addition to the compensation and benefits provided under an accompanying employment or independent contractor agreement.

Financial incentives offered under a recruitment agreement may include (1) a signing bonus; (2) reimbursement for reasonable moving expenses up to a certain dollar amount; (3) a housing allowance for a specified period; (4) reimbursement for previously incurred or ongoing educational expenses; (5) payment of malpractice, life, or disability insurance premiums; (6) a low-interest or interest-free loan; (7) a practice income guarantee for a specified period, in which the hospital pays the physician the difference between the anticipated and the actual income produced by the physician's practice; (8) an office space or equipment lease arrangement at below fair market value; (9) an automobile, cellular telephone, or pager allowance; or (10) other incentives specifically negotiated by the recruited physician.* Typically the hospital or other recruiter pays the physician such incentives on the condition that the value of the incentives is to be paid back, either in cash or in the form of services rendered by the physician to the hospital, recruiter, or patient community over a specified time.

FORGIVENESS

Recruitment incentives are often treated as loans, which must be paid back, unless "forgiven" over a period set forth in the recruitment agreement, usually on a monthly or yearly basis. Forgiveness of the value of the incentives may begin immediately upon signing the agreement or commencing the performance of services. In some instances, repayment does not begin until the physician completes an initial term of an employment or independent practice agreement.

RECRUITMENT VERSUS EMPLOYMENT INCENTIVES

Recruitment incentives may be offered in many circumstances, both with and without a separate professional services agreement. It is often difficult to draw a distinction between financial benefits in an employment agreement (which are intended as compensation for services) and financial benefits in a recruitment agreement (which are intended as incentives for the physician to relocate and render services in a community for a certain period). For example, when a group of physicians offers employment to a physician who would be required to relocate to the group's service area, the group may offer to reimburse the new employee's moving expenses. The same incentive is typically found in a recruitment agreement.

WHAT TO EXPECT

One frequently asked question is which recruitment incentives and what amount of recruitment incentives are considered reasonable and appropriate in particular circumstances and which are considered excessive or inappropriate.

---

* Nothing in this section or this chapter is intended to represent or recommend the appropriateness or legality of any form of recruitment incentive. This discussion is intended solely to assist the physician in understanding commonly encountered recruitment incentives and arrangements.

For the most part, the answer depends on the extent of the need within the community for the physician's services, the fair market value of the services rendered by the physician for or on behalf of the hospital or other recruiter, and the parties' intent. In many instances, however, the answer also depends on the the type of relationship between the physician and the recruiter, because certain physician recruitment incentives may be appropriate when offered in connection with one type of relationship and inappropriate when offered in connection with the other.

The importance of distinguishing between an employment agreement and an independent contractor agreement when either is accompanied by a recruitment agreement or recruitment incentives is to ensure that the recruitment incentives are consistent with the type of relationship. That is to say, some recruitment incentives are unique to the type of relationship between the parties. For example, it probably would be inappropriate for a hospital to offer a physician an office space and equipment allowance, a practice start-up loan, or a practice income guarantee under a recruitment agreement accompanied by an employment agreement from the same hospital. An employment agreement would require the physician to perform professional medical services for and on behalf of the hospital for a salary, with the hospital providing the space and equipment necessary to perform medical services. These same recruitment incentives may be appropriate, however, in conjunction with an independent practice agreement, in which the physician will maintain office space at his or her own expense and look primarily to the patient or a third party rather than to the hospital for compensation for services rendered.

Physicians also frequently ask when recruitment incentives must be paid back to the other party and when they may be retained by the physician. The answer depends upon the purposes served by the incentives. Health care organizations typically use recruitment incentives not only to attract physicians to a particular community but also to retain physicians within that community for a specific period. If the physician leaves the community before the agreed-upon period, the other party generally requires repayment of the recruitment incentives. Thus, the repayment obligation also serves as a retention device.

If the other party does not require repayment of the recruitment incentives under any circumstances, the recruitment incentives, in essence, are compensation to the physician for services rendered. The issue then becomes whether, as a whole, the compensation paid to the physician under the agreement is in accordance with fair market value and reasonable (not excessive) in relation to the services provided to the other party in return.

EXCESSIVE INCENTIVES

Physicians should be aware of the appropriateness or inappropriateness of various recruitment incentives for a number of reasons. When a physician accepts or is offered a financial incentive that is inconsistent with the type of relationship created by the professional services agreement, the payment sometimes can be considered to be excessive. Excessive payments to a physician by a hospital or other health care organization should be avoided. First, excessive payments may raise concerns about whether the payment was made for another purpose, such as payment for patient referrals. As discussed later in this chapter, the solicitation, receipt, offer, or payment of anything of value in exchange for a patient referral may subject both parties to criminal as well as civil liability. Second, as discussed in further detail at the end of this chapter, the receipt of excessive benefits from a not-for-profit hospital that is tax-exempt under Section 501(c)(3) of the Internal Revenue Code may subject the physician to substantial penalties in the form of excise taxes.

NEGOTIATION

THE IMPORTANCE OF BARGAINING POSITION

In any negotiation, the relative bargaining strength of the parties is a major determinant. The following factors increase the physician's bargaining strength:

1. Few competitors in the relevant geographic or specialty area (strong community need for physician's specialty)

2. Physician's integration or alliance with other service providers

3. Practice that otherwise represents a significant segment of the relevant market

4. Large geographic and specialty distribution within the relevant market

5. Competitive pricing

6. History of efficient utilization of services

7. High patient demand for physician's services (physician has high name recognition, and patients' perception of the quality of physician's services is high)

8. Professionally managed practice

9. Physician who is quick to react and easy to deal with

The following factors decrease the physician's bargaining strength:

1. Many competitors in the relevant geographic or specialty area (lack of community need for physician's specialty)

2. Stand-alone facility or solo practice

3. Lack of competitive pricing

4. History of high utilization of services

5. Average or low patient demand for physician's services (physician has average or low name recognition, and patients' perception of the quality of physician's services is average or low)

6. Management of practice by a clinician

7. Physician who is slow to act on opportunities and difficult to do business with

The physician should ask himself or herself: Do I need them more than they need me? If the answer is yes, the physician's bargaining position is weak. If, however, the answer is no, the physician's bargaining position is strong. The amount of time and effort that a physician puts into negotiating a professional services agreement and his or her expectations in the negotiation should be determined by the physician's candid evaluation of his or her bargaining position. If the physician has leverage, he or she, of course, should use it. If the physician does not have leverage, the physician should adjust his or her expectations, do his or her best, and make a business judgment about the value of the agreement in light of its shortcomings.

This is not to say that every physician in a weak bargaining position is doomed. Well-run health care organizations are often willing to make reasonable sacrifices for the sake of good physician relations. In the long term, however, as the going gets tougher, physicians should consider all viable alternatives for increasing their bargaining strength.

USING AN ATTORNEY

Employment and independent contractor agreements normally begin with oral discussions between the parties. Managed care contract discussions, on the other hand, are usually begun with reference to a standard form of provider agreement prepared by the managed care organization or third-party payor. In either case, it is important that the written agreement (1) accurately reflect the physician's understanding of the entire arrangement and (2) not shift legal risks inappropriately to the physician. An attorney can be helpful in achieving these results.

In choosing a lawyer to assist you in preparing, reviewing, or negotiating your contract, ask other physicians, your local or state medical society, the American Medical Association, your national specialty society, or a hospital's or university's in-house lawyer (assuming that the hospital or university is not a party to the contract) for recommendations. Your goal is to get a well-trained lawyer who has experience with the type of agreement you are negotiating. If you are an employer, independent contractor, managed care company, or practice management company, you normally will assume the burden of producing the initial draft of the agreement. If you are an employee, a principal contracting for the services of an independent contractor, a physician considering participation in a managed care plan, or a physician or group considering a practice management proposal, you normally will review a form of agreement proposed by the other party. Either way, the more agreements of these types your lawyer has prepared or reviewed, the more insightful and efficient he or she should be.

Lawyers usually work by the hour measured in one-tenth or quarter-hour increments. Rates vary widely, according to the lawyer's experience and locale. You will be doing yourself and the lawyer a favor by asking for a full explanation of the billing arrangement up front—a misunderstanding of the contract for legal services is the last thing that either of you wants. Most lawyers will provide you with an engagement letter that explains the lawyer's understanding of what he or she has been asked to do and your obligations with respect to payment for services. As in obtaining the services of any professional, the most important factor is to hire a lawyer that you think is competent and trustworthy.

An initial review of the proposed agreement by an attorney should provide the physician with enough information to decide whether the agreement accurately reflects the physician's understanding of the transaction and whether it poses unacceptable levels of risk for the physician. If revisions are needed, the attorney should be able to provide an estimate of the additional time and expense that probably would be necessary to negotiate an acceptable agreement.

Based on an initial review by an attorney, the physician may choose to negotiate changes in the agreement with the other party directly, depending on the complexity of the legal issues to be resolved, the physician's level of comfort in doing so, and the closeness of his or her relationship with the other party. If the physician chooses to have an attorney negotiate changes in the agreement, the physician should provide the attorney with specific goals and objectives and inform the attorney of time or expense limitations. The physician should ask the attorney to explain any provision of the proposed agreement that is not clear to the physician and should identify any provision of the agreement that is unacceptable to the physician as presented.

FORM CONTRACTS

Frequently, when a physician is considering a future business relationship with another physician or a health care organization, the other party proposes a standard "form contract" to the physician as an offer to contract or as a starting point for negotiation. In most instances, it is necessary to modify the standard form to account for the details of the individual agreement. A physician should not sign a form contract if it does not accurately and completely describe his or her understanding of the agreement. A physician may be told that the standard form has been signed "as is" by many other physicians and that modifications will not be allowed, but in our experience this is seldom the case. Once employers or other parties fully understand the need for change, they are usually amenable to adopting an accurate description of the parties' relationship. A clear, complete, and accurate statement of the agreement is to the benefit of both parties. One should never count on an ambiguity being interpreted to one's own advantage.

In some cases, the physician may be told by the other party that a particular provision of the standard form does not apply to him or her or is simply standard contract language. The other party also may insist that certain provisions mean something other than what they plainly say. Each of these circumstances is an indication that modifications to the standard form of agreement are probably needed.

The other party may have made oral promises that are not clearly stated in the written agreement. The physician may be told that these additional oral promises will be fulfilled outside the written agreement or added to the contract at a later time. If this situation arises, the physician should consider whether he or she is willing to enter into the agreement without the benefit of whatever was promised orally but not contained in the standard form of agreement. If the physician would not be willing to do so, he or she should insist that the standard form be modified to include the oral promise in writing before signing the agreement. The physician, of course, should consider the parties' relative bargaining positions, as discussed earlier, to determine whether insistence on modifications to the standard form would jeopardize the offer or the parties' future relationship.

Sometimes a contracting party may not be willing to modify a standard form agreement for reasons that have at least some validity, such as ensuring that contracts remain uniform and fair throughout an organization or abiding by the board of directors' instructions that no modifications be made without its prior approval. However, before signing a standard form agreement without modifications, the physician should consider whether the other party's rigid adherence to a standard form is an indication that his or her future relationship with the party will be similarly inflexible.[2]

SIGNIFICANT REGULATORY ISSUES

The business of medicine has become a heavily regulated field. Below is a summary of some of the most significant laws and regulations that govern the business relationships between physicians and other health care providers. No summary can be considered comprehensive, and the effect of the law summarized below on any particular physician will depend on all of the relevant facts and circumstances. In addition, much of the law discussed below is relatively new and subject to rapidly changing interpretations. Therefore, physicians should consult an attorney to gain a reliable appreciation of the legal effect of regulatory issues on a professional services agreement before signing.

ANTIKICKBACK LAWS

In recent years, federal and state governments have increased efforts to control rising health care costs by strengthening existing legislation and passing new legislation designed to curtail fraud and abuse in the health care system.

Among the most notable are the antikickback provisions of the federal fraud and abuse laws, which are aimed at eliminating financial incentives for physicians to prescribe or deliver unnecessary health care services. The federal statute prohibits, among other things, the knowing and willful solicitation, offer, payment, or receipt of "any remuneration (including any kickback, bribe, or rebate) directly or indirectly, overtly or covertly, in cash or in kind" in return for referring a patient for health care services or supplies for which payment may be made in whole or in part under any federally funded health care program (Social Security Act §1128B, 42 U.S.C. §1320a–7b). The statute extends to physicians and nonphysicians alike. At the state level, laws and regulations that prohibit the offer, payment, solicitation, or receipt of kickbacks in exchange for patient referrals may use terms such as *bribes, rebates, commissions,* or *fee-splitting* to describe the same prohibited conduct. The Health Insurance Portability and Accountability Act of 1996 (HIPAA), popularly known as the Kennedy-Kassebaum bill, has greatly expanded the federal and state governments' enforcement capabilities by creating a national program, with significantly increased funding, aimed at combating health care fraud and abuse.

Whenever a physician enters into a professional services agreement or any other business relationship with another health care provider in which the physician is in a position to make referrals to that provider, any benefit flowing to the physician under the agreement must be examined to ensure that it does not run afoul of state or federal antikickback laws.

SELF-REFERRAL LAWS

Like antikickback laws, state and federal self-referral laws are aimed at curtailing overutilization of health care services and supplies. Whereas the antikickback laws are focused on financial incentives relating to referrals between and among providers and others who refer to one another, the self-referral laws are concerned with the financial incentives relating to referrals by providers to themselves.

Most notable among the self-referral laws is the federal Stark II law. Stark II generally prohibits a physician (or physician's family) who has an ownership or investment interest in or a compensation arrangement with an entity from making a referral to that entity for eleven "designated health services" for which payment may be made in whole or in part under Medicare (Social Security Act §1877, 42 U.S.C. §1395nn). In addition, no funding will be provided to a state under Medicaid to compensate for a referral that would be prohibited under Stark II if it were a service compensable under Medicare [Social Security Act §1903(s), 42 U.S.C. §1396b(s)].

The term *designated health services* includes the following health care items or services: (1) clinical laboratory; (2) physical therapy; (3) occupational therapy; (4) radiology, including magnetic resonance imaging, computed tomography, and ultrasound services; (5) radiation therapy and supplies; (6) durable medical equipment and supplies; (7) parenteral and enteral nutrients, equipment, and supplies; (8) prosthetics, orthotics, and prosthetic devices and supplies; (9) home health; (10) outpatient prescription drugs; and (11) inpatient and outpatient hospital services [Social Security Act §1877(h)(6), 42 U.S.C. §1395nn(h)(6)].

Stark II may be implicated in a professional services agreement whenever there is a "financial relationship" between the physician and another health care provider that provides one of the above-listed designated health services. "Financial relationship" is defined broadly by the statute to include, with a few exceptions, an "ownership or investment interest" with an entity or a "compensation arrangement" between an entity and "a physician (or an immediate family member of such physician)" [Social Security Act §1877(a)(2), 42 U.S.C. §1395nn(a)(2)]. Although Stark II contains a number of technical definitions and exceptions, which continue to cause confusion in determining its exact scope and applicability in specific circumstances, federal enforcement agencies have made it clear that they intend to enforce the Stark II self-referral prohibitions vigorously.

CORPORATE PRACTICE OF MEDICINE LAWS

State corporate practice of medicine laws generally prohibit corporations and other business organizations from engaging in the practice of medicine by employing physicians to deliver medical services on behalf of the corporation or other organization. Exceptions are recognized for professional corporations and other medical practice entities, but state laws typically prohibit an individual who is not licensed to practice medicine from being a partner or shareholder in a medical practice. Despite a great deal of criticism, corporate practice of medicine laws are still in effect in most states.

Corporate practice of medicine laws may be implicated whenever a physician considers entering into a professional services agreement with another individual or entity who is not licensed to practice medicine. In some cases, the written form of the professional services agreement may be entitled or declared by the parties to be an independent contractor agreement when, according to its terms and conditions, it is in fact an employment agreement. If the state in which the performance of the contract is to take place prohibits the corporate practice of medicine, in addition to any sanctions that might apply under that law, the disguised employment agreement may be construed by a court of law to be an illegal agreement, rendering its terms unenforceable by either party.

INTERNAL REVENUE SERVICE INTERMEDIATE SANCTIONS

Physicians often enter into business relationships with nonprofit health care organizations, such as hospitals, which are tax-exempt charitable entities under Section 501(c)(3) of the Internal Revenue Code. This form of tax-exempt status affords the organization with a number of benefits, including the following: (1) exemption from federal income taxation; (2) tax-deductible contributions from individuals and businesses; (3) reduced postal rates; and (4) favorable tax treatment for certain employee benefit plans.[3] Tax-exempt status is often considered to be vital to the existence of such organizations. One of the preconditions to qualifying for and maintaining tax-exempt status is that the organization must ensure that "no part of . . . [its] net earnings . . . inures to the benefit of any private shareholder or individual" [Internal Revenue Code §501(c)(3)]. This requirement is generally referred to as a proscription against "private inurement" and "private benefit."

There is a great deal of confusion over exactly what constitutes private inurement and private benefit. In general, however, the prohibition against private benefit pertains to the notion that a tax-exempt organization must serve public rather than private interests. Thus, if more than an insubstantial amount of the organization's operations or funding is devoted to noncharitable purposes, such as operating an unrelated business, private benefit exists and the organization ceases to qualify for tax-exempt status under Section 501(c)(3).

The proscription against private inurement is a narrower form of private benefit that pertains to the transfer of any amount of the financial resources of the tax-exempt organization to an insider of the organization, such as an officer, director, manager, or employee, based solely on that person's relationship with or influence over the organization and not in furtherance of a tax-exempt purpose. Although reasonable compensation for services rendered does not result in private inurement, excessive compensation is considered the most common form of private inurement. For many years, physicians on the medical staff of a tax-exempt hospital were automatically considered to be insiders, in part because of their ability to influence patient referrals, although this view seems to be changing.

Physicians should be concerned about avoiding private inurement when entering into a professional services agreement with a tax-exempt organization for a number of reasons. First, if the physician's compensation, including recruitment incentives, under a professional services agreement with a tax-exempt organization is deemed excessive by the IRS, not only may the organization potentially lose its tax-exempt status, but the physician and organization managers involved in negotiating the agreement may be subject to substantial penalties in the form of excise taxes. Excise taxes were recently introduced by the IRS as *intermediate sanctions* (Internal Revenue Code §4958) to provide an alternative and additional sanction for violations of the private inurement and private benefit proscriptions. Previously, the sole remedy for such violations was revocation of the organization's tax-exempt status.

The IRS intermediate sanctions provide that penalty excise taxes may be imposed on disqualified persons and organizational managers who knowingly participate in excess benefit transactions. The term "disqualified person" is similar to the term "insider" and refers to any person who (or whose family member) is or was, at any time within a five-year period before a transaction, in a position to "exercise substantial influence over the affairs of the organization." The term "excess benefit transaction" is similar to the terms "private benefit" and "private inurement" and refers to a transaction in which a disqualified person receives an economic benefit from the tax-exempt organization that exceeds the value received by the organization in exchange.

Under the intermediate sanctions provisions, physicians are not automatically considered to be disqualified persons. A physician is considered to be a disqualified person only if he or she (or his or her family member) was in a position to exercise substantial influence over the affairs of the organization at any time within the five years preceding the transaction under review. Thus, a newly recruited physician who has just finished his or her residency should not be considered a disqualified person under the intermediate sanction provisions, because he or she generally will not have been in a position to exercise substantial influence over the affairs of the recruiting organization before joining it. Nevertheless, a physician entering into a professional services agreement with a tax-exempt organization must be aware of the potential applicability of intermediate sanctions to any compensation (including recruitment incentives) deemed by the IRS to be excessive.

Furthermore, if the physician's compensation under a professional services agreement with a tax-exempt organization is deemed to be excessive, the IRS determination will normally be made known to the Office of Inspector General (OIG) of the United States Department of Health and Human Services, which is responsible for the administration of the Medicare and Medicaid programs. The OIG would be expected to investigate the possibility that the excess compensation actually was an illegal kickback to the physician in exchange for patient referrals to the tax-exempt organization.

MEDICARE ASSIGNMENT AND REASSIGNMENT

Whenever a physician enters into a service agreement in which the physician will be compensated for his or her services by the other party, the agreement generally contains an assignment-of-fees provision. Such a provision requires that instead of billing and collecting from the patient or third-party payor for services rendered, the physician assigns his or her rights to the payments to the other party in exchange for a guaranteed salary or other compensation.

The physician's assignment of fees to the other party implies that the other party possesses the right to determine the physician's fees for services, or such a right may be explicitly stated in the assignment-of-fees provision. Although an assignment-of-fees provision is more common in an employment agreement, such a provision can be included in an independent contractor agreement, in which the other party acts as the physician's billing agent.

Both parties must be careful to abide by the Medicare assignment and re-assignment provisions when entering into an assignment-of-fees provision. With a few exceptions, the Medicare laws and regulations generally prohibit the assignment of Medicare Part A benefits and the reassignment of Medicare Part B benefits that have been assigned to the provider by the beneficiary (Social Security Act §§1815(c), 1842(b)(6), 42 U.S.C. §§1395g, 1395u(b)(6); 42 C.F.R. §§424.70–424.90). Exceptions in which Medicare will make payment to someone other than the provider include certain employment agreements and agreements for billing and collection services [see 42 C.F.R. §§424.73(b)(3), 424.80(b)(6)]. A physician may be subject to administrative sanctions, civil monetary penalties, and/or criminal penalties for violating Medicare assignment and reassignment laws.

ANTITRUST LAWS

In the health field, "antitrust laws" refer primarily to a body of federal statutory and case law concerning the preservation of competition in interstate markets. The antitrust laws may be implicated in a professional services agreement under which, for example, the physician implicitly or explicitly agrees to engage in conduct with other physicians or health care providers that is designed to harm (or actually harms) competition in a particular health care market. Because the agencies charged with enforcing the federal antitrust laws do not have the authority to promulgate regulations, the courts play the primary role in construing the statutes and judicial precedent.

One of the earliest pieces of federal antitrust legislation was the Sherman Act. Section 1 of the Sherman Act (15 U.S.C. §1) provides in part: "Every contract, combination, . . . or conspiracy in restraint of trade or commerce . . . is declared to be illegal." Soon after the adoption of the Sherman Act, the courts recognized that it cannot be read literally but must be understood to prohibit only "unreasonable" restraints of trade [*Board of Trade of City of Chicago v. United States*, 246 U.S. 231, 238 (1918)]. An "unreasonable" restraint of trade is one that damages competition [see, e.g., *Jefferson Parish Hospital v. Hyde*, 466 U.S. 2, 31 (1984)]. Certain types of conduct came to be viewed by the courts as always damaging to competition and thus per se unlawful under the Sherman Act, including price fixing, group boycotts, and market divisions (*Arizona v. Maricopa County Medical Society*, 457 U.S. 322 (1982) [price fixing]; *Wilk v. American Medical Ass'n*, 111 S. Ct. 513 (1990)[group boycott]; and *Bloom v. Hennepin County*, 783 F. Supp. 418 (D. Minn 1992) [market division]).

Price fixing occurs whenever competitors enter into an agreement (express or implied) to in any way affect price, e.g., boost prices, keep prices down, or stabilize prices. Agreements affecting price are inherently harmful to competition, and thus per se unlawful.

A group boycott, more precisely referred to as a "concerted refusal to deal," arises when two or more parties act in concert to exclude a competitor from a market. For example, a group of unaffiliated physicians in a single specialty conspire to keep another physician in the same specialty from establishing a practice in the local market by working unfairly against the new physician's application for privileges at the only local hospital, by refusing to provide call coverage for the new physician, and by discouraging landlords from leasing to the new physician.

Market divisions are agreements among competitors not to compete, but instead to carve up the market into multiple exclusive territories. Examples of per se unlawful price fixing, group boycott, and market division activity are plentiful in health care, especially among physicians.

The categorization of conduct as per se unlawful means that the courts will not consider the potentially procompetitive consequences of the arrangement but will conclude that the activity is unlawful by its very existence [see, e.g., *Arizona v. Maricopa County Medical Society*, 457 U.S. 332 (1982)]. Absent per se classification, the courts will find conduct to be permissible if the net effect of the conduct is to promote rather than to discourage competition [see, e.g., *Wilk v. American Medical Ass'n*, 895 F.2d 352 (7th Cir. 1989), *cert. denied*, 111 S. Ct. 513 (1990); *Patrick v. Burget*, 486 U.S. 94 (1988); *National Society of Professional Engineers v. United States*, 435 U.S. 679 (1978)].

The federal antitrust laws may be enforced through various mechanisms, including criminal enforcement, civil actions for damages, and civil actions seeking injunctive relief (15 U.S.C. §§1–3, 15, 26). Criminal enforcement actions against health care providers have been rare and are triggered only by the most egregious and flagrant violations. Although the prospect of criminal enforcement should not be ignored, it is not the principal risk. Civil actions brought by the Federal Trade Commission (FTC) or United States Department of Justice and private civil actions brought by persons injured by anticompetitive conduct are far more common.

A civil action for damages may be brought under the antitrust laws by any person or entity who sustains competitive injury as result of the collusive conduct of competing physicians (15 U.S.C. §15). Potential private plaintiffs may include competing health care providers, patients, or third-party payors. In a private civil action under the antitrust laws, the successful private plaintiff is awarded three times its actual damages plus costs and reasonable attorneys' fees sustained in bringing the action (15 U.S.C. §15). The treble damages provisions of the law are intended to encourage private enforcement.

The FTC has the authority to act to prohibit "unfair methods of competition," which broadly include price fixing and other common antitrust claims. The FTC has no criminal enforcement authority and usually acts by seeking to enjoin anticompetitive conduct (by the use of cease-and-desist orders). The United States Department of Justice similarly has broad enforcement authority and commonly acts through the use of consent decrees, whereby the defendants consent to stop the objectionable conduct and to other remedial measures dictated by the Justice Department.

CONCLUSION

Professional services agreements often have a critical impact on the financial success or failure of a physician's medical practice. Before signing the contract, the physician himself or herself should review carefully the proposed written agreement (including all exhibits or other documents incorporated by reference in the agreement) and prepare a list of questions and comments about anything he or she does not fully understand to present to an attorney or other business advisors.

Consulting this chapter for an explanation of various terms and conditions in the agreement should enhance the physician's understanding of the agreement and assist in refining areas of uncertainty. Depending on the physician's own assessment of his or her bargaining strength, the complexity of the legal issues to be resolved, and other factors, the physician may wish to negotiate changes to the written agreement, either himself or herself or through an attorney.

Once the physician is confident that he or she fully understands the written agreement and that the agreement poses no unacceptable levels of legal or business risk, he or she is prepared to sign the agreement. Before signing the contract, the physician should ensure that all blank spaces in the contract have been filled in. Once it is signed, the physician should keep a complete, signed original of the agreement in a secure location.

REFERENCES

1. Aynah V, Askanas JD: Physician's Managed Care Manual. San Francisco, California Medical Association, 1995, pp 9–10.
2. Hirsh BD, Wilcox DP: How to Negotiate a Physician Employment Contract. Chicago, American Medical Association, 1995, p 2.
3. Hyatt TK, Hopkins BR: The Law of Tax-Exempt Healthcare Organizations. New York, John Wiley & Sons, 1995, pp 21–23, 445.

FRANCIS X. CAMPION, MD

MICHAEL D. KNEELAND, MD, MPH

6

Malpractice

The topic of professional liability is one that most physicians would rather avoid. Given the expanse of scientific information to be assimilated and the long hours of practicing clinical skills, physicians tend to receive little formal education about medical malpractice. As with other aspects of the business of medicine, a lack of familiarity with the fundamental facts of malpractice can breed anxiety, which may lead to poor decision making about the selection of professional liability insurance and appropriate practice infrastructure to manage the risk of medical malpractice that faces every practicing physician. More than 40% of (nonfederal) practicing physicians report being sued at least one time in their careers, and 6–8% of physicians are sued for malpractice each year.[1] The facts are understandable, and the principles of risk management are the same as the principles defining high-quality medical care and a healthy physician–patient relationship.

DEFINITION OF NEGLIGENCE

All health care providers are exposed to potential medical malpractice claims. The law defines the four necessary elements that must be present to constitute medical malpractice for physicians (Table 1). First, a **physician–patient relationship** must exist so that the physician has a duty to treat the patient. There must then be a **breach of care**, which violates the standard of care expected of an average qualified physician practicing the specialty of the physician defendant at the time of the alleged incident. There must be **injury** to the patient that is **causally related** to the breach of care.

During a medical malpractice trial, which is a civil proceeding, the defense attorney pays close attention to determine whether the plaintiff attorney has adequately addressed all of the legal requirements for medical malpractice. After the plaintiff attorney rests his case, the defense attorney has an opportunity to

---

TABLE 1. Elements of Medical Malpractice

- Physician–patient relationship
- Breach of standard of care
- Injury to patient
- Injury caused by breach of care

---

ask the judge for a directed verdict for the defense if any of the elements constituting medical malpractice have not been properly presented. If the motion for a directed verdict is allowed, judgment is entered for the defendant. If the judge denies the motion, the defense has an opportunity to present its case.

The physician's duty to treat the patient is not commonly contested during a trial because the allegations usually involve physicians caring for the patient in question. During the trial, both plaintiff and defense attorneys present expert witnesses who express their opinions about whether there was a breach in the standard of care expected of an average qualified physician practicing the specialty of the physician at the time of the alleged incident. Expert witnesses are almost always required because the issues are generally beyond the realm of the common knowledge and experience of a jury. In certain instances, a plaintiff expert witness is not required. In *Lipman v. Lustig*, 342 Mass. 182, 190 N.E. 2d 675 (1961), the court held that expert testimony was not required in a suit filed against a dentist who had dropped an instrument in the patient's mouth and inflicted injury that required surgery. The court recognized that expert testimony was not necessary for the jury to determine whether there had been a deviation from the accepted standard of care and whether the deviation had caused harm to the patient.

Generally, an expert witness is relied on to testify whether any alleged deviation from the accepted standard of care more probably than not caused harm to the patient. In addition to the expert's own experiences, supporting arguments may be drawn from textbooks and medical literature. Attorneys from each side attempt to discredit the opposing expert's testimony during cross-examinations. In the past, expert witnesses were generally required to be from the same locality as the defendant physician. During the past 30 years this locality rule, which suggested that each area has its own standard of care, has eroded. In an emerging era of mass communication that allows physicians access to the latest medical literature and physician specialty examinations that are national in scope, several courts ruled that a national standard of care had developed and that the locality rule was no longer applicable. As a result of these rulings, plaintiff expert witnesses are no longer limited to physicians from the same locality as the defendant physician, and there is general recognition of a national standard of care. The jury weighs all of the evidence presented during the trial to determine whether medical malpractice occurred.

Physicians are not the only health care providers who can be sued for medical malpractice. As nurses assume more responsibilities for patient care, they face a greater risk of being sued. Nurses and allied health professionals, such as physician assistants and nurse practitioners, are held to the standards of care of their own professions. As with physician defendants, expert witnesses in these fields of medicine testify in malpractice trials if a claim is filed against such a provider. Physicians can be sued for negligent supervision of allied health professionals. It is therefore important that supervising physicians give clear guidance to their allied health professionals about how to treat patients. This guidance should detail the situations when the physician must be consulted before treatment decisions are made by the allied health professional. Such patient presentations often include chest pain, shortness of breath, high fevers, severe headache, abdominal pain, and markedly abnormal laboratory values. Signed agreements between the physician and allied health professional detailing the above are excellent quality and risk management tools for both the physician and allied health professional.

Hospitals can be sued under several theories of negligence. *Darling v. Charleston Community Memorial Hospital*, one of the most significant medical malpractice cases during the 1960s, addressed the responsibilities of hospitals for the kind of care provided by medical professionals.[2] The case involved the alleged negligent care of an 18-year-old man who presented with a fractured leg that was placed in a cast by an emergency department physician who continued to care for the patient while the patient was in the hospital. The leg became infected, and the patient eventually required a below-the-knee amputation. The plaintiff sued the hospital, claiming that it was negligent in permitting the attending physician to perform the kind of care required for the patient. In its defense, the hospital argued that it is "powerless under the law to forbid or command any act by a physician or surgeon in the practice of his profession." The hospital argued further that "the extent of the duty of a hospital with respect to actual medical care of a professional nature such as is furnished by a physician is to use reasonable care in selecting medical doctors." The court ruled for the plaintiff, holding the hospital liable for negligently allowing the attending physician to treat the type of injury suffered by the patient.

PROFESSIONAL LIABILITY INSURANCE

Before the mid-1970s, physicians could purchase professional liability policies at a relatively low cost from many commercial insurance companies. During the following 10 years the number of suits filed against physicians increased and the average judgment award escalated. According to the American Medical Association (AMA), the number of claims filed against physicians increased from an average annual rate of 3.0 per 100 physicians before 1980 to 10.2 per 100 physicians in 1985.[3] During this "crisis" period, some commercial insurance carriers stopped offering professional liability coverage altogether, and others became highly selective in the type and amount of malpractice coverage that they offered physicians.[4] The cost of malpractice insurance predictably increased.

In an effort to stabilize insurance premiums, some hospitals have created their own self-insurance companies, sometimes called captives, to provide medical professional liability coverage for their employees and staff physicians. In some cases, groups of hospitals have jointly formed a captive insurance company. Creating a self-insurance program is especially appealing if hospitals believe that the malpractice experience of their employees and insured physicians will be favorable. In this scenario, captive insurance companies are profitable and malpractice premiums remain stable for participating hospitals and physicians. In addition, hospitals insured by their captive insurance companies can write policy language to meet their own particular insurance needs, a task that can be difficult and costly with commercial insurance companies. For a variety of reasons, including favorable capitalization requirements, many captive insurance companies are formed, or domiciled, in Grand Cayman or Bermuda.

TYPES OF MALPRACTICE POLICIES

All malpractice policies are not the same. In fact, malpractice policies issued by the same insurance company may differ. Physicians should carefully review their malpractice policy each year with a knowledgeable person such as an attorney or insurance consultant.

Typically physicians can purchase two types of professional liability (medical malpractice) insurance policies: occurrence and claims made. An occurrence policy covers physicians for claims arising from medical incidents occurring between the policy's inception date and expiration date. It does not matter when the claim is actually filed against the physician as long as it pertains to a medical incident that occurred during the policy period. For example, an occurrence policy with an inception date of January 1, 1996, and an expiration date of January 1, 1997, would respond to a claim filed two years after the expiration date as long as the medical incident occurred during the coverage period.

A claims made policy, however, responds only if the claim arises from a medical incident that occurred after the inception date and before the expiration date of the policy *and* the claim itself is filed during the same period. For example, a claims made policy with an inception date of January 1, 1996, and an expiration date of January 1, 1997, would not respond to a claim filed January 2, 1997, even if the medical incident occurred during the coverage year. As claims made policies are renewed from year to year, the first date of claims made coverage, the retroactive date, is continued. A claims made policy with an effective date of January 1, 1996, an expiration date of July 1, 1997, and a retroactive date of July 1, 1995, would respond to a claim made in 1996 for a medical incident that occurred on August 1, 1995. As long as claims made policies are renewed with the same retroactive date, there should be no coverage gaps. If claims made coverage is canceled or not renewed or if claims made coverage is replaced with occurrence coverage, there will be a gap for claims made against the physician after the end of the claims period for any medical incident that occurred before the end of the claims made period. To avoid this gap, physicians can purchase "tail" insurance when canceling a claims made policy. Tail coverage provides the physician with coverage for medical incidents occurring between the policy's retroactive and expiration dates even if the claim is filed after the expiration date. Physicians should be certain that they are purchasing a lifelong tail policy that will respond whenever the claim is filed rather than a tail policy with a finite time of coverage, such as a tail extending only one year beyond the policy's cancellation date. There is, of course, no coverage for alleged negligence occurring either before a policy's retroactive date or after its expiration date.

Table 2 shows an example of premium costs by specialty for an occurrence policy of $1 million/$3 million, the abbreviation for a policy with a cap of $1 million per incident and $3 million annual aggregate.

TABLE 2. Example of Premium Class and Cost for $1 Million/$3 Million Occurrence Policy*

Premium Class	Price	Types of Specialties Included in Class
1	$ 2,100	Physiatry, psychiatry (no ECT), occupational medicine
2	$ 3,000	Pathology, psychiatry with ECT, nuclear medicine
3	$ 3,700	Pediatrics
4	$ 4,400	Internal medicine
5	$ 5,200	Radiology, ophthalmology
6	$ 5,300	Internal medicine subspecialists
7	$ 6,400	Cardiology with catheterizations
8	$ 8,700	Anesthesiology
9	$ 9,500	General surgery, emergency medicine
10	$15,300	Plastic surgery
11	$16,000	General surgery, gynecologic surgery, hand surgery
12	$18,000	Cardiothoracic surgery, vascular surgery
13	$23,000	Orthopedic surgery, no spinal surgery
14	$29,000	Orthopedic surgery, with spinal surgery
15	$36,000	Neurosurgery
16	$39,700	Obstetrics

ECT = electroconvulsive therapy.
* Premiums vary significantly by region and by insurance carrier.

MALPRACTICE POLICY LIMITS

There is no ideal way to determine how much professional liability coverage to purchase. Such decisions should include policy cost, the liability exposure in one's practice, and the area of the country in which the physician is practicing. Some states require physicians to carry a specified minimal amount of coverage. A hospital's medical staff may increase the amount of required coverage through its bylaws. Some physicians are comfortable carrying lower limits of coverage, whereas others want the highest coverage limits that they can purchase. It is possible, however, that carrying an amount of coverage higher than others may actually increase one's likelihood of being sued. This is the so-called "deep pocket" theory. Because plaintiff attorneys can obtain, or discover, the amount of insurance coverage carried by physicians involved in an untoward incident, those with higher levels of coverage sometimes become more attractive financial targets for the plaintiff. The plaintiff may then fashion a theory of negligence against such a physician, an effort that might not be made if the physician had a lower policy limit. On the other hand, physicians should purchase adequate policy limits to protect their assets.

An advice of insurance is a document issued by the insurance company to the insured physician as evidence of coverage. A certificate of insurance is a document sent from the insurance company to a third party that provides evidence that the physician has insurance coverage. Medical staffs, managed care entities, and third-party payors generally require the physician to send them a copy of the advice of insurance during the credentialing process. The advice of insurance specifies the amount of coverage that the clinician has purchased or bound. If a physician with $1 million/$3 million coverage loses or settles a claim for $1.2 million, the insurance company is obligated to pay only $1 million of the award. If a physician were to lose or settle multiple cases during a policy year for a total of $4 million, the insurance is responsible for paying only a maximum of $3 million and no more than $1 million for any single claim. Physicians purchasing a medical malpractice policy should ask the insurance carrier whether the coverage amounts include or exclude expenses incurred to defend the physician in the malpractice action, such as attorney fees.

Malpractice premiums are usually assigned according to the physician's field of medicine. Actuaries advise the insurance company on how much premium to charge by physician category. Their methods are complicated to the layman, but they include factors relating to the amount of jury judgments or out-of-court settlements for malpractice claims paid on behalf of physicians in various categories, return on company financial investments, and anticipated future losses. By this method, general internists can be expected to have lower premium rates than emergency department physicians. Although internist Smith will pay the same amount of premium as internist Jones, assuming that they have the same type of policy, factors such as the geographic location of the physician's practice, participation or nonparticipation in a group practice, or participation in certain risk management courses may affect the price of the individual physician's final premium. Most insurance carriers have developed programs to identify physicians who are outliers—the insurance carrier has paid many more claims on their behalf compared with other physicians in the same category. The insurance carrier may place such physicians in a special category, requiring them to pay higher premiums, or surcharges, than other physicians in their coverage class. Commercial insurance carriers also can cancel the policies of physicians because of their claims histories.

Physicians are categorized into premium classes so that lower classes pay lower premiums than higher classes. Physicians must understand the types of clinical activities within their premium class that are covered by the insurance. This issue may arise, for example, if a general internist also works in an emergency department or assists during surgery. Insurance carriers have different approaches to this issue. Some provide coverage if other activities account for less than a specified amount of time, whereas others require the physician to purchase additional coverage. Some insurance carriers offer moonlighting policies that cover the activities of physicians working in an area of medicine outside their premium class.

For a better understanding of coverage issues, physicians should ask their insurance carriers to send them a copy of the full policy, not just an advice of insurance. Because the insurance business has its own jargon, it may require a knowledgeable person to interpret the policy's language. The hospital risk manager may be able to provide such advice. Physicians should pay particular attention to the kind of events that are excluded from coverage, such as willful and intentional negligence. Some professional liability policies specifically exclude from coverage utilization review activities made in behalf of third-party payors. Physicians performing such activities should consult their attorney or insurance adviser about the need to purchase a so-called managed care errors and omission policy. Professional liability policies also may exclude coverage for indemnification agreements with some other party, such as a managed care entity. Indemnification language in managed care contracts may require the physician to be responsible for paying the defense and resulting award against the managed care entity if a claim arises because of some activity by the physician. Some managed care contracts stipulate that the physician is responsible for claims if the managed care entity is sued because of utilization review decisions made by the managed care entity. These examples emphasize the importance of proper review of all contracts. Some insurance carriers offer contractual liability or managed care policies to cover some forms of agreements made by physicians with managed care entities. Contractual liability policies may be broad in coverage, covering the entire language of the contract, whereas others can be narrowly written, providing more limited coverage. The premiums for such coverage are often set at a percentage of the physician's professional liability policy premium.

TABLE 5.   Improper Treatment

Top Five Allegations	Number of Claims	Cost of Claims ($)
Improper treatment—birth-related	346	132,800
Improper treatment—drug side effect	194	72,700
Improper treatment—infection	164	63,100
Improper treatment—fracture/dislocation	120	65,300
Improper treatment—incorrect drug	112	105,900

Summary of claims reported between July 1993 and June 1995, evaluated as of June 1995. The cost of claims includes defense costs, settlement awards, and jury verdict awards. (From St. Paul Companies: Physicians and Surgeons Update: 1995 Year-End Report. St. Paul, MN, St. Paul Companies, 1995, with permission.)

MANAGED CARE

The era of managed care and the role of the primary care provider as the "gatekeeper" raise concerns that the frequency of malpractice claims will increase. In an effort to maintain a favorable profile with the managed care organization, the primary care provider may be tempted to care for patients with conditions that he or she may ordinarily refer to a subspecialist under a fee-for-service plan. This risk is heightened if physicians are concerned that they will be removed as providers in managed care plans because of "high" utilization rates and economic credentialing. From a risk management perspective, physicians must treat and refer patients in the same manner, regardless of the method of payment. Attorney James Rosenblum notes that under managed care, plaintiff lawyers are "licking their lips."[6] As managed care plans increase the emphasis on reducing utilization, physicians are still accountable for errors in treatment decisions. He highlights these issues in a hypothetical courtroom scene:

Q: Doctor, would further testing have been worthwhile for the patient?
A: Well . . .
Q: Doctor, can't you answer that simple question with a simple yes or no?
A: Well, yes, it probably would have been worthwhile, but . . .
Q: So that answer is yes?
A: Yes.
Q: And doctor, would further information about the patient's condition have been valuable in assessing his condition?
A: Yes, in retrospect, it would have been valuable, but . . .
Q: Doctor, you're not going to deny that further testing was valuable, are you?
A: No.
Q: And doctor, your own organization, indeed, even your little coffee mugs, all say you put patients first, correct?
A: Absolutely.
Q: And putting patients first means putting their needs and concerns above financial concerns, like saving a few dollars at the patient's expense.
A: Well, it's more complicated.

Q: You're not saying that your goal is to save a few bucks, at the expense of your patient's life, are you?

A: No, of course not.

Q: So, if a test is worthwhile, and the information is valuable, you would have to do that test?

A: Yes, but . . .

Rosenblum believes that physicians can minimize their risks in caring for managed care patients by not letting financially based rules interfere with patient decisions.

In a capitated contract, physicians assume varying degrees of financial risk for the patient's care. Even more than physicians caring for patients in a managed care plan, physicians caring for capitated patients must take particular cautions to ensure that they cannot be successfully accused of withholding necessary care, whether it be diagnostic tests or referrals, because of the financial risk to the physician. Judges may allow juries to consider physician financial incentives in medical malpractice cases.

In 1996 several state legislatures considered reform of medical malpractice liability laws as they relate to managed care organizations and insurers. Texas became the first state to subject managed care insurers to malpractice liability for clinical care decisions related to utilization review. At a federal level, Congress is considering changes in the Employee Retirement Income Security Act (ERISA), which currently protects self-insured (for health care coverage) businesses from liability.

RISK MANAGEMENT

Risk management is a set of practice behaviors designed to reduce the possibility of being sued. Fundamentally, risk management is about practicing good medicine, documenting the care, maintaining good relationships with patients and their families, and responding properly to adverse events when they occur.

ROLE OF THE RISK MANAGER

Hospital risk managers are a medicolegal resource for physicians. Risk managers educate and advise physicians about how to avoid claims and how to handle difficult situations. A good risk manager maintains an excellent and visible relationship with the medical staff. Risk managers are usually responsible for processing incident reports, which are vital to the hospital's ability to optimize patient care. A sharp risk manager can identify adverse trends and work with the clinical staff to reduce their occurrence.

It is important that discussions with the risk manager remain confidential. A properly designed risk management program minimizes the likelihood that discussions and correspondence with clinicians are subject to plaintiff discovery. How confidentiality is achieved depends on each state's statutes. Physicians new to a medical staff should meet the risk manager and ask what precautions are taken to maintain confidentiality of communications.

Risk managers come from a variety of professional backgrounds. Ideally, a risk manager not only understands medicolegal issues but also has a background in clinical medicine. Some risk managers are nurses, some are attorneys with or without clinical backgrounds, and others have no clinical training at all. Although risk managers can be valuable resources for physicians, practicing good medicine and avoiding errors are the best risk management tools.

ADVERSE EVENTS AND NEGLIGENCE

In a study that continues to receive much attention, Leape et al. reviewed 30,195 randomly selected medical records of patients hospitalized in 51 hospitals in the state of New York.[7] They defined an adverse event as an unintended injury that was caused by medical management and resulted in measurable disability. Negligence was defined as failure to meet the standard of care reasonably expected of an average physician qualified to take care of the patient in question. They found that 3.7% of patients had injuries and that negligent care was responsible for 28% of these adverse events. Extrapolating their findings to the entire country, more than a million patients are injured in hospitals each year, and some 180,000 die annually as a result of these injuries.[8] This number, if correct, would account for more deaths than all other accidents combined, including automobile accidents.

In a follow-up analysis, Leape et al. analyzed the adverse events and their relation to error, negligence and disability.[9] They found that 48% of adverse events pertained to a surgical procedure and that 17% of these were due to negligence. Fifty-two percent of the adverse events were nonoperative, 37% of which were due to negligence. Analyzing both groups together, drug complications were the most common type of adverse event (19%), followed by wound infections (14%). They also concluded that 58% of the adverse events were due to errors in management, and nearly one-half were attributed to negligence. The authors concluded that most adverse events are preventable and that errors in medical practice are common. The classification of errors is shown in Table 6.

ADVERSE DRUG EVENTS

In another landmark study, Bates et al. assessed the incidence and preventability of adverse drug events (ADEs) and potential ADEs in 4,301 adult admissions in two Boston tertiary care teaching hospitals during a 6-month period.[8] They identified 247 ADEs, of which 28% were believed to be preventable. Of the life-threatening and serious ADEs, they concluded that 42% were preventable.

TABLE 6. Classification of Errors in Medical Practice

Type of Error	% of All Errors	% Judged Negligent
Performance	35.2	28.1
Prevention	21.9	59.6
Diagnosis	13.8	74.7
Drug treatment	8.9	52.8
System and other	2.4	66.0
Unclassified	17.9	43.4

They noted that among the 264 preventable ADEs and potential ADEs, 49% involved the ordering stage, 26% the administration stage, 14% the dispensing stage, and the remaining 11% the transcription stage. The authors suggested that computer order entry approaches are well suited to prevent medication errors, such as overdoses and patients receiving drugs to which they have known allergies. Rind et al. reported in 1994 that hospital computer-based alert systems which track patients with rising creatinine levels affect physician behavior, prevent serious renal impairment, and preserve renal function.[10]

Leape notes that physician and nursing cultures typically use blame to encourage proper performance and that errors are regarded as someone's fault.[11] He points out that although the proximal error leading to an accident is usually human error, the causes of that error are often well beyond the individual's control. "All humans err frequently," Leape says, adding that "systems that rely on error-free performance are doomed to fail." He therefore recommends that the primary objective of system design for safety is to make it difficult for people to err. "Ideally," he says, "the system will automatically correct errors when they occur. If that is impossible, mechanisms should be in place to at least detect errors in time for corrective action."

In 1996 the AMA announced the formation of the National Patient Safety Foundation (NPSF) with a goal of ensuring that all patients in all settings receive health care services safely.[12] The NPSF will serve as a center and clearinghouse for information, education, and research related to the improvement of patient safety relevant to physician offices, hospitals, and other settings.

CONFIDENTIALITY

Physicians have a legal obligation to respect the privacy of patients pertaining to their privileged communications. The patient's medical record is not a public document to be shared with individuals who have no authority to review the information contained in it. In a hospital setting, only individuals with a need to know the information in the medical record should be allowed access. This confidentiality may be breached, for example, if a well-known patient enters the data drawn from other geographic areas. In many cases, the limitations were set differentially by specialty so that physicians performing the same procedure could be paid substantially different amounts depending on their specialty area. In addition, new physicians—i.e., those recently out of training and/or entering practice in the area—could often set their fees at or near the top of the range, whereas physicians with longer histories were often limited by their own historical fee patterns.[1]

The UCR fee limitations imposed by Medicare, BCBS plans, and commercial insurers were relatively weak and generally affected only those fees at or near the top of the fee pyramid. For example, many BCBS and commercial insurers used a 90th percentile cutoff for determining payments to physicians under their indemnity plans. Thus, a physician would be paid his or her actual fee unless it was higher than the fees submitted by 90% or more of the other physicians billing for the same procedures or services in the same locality. The impact of the limits was primarily on extreme "outliers" rather than on most fees or physicians.

The rapid escalation of public and private health care costs in the 1970s and 1980s, fueled by runaway general inflation and increases in the volume and complexity of medical services, led the federal government and private employers to exert increasing amounts of pressure on hospital rates, physician fees, and other provider payment levels.[2,3] In 1983 Medicare introduced a comprehensive set of limitations on hospital inpatient rates, based on diagnosis-related groups (DRGs).[4] In addition, BCBS plans and insurers began building preferred provider organizations (PPOs) to respond to demands from major corporate accounts for lower costs. In PPO arrangements, hospitals and physicians were asked to give discounts from their usual fees in exchange for inclusion in the PPO provider networks. In theory, physicians and hospitals that accepted lower fees would benefit from PPO incentives (e.g,. lower deductibles and/or coinsurance obligations) that would encourage PPO subscribers to use participating PPO physicians and other providers. In some instances, the physicians who joined PPOs saw increases in their volume of patients; however, in most cases, acceptance of the lower PPO fee levels simply enabled the providers to avoid losing patients who enrolled in the new PPO plans.[5]

PPO enrollments grew rapidly during the latter half of the 1980s. Many PPOs imposed UCR-type limitations at the 60th or 70th percentile level. Substantial discounts were also negotiated with hospitals, often on the basis of discounts from charges or per diem inpatient rate structures. However, PPOs did not incorporate financial incentives to limit the volume of services (e.g., hospital days, laboratory tests, surgical operations, radiologic procedures) rendered to PPO enrollees. Instead, they relied on administrative forms of utilization management (UM), including precertification, second surgical opinions, and concurrent review. As PPOs increased their number of members, fee discounting became more common and the UM scrutiny faced by physicians became more intense.

The perceived lack of effective volume controls in PPOs led to the expansion of HMOs in the late 1980s and 1990s. In theory, an HMO plan incorporates financial incentives, as well as traditional UM methods, that are designed to keep enrollees healthy and to reduce the unnecessary use of services. HMOs are more likely to negotiate fee schedules, rather than UCR-type limits or discount arrangements with physicians. As discussed below, they also enter into capitated payment arrangements, especially with primary care physicians (PCPs). In HMOs, physicians are often given financial rewards for achieving certain cost or utilization objectives, such as fewer hospital days per 1000 members.

HMO enrollments have ballooned over the past ten years, largely through the growth of point of service (POS) products that allow members to refer themselves for care, and they appear at least to have moderated the growth of health care costs.[6,7] As of July 1997, the Medicare program had approximately 10% of its total enrollment in Medicare HMOs, with an additional 80,000 beneficiaries joining each month, and at least seventeen states had converted or were in the process of converting their Medicaid plans into competitively priced, privately operated HMO-type delivery systems. This wholesale conversion is occurring despite physician and member objections to the growing amount of red tape involved in managed care programs. In addition, there is considerable debate about the extent to which HMO cost savings come from more effective management or from their ability to attract younger, healthier populations with lower illness burdens.

In philosophic, conceptual, and economic terms, managed care is now the dominant form of health care payment and service delivery in the United States. Although PPOs have lost some luster in comparison with HMOs, they still account for as many or more enrollees because many employers have found it difficult to persuade their employees to accept the smaller provider networks and more complicated referral procedures of HMOs. The distinctions between PPOs, HMOs, POS, and other types of plans are blurring as each attempts to mimic the most attractive or cost-effective features of the others. In addition, new ideas—or, more often, variations of well-established or previously tried reimbursement and UM strategies—are constantly being introduced by plans seeking to reverse previous mistakes, correct existing weaknesses, or gain a special cost or marketing advantage. The turmoil is heightened by the quarter-to-quarter pressures faced by publicly traded HMOs and insurers to meet the growth and earnings expectations imposed by the investment community.

Thus, the typical physician is now confronted with the task of evaluating a wide range of conceptually diverse and technically abstruse proposals from HMOs and insurers that account for a rapidly increasing proportion of all public and private patients. These proposals present a complex maze of financial risks and opportunities. Physicians must evaluate them quickly and competently if lower fees are supposedly justified by some market "exclusivity" conferred on the physician. In most instances, the new products never reach their marketing projections, and the lower fees accepted by participating physicians become a target to be matched by the more established plans. Thus, physicians who are too resistant can suffer the loss of large shares of their patient base if they are dropped by a major HMO or insurer, and physicians who are too cooperative can precipitate downward fee spirals in which the purchasers use the weakest, most economically desperate physicians to drive general fee schedules to lower and lower levels.

This predicament is more and more typical in the United States. It is the primary force leading physicians to organize themselves into larger groups. The overhead costs of medical practice are rising inexorably in reaction to the increasingly burdensome administrative requirements of managed care. Individual physicians and small groups are finding it impossible to meet these costs while also absorbing fee reductions. The loss of autonomy that inevitably accompanies, to a greater or lesser degree, the abandonment of solo or small group practice is offset by the greater ability to spread overhead and the increased bargaining leverage gained by physicians when they join larger units. Large practices, whether they are of multispecialty or single-specialty orientation, can negotiate on a more equal footing with managed care plans. The importance of this bargaining leverage is greatest in the negotiation of at-risk compensation arrangements because the potential rewards and penalties of such arrangements can be much larger than those associated with nonrisk arrangements.

AT-RISK COMPENSATION ARRANGEMENTS: OVERVIEW

In an at-risk compensation arrangement, as defined in this chapter, the payments due to an individual physician or group of physicians from the payor—typically an HMO—are at least partially related to the performance of the physician in managing costs, meeting utilization objectives, and achieving other goals such as patient satisfaction or quality targets. In such arrangements, physicians may face only positive incentives, whereby compensation can only increase above a baseline level, or they also may face negative incentives, whereby compensation may be reduced below baseline levels, depending on their performance relative to the stated objectives of the plan. The incentive component of the at-risk arrangement may relate only to services provided directly by the physician or physician group, or it may extend to services provided by other physicians, freestanding ambulatory care facilities, and/or hospitals. As the at-risk arrangements become more encompassing, they increase the risks but also the potential rewards available to physicians who choose to participate in them.

The main types of at-risk physician compensation arrangements, presented in order of increasing complexity, risk, and comprehensiveness, are the following:

- Primary care capitation
- Single-specialty capitation (professional services only)
- Single-specialty global capitation (professional and facility services)
- Multispecialty capitation (professional services only)
- Multispecialty global capitation (professional and facility services)
- Full capitation/percent of premium arrangements covering all or most professional and facility services

Primary care capitation is by far the most common form of at-risk physician compensation arrangements. It is closely allied to the PCP gatekeeper model in which an HMO uses a PCP to manage the use of medical services. The PCP acts as a gatekeeper by evaluating the needs of members who have chosen him or her as their primary care physician and referring them for needed specialty professional and facility services.

Primary care capitation is a cornerstone of the utilization management and incentive structures of many HMOs, but it has recently been subjected to a wave of criticism. In particular, the PCP gatekeeper approach is associated in the minds of the public and, to a considerable degree, in the consciousness of the medical profession with the complex tangle of referral requirements and other utilization management controls that is threatening to strangle the medical delivery system. Specialists, in particular, resent the notion that PCPs are equipped to diagnose and, in some instances, to treat medical problems for which specialists may have superior training and experience. In addition, the evidence that PCP gatekeeper models reduce costs below those achieved in plans where access to specialists is more direct is not compelling. However, the poor design of many gatekeeper models, the lack of comparability in the gatekeeper approaches implemented by various HMOs, the absence of timely, comparable information about the populations at risk and their costs, and the relatively small amount of resources devoted to rigorous performance studies by many HMOs reduce most criticisms of gatekeeper models to an anecdotal level. Nevertheless, a number of major HMOs, including United HealthCare and Oxford Health Plans, have recently moved away from the PCP gatekeeper approach to models that provide members with more direct access to specialists.[15]

During the first half of the 1990s, the second most common form of at-risk physician compensation arrangements was the single-specialty, professional services-only model (described in a later section). More recently, networks of specialists (e.g., cardiologists, cardiovascular surgeons, orthopedists) have begun to offer HMOs and insurers global fee packages that cover either or both professional and facility services for specified medical treatments. Finally, full capitation or similar percent of premium arrangements—in which a physician group, usually in cooperation with a hospital or group of hospitals, accepts the risk for the cost of all or virtually all medical services for an enrolled population—have started to establish themselves in various parts of the United States.

The following sections discuss each type of at-risk arrangement. A separate section presents an itemized list of particular contractual issues that are common to all or most types of at-risk arrangements.

PRIMARY CARE CAPITATION

The most widespread and best-established form of at-risk physician compensation is primary care capitation. In a typical primary care capitation arrangement, the members of an HMO are asked to select a participating primary care physician. Usually the HMO defines the category of PCP to include internists, family and general practitioners, and pediatricians; occasionally women are allowed to choose a gynecologist as their PCP. The HMO establishes a schedule of per-member per-month (PMPM) amounts that it pays on a monthly basis to each participating PCP in exchange for delivery of primary care services and management of needed specialty referrals. Under primary care capitation, the monthly revenue of the PCP becomes highly predictable because it is a function of the number of HMO members who have chosen him or her and the PMPM amounts paid by the HMO.

A variant of the primary care capitation model is an approach in which the PCP serves as a gatekeeper and has an incentive-based interest in controlling overall costs and utilization but is paid on a fee-for-service rather than a capitated basis. For example, PCPs may receive CPT-based payments for the medical services that they provide directly plus a PMPM management fee for each member in their patient panel. The management fee is periodically adjusted up or down by the HMO, depending on the success of the PCP (or PCP group) in managing costs, controlling utilization, and/or meeting other HMO objectives. The advantages of this model to the HMO and PCP can be considerable. For example, the use of fee-for-service payments encourages the PCP to provide services. This incentive allows the PCP to raise his or her income by substituting for the role of specialists. Fee-for-service payments also eliminate the worry that capitation arrangements dispose physicians to ignore patient needs. If the incentive payments that PCPs can earn are considerable, PCPs in this type of noncapitated but budgetarily responsible framework can be highly motivated to meet the HMO's objectives.

PCPs should weigh the relative attractiveness of fee-for-service compensation with a management fee kind of incentive vs. primary care capitation with incentives tied to similar budgetary and other performance criteria. The most important considerations in evaluating these options are the fairness of the targets, the structure of the incentive model, and the size of the incentive payments that are realistically available to PCPs as a reward for good performance.

The relative predominance of the capitated PCP gatekeeper approach makes it efficient to concentrate on that model rather than the fee-for-service budget incentive model for the remainder of this section. However, most issues and suggestions are pertinent to either approach. Individual PCPs and PCP groups differ in their preferences for one or the other model, and particular HMOs have their own strong preferences. Nevertheless, it is sometimes possible to blend some aspects of the approaches—for example, by paying some services on a capitated basis and others on a fee-for-service basis—to achieve a mutually acceptable balance between the needs of the PCPs and the needs of the HMO.

In a capitated primary care arrangement, the predictability of cash flow is often a significant inducement to participation by PCPs. Of course, the attractiveness of the cash flow is directly related to the level of the PMPM allowances in relation to the range of services included in the capitation and the likely demand for services by capitated members. PCPs entering into a primary care capitation arrangement should press the HMO for a specific listing of services covered by the capitation payments and services billable on a fee-for-service basis. For example, hospital visits are sometimes excluded from the list of capitated services; basic laboratory tests, electrocardiographic tracings, and other minor diagnostic procedures may or may not be included in the capitation service listings. Obviously, the attractiveness of the PMPM fees increases or decreases based on the scope of services that must be provided without additional compensation.

In some instances, HMOs are trying to expand the list of services that must be provided within the capitated allowances. If services that were formerly provided mostly or exclusively by specialists are included in the capitation, PCPs must determine whether they feel competent to provide such services and whether the PMPM allowances reflect their addition. In particular, PCPs should find out whether the HMO will charge them—by reducing their PMPM allowance or some other means—if a specialist happens to perform one of the services listed as a capitated service.

The presence and size of an office visit copayment also affect the attractiveness of the PMPM fees. The base PMPM allowances and the expected out-of-pocket payments by members when they receive services must be added together before the base compensation level offered by the HMO can be judged. The higher the office copayment, the less likely the members are to use primary care services and the higher the PCP's direct compensation for such visits. However, if the office copayments are too high, members may not come for needed care on a timely basis, and the PCP may be faced with the need to provide or arrange more time-consuming and costly services at a later date. In general, office copayments should be high enough (e.g., $10–15 per visit) to discourage frivolous utilization but not so high that they interfere with timely care or with the development of a strong rapport and mutual trust between the PCP and his or her patients.

The fairness of a primary care capitation arrangement to all parties—PCP, HMO, and members—is an essential ingredient in its long-term success. It is particularly important to the equity of a primary care capitation arrangement to have a schedule of PMPM amounts that is differentiated by sex and by broad age classes (e.g., 0–1, 1–5, 6–13, 14–24, 25–34, 35–44, 45–54, 55–64, 65–74, 75–79, 80–84, and 85+) because the need for services varies systematically on average with these demographic features. Without such adjustments, some PCPs may be overpaid because they attract a relatively young patient population (perhaps because their office is located in a neighborhood that appeals to a younger population), whereas others may be underpaid because they are more established and have a patient population that has aged with them.

The average PMPM payment varies substantially under primary care capitation but is usually $10–15 for private sector patients. These amounts are consistent with the fact that primary care services typically account for approximately 10–15% of total health care costs in the private sector. In Medicare risk plans, if primary care capitation is used, the PMPM amount is usually in the $25–30 range, which is consistent with the fact that primary care services account for only 5–10% of total Medicare costs. In 1997, Medicare costs averaged approximately $460 PMPM for the aged, nondisabled class of beneficiaries who are most likely to join HMO plans.

Primary care capitation arrangements vary in the extent to which they carry significant opportunities for PCPs to earn incentive compensation. Some HMOs, like U.S. Healthcare, have established relatively elaborate criteria to measure a PCP's overall performance across a range of factors, including patient satisfaction, availability to new patients, appearance and condition of office facilities, appropriateness and quality of medical care based on chart reviews, and cost control based on hospital days and other utilization statistics. PCPs who achieve relatively high scores receive additional compensation that supplements their PMPM allowances. Many other HMOs use similar types of incentives to encourage PCPs to take an active role in managing health care services and meeting enrollee expectations.

In assessing a primary care capitation proposal that includes an incentive payment component, a PCP or group of PCPs should consider the following questions:

1. What is the PMPM allowance? How is it structured—e.g., does it incorporate age and sex adjustments? What services does it encompass? Can the allowance or the list of services covered by it be changed unilaterally by the health plan?

2. Are the criteria to which the incentive compensation is tied and the methods used to compute it clearly described in the agreement? Will the necessary data be available and reliable? Are the measures primarily objective or subjective? How much relative weight is given to such matters as patient satisfaction, cost control, and quality of care? Are the emphases of the HMO compatible with those of PCPs?

3. What services are included in the incentive arrangement? Will the PCP be measured by his or her ability to manage total costs and utilization not only for primary care but also for specialty professional care, outpatient facilities, and inpatient hospital care? Broader responsibilities generally involve larger incentive compensation potentials and give the PCPs more opportunity to exercise a significant medical management function. However, they can also increase risk.

4. Is the incentive program structured to be only positive—i.e., is it set up so that PCPs never receive less than their PMPM allowances but are able to receive more through the incentive? Or does it also include a negative component whereby PCPs may find their PMPM allowances reduced as a result of a poor showing on the incentive measures? How large, in absolute and percentage terms, are the potential incentive payments (both positive and negative) relative to the base PMPM allowances? Are the amounts significant enough to make it worthwhile for PCPs to make a special effort to achieve the objectives specified by the HMO? Trivial incentives, such as a maximal bonus of 5–10% of the PMPM allowances, are obviously not an important consideration, especially when some portion of the bonus may be either virtually assured or unattainable. In contrast, large potential incentives (e.g., 25% of base compensation) are a significant matter, especially if the potential negative adjustment is substantial relative to base payment levels.

5. How are the incentive targets established? Are they set prospectively or retroactively? Are the targets fixed and preestablished or relative? For example, will a PCP group know in advance that it will receive an incentive payment for holding hospital days below a specified level (e.g., 250 days/1000) or only that it will receive an incentive payment if its level of hospital days per 1000 is below the average across all PCP groups included in the incentive calculations? What proportion of all PCPs or PCP groups participating in the HMO in a prior period (e.g., past year) received what levels of incentive payments? It is much easier to evaluate targets that are stated explicitly in advance in absolute rather than relative terms. Prior experience also provides a useful indication of the likely impact of the incentive plan.

6. Are the incentive measures computed on a PCP-specific basis or on a group basis? To the extent that they will be computed on a group basis, how is the group defined by the HMO? Does it include only PCPs in the same medical practice? Or does it include other PCPs with whom the particular PCP may or may not be acquainted or comfortable? How large are the groups defined by the HMO for incentive compensation determination? Does the individual PCP's performance significantly affect his or her rating by the HMO, or is it likely to be lost in an averaging of performance across a large number of PCPs grouped together by the HMO for calculation purposes? In general, PCPs

SINGLE-SPECIALTY AND MULTISPECIALTY PROFESSIONAL AND FACILITY SERVICE MODELS

It is still relatively unusual for physicians in any specialty or in a combination of specialties to be asked or to offer to accept risk for both professional and facility services on a fully capitated or substantially capitated basis. When such arrangements are in place, they are likely to include outpatient facility services (e.g., ambulatory surgery facility services) but not inpatient facility services. The more frequent inclusion of outpatient facility services is driven by two risk-mitigating factors: (1) because the complexity of outpatient services is relatively low, the attendant facility costs are usually not especially large, and (2) physicians are often full or partial owners of the outpatient facility and therefore have more direct control over the costs and charges billed to them.

In the case of capitation arrangements that include inpatient facility costs, the importance of facility services in relation to professional services varies greatly across the specialties. For example, the facility component of costs in a capitated psychiatry arrangement would be small in relation to professional costs, whereas the facility component of total costs would loom large for orthopedics and much larger still for cardiovascular surgery. The inclusion of inpatient facility costs in the capitated or otherwise at-risk arrangement greatly increases the risks posed to physicians in any specialty that involves a substantial amount of facility-based services. Physicians entering into such arrangements should work out cooperative arrangements with facilities that are willing to share a substantial proportion (and frequently the majority) of the financial risks associated with hospital or other facility costs that exceed the preestablished budget. Stop-loss arrangements can reduce some of the risks, but the cost of such reinsurance may be prohibitive if the physician group has not contracted with facilities that are willing to provide services at a reasonable cost. The more risk a cooperative facility will share with the physicians, the less need there will be for reinsurance and the lower will be the total cost of obtaining the necessary economic protections against catastrophic losses.

There is great variation in payment methods, incentive arrangements, and administrative requirements embedded in the single-specialty and multispecialty professional and/or facility services models that are offered and operated by HMOs. However, the questions that should be raised by physicians are quite similar, regardless of the model. Accordingly, physicians who are confronted with or interested in pursuing such arrangements are urged to ask the following questions in addition to those posed in the general checklist at the end of the chapter:

1. What services are covered by the PMPM allowance? In particular, are facility services included? What kinds of facility services? Physicians should be wary of accepting capitated risk for outpatient services without an adjustment for the movement of inpatient services into the outpatient setting. How does the PMPM allowance compare with the fee-for-service payments that the physician or physician group would normally receive? Will the PMPM amounts cover the facility services that are likely to be needed? Does the physician or physician group have the ability to estimate reliably the facility component of costs? Who will be responsible for the cost of hospital-based physicians?

2. Are the PMPM allowances adjusted to reflect differences in age, sex, and other characteristics of the enrolled population? Without sex and age adjustments, at a minimum, physicians may be responsible for providing services to a much sicker than expected population without an increase in compensation above the negotiated PMPM allowance. How will the PMPM allowances be adjusted on a periodic (e.g., annual) basis? Is an inflator specifically included? How will it be computed? If the HMO grants fee increases to some types of providers, such as hospitals, will the PMPM allowances be adjusted to reflect such increases? Or will the physicians be expected to absorb them through utilization reductions or other efficiencies?

3. How will the at-risk group identify the members who are covered by the capitated or otherwise at-risk arrangement? Will they carry membership cards? Will there be a way of checking eligibility by telephone or through a computer? And will the HMO be responsible for payment if it authorizes services for a member who is later determined to have been ineligible at the time that services were delivered?

4. Is the number of members covered by the capitated arrangement large enough for their expenses and utilization levels to be reasonably predicted? Is the HMO able and willing to share historical cost and utilization information about its members with the physician group or network? Will the HMO agree to risk-sharing provisions whereby the HMO will absorb part of the excessive cost if the medical services needed by the enrolled population substantially exceed the targeted levels? Are explicit forms of risk limitation, such as individual and aggregate stop-loss insurance, available from the HMO? Is the charge for such protections reasonable? Does the physician group have the right to reject the HMO's reinsurance coverage and obtain its own?

5. In general, are the utilization management practices imposed by the HMO helpful or harmful to the physicians in managing the demand for their services and overall cost and utilization levels? What are the referral procedures and other utilization management techniques imposed by the HMO or by the provider network or management firm? Are they administratively onerous? In particular, if facility costs are not included in the capitation, will precertification of outpatient surgical operations, significant diagnostic procedures, and/or hospital admissions be required? How far in advance? By telephone? By modem? Will a PCP authorization be required? How will such authorizations be compiled, tracked, and made available to individual physicians? What penalties apply to a physician who provides a service without authorization—full loss of

full capitation and percent of premium arrangements. At the risk of some redundancy, we strongly urge any physicians or other providers contemplating
participation in such arrangements to consider the following list of questions:

1. What is the local reputation of the HMO for honesty, administrative efficiency, and marketing effectiveness? How long has it been operating in the
local market? Regionally? Nationally? What is its financial position in terms of
profitability, liquidity, capital reserves, and debt capacity? Does it have a record
of timely payments to providers? Is its utilization management program reasonable? Can it provide useful information in a timely manner? Does it have a
fair and equitable procedure for resolving medical and administrative disputes?

2. What medical services are included in the at-risk arrangement? What
services are carved out and treated as the financial responsibility of the HMO?
Out-of-area services? Emergency services? Transplants? Burn cases? Pharmacy?
Mental health? Was the provider group consulted before such services were included or carved out? Is the HMO flexible in how they are handled? For example, can the risk be shared for some of these services between the HMO and
provider group?

3. What administrative services are provided by the HMO? By the provider
group? If required to provide an array of administrative services, is the provider
group adequately compensated? Does the provider group have these capabilities?

4. Is the schedule of PMPM allowances (or the premium structure) established by the HMO sensitive to differences in the age and sex of enrollees?
Will individual and family contracts be counted differently? How will the
amounts credited to the provider group be determined? Will the PMPM allowances and/or premium structure of the HMO be adjusted, depending on
whether certain benefits (e.g., prescription drugs) are included? Will the
HMO adjust the PMPM allowances or premium credits assigned to the provider group if it changes the covered medical services and/or the cost sharing
(i.e., deductible and coinsurance/copayment) obligations of enrollees? Providers should avoid being held responsible for providing an expanding set of
services to a population whose expected costs are not reasonably reflected in
the PMPM allowances or premium credits.

5. How will the PMPM allowances be adjusted throughout the term of the
agreement? Is there a specified inflator? Will the HMO adjust the PMPM allowances to reflect any fee increases that it grants to various provider groups?
Or will the physicians be placed at risk for such fee increases? In percent of
premium arrangements in which the HMO retains some underwriting responsibility (i.e., a share of any gains or losses), the PMPM allowances automatically
adjust with changes in the premium levels.

6. Will the HMO do medical underwriting? In other words, will it screen
the population applying for coverage to identify individuals who have or are
likely to develop major illnesses? Or will it offer coverage on an open enrollment basis? Whatever the social view of the provider group with regard to the

appropriateness of medical underwriting, it needs to protect itself from potentially disastrous financial commitments. If the HMO does not do medical underwriting and if the provider group is at risk for the cost of medical services, it may absorb large losses even if the PMPM allowances or premium credits are designed to reflect differences in age, sex, and other demographic characteristics. An HMO that has shifted the responsibility for health care costs to an at-risk provider group has little reason to screen potential members. Therefore, if historically the HMO has done medical medical underwriting and if the experience data used to establish the PMPM allowances or premium credits reflect that medical underwriting, the arrangement with the HMO should provide that changes in underwriting practices will be grounds for renegotiation of the PMPM allowances or premium credits.

7. Is any requirement placed on the HMO to keep its premiums reasonably in line with those charged by other HMOs in the market for similar products? Similarly, does the HMO bear any risk for losses generated by excessive medical costs? As noted above, if the HMO does not participate in underwriting losses, it will have little interest in making sure that its underwriting practices (e.g., premium setting, risk assessment, risk management) are designed to prevent such losses.

8. Is stop-loss coverage available in the agreement from the HMO? Does it cover individual cases (e.g., individuals with medical expenses greater than $25,000 in any contract year)? Is aggregate stop loss also available? At what attachment point(s) are the individual stop-loss (ISL) and aggregate stop-loss (ASL) protections available? For what proportion of costs, if any, is the provider group responsible above the attachment point(s)? How are the medical costs counted or accumulated for the purpose of determining the recovery due under the stop-loss policy? Is there an explicit charge to the provider group? Is the reinsurance coverage adequately described? Does the HMO give a copy of the reinsurance policy or its provisions to the provider group? Is the provider group free to obtain its own reinsurance coverage and to eliminate any charge for such coverage that otherwise would be levied by the HMO?

9. In establishing the capitated or percent of premium budgets, does the HMO set a single integrated budget (i.e., one covering all at-risk services), or does it establish separate pools for hospital vs. professional and other services or similar components? Why? And on what basis is the allocation of funds to the various pools determined? What shares of surpluses or losses are assigned to the HMO and to the provider group? Do these shares differ across the pools? Why? Can the HMO change the allocations to these pools during the contract term? On what bases? Does the provider group have to agree to such changes? If losses occur, how is the provider group required to pay them back? By check? By means of reductions in future PMPM allowances or premium credits? How frequently are surpluses and losses computed, and in what time frames are associated rewards rewards and penalties applied? Is the HMO or or treatments? Are these criteria well-recognized and available to the physicians or developed by the HMO? Will local physicians have input into these criteria? Will the HMO have the right to make retroactive denials of services? Will UM decisions be made by physicians? Under what circumstances? Will UM responsibilities be delegated to the provider network?

Quality management. What quality management methods will be used by the HMO? What is the source of any quality standards? What will be the responsibility of the physicians? Will they be paid for participation on quality management or other committees? Can some aspects of the quality management function be delegated to the providers? How will differences in quality be measured? Rewarded? Penalized?

Professional liability insurance. How much professional insurance will the individual physicians be required to maintain? Is the requirement reasonable?

Information. What information will the HMO regularly provide to the physicians or provider group? Will it be provided in hard copy or computer-readable form? Will the HMO assure its reliability? What information will the physicians be required to provide to the HMO?

Appeals, grievances, and disputes. Does the HMO offer fair and reasonable and timely processes for resolution of differences between parties over medical services and administrative issues? Who makes the final decision? Is arbitration available through an independent body?

Audits. Does the physician or provider group have access to the books and records of the HMO as needed to verify the accuracy of PMPM allowances, premium credits, claims payments and utilization levels, allocations of losses, and surpluses? Otherwise, how can the providers be sure that they receive fair treatment?

Assignment. Does either party have the right to assign the agreement to another entity without the approval of the other party? Under what circumstances? Are any assignment rights reciprocal between the parties?

The checklist provided above certainly does not substitute for a detailed and thorough review of a proposed contract by an experienced health care attorney and by other persons trained in the financing and delivery of health care services in the managed care environment. However, the checklist and the previous discussions supply useful insights into the most important features, risks, and potential rewards of at-risk managed care contracts.

REFERENCES

1. Office of Technology Assessment: Payment for Physician Services: Strategies for Medicare. Washington, DC, U.S. Government Printing Office, 1986.
2. Zubkoff M, Raskin IE, Hanfft R (eds): Hospital Cost Containment: Selected Notes for Future Policy. New York, Prodist, 1978.
3. Fielding JE: Corporate Health Management.Reading, MA, Addison-Wesley, 1984.

4. Office of Technology Assessment: Medicare's Prospective Payment System: Strategies for Evaluating Cost, Quality, and Medical Technology. Washington, DC, U.S. Government Printing Office, 1985.

5. Cowan DH: Preferred Provider Organizations: Planning, Structure, and Organization. Germantown, MD, Aspen Systems, 1985.

6. Lewin Group: Managed Care Savings for Employers and Households: 1990 through 2000. Washington, DC, The Lewin Group, 1997.

7. Winslow R: Employee health care costs were steady last year. Wall Street J January 30, 1996.

8. American Medical Association: Negotiating and Contracting in Managed Care. Chicago, American Medical Association, 1993.

9. American Medical Association: Physicians' Current Procedural Terminology, 4th ed. Chicago, American Medical Association, 1996.

10. American Medical Association: Medicare RBRVS: The Physician's Guide. Chicago, American Medical Association, 1996.

11. CPT Guidebook for Managed Care. Reston, VA, St. Anthony, 1996.

12. Managed Care Industry Overview. Baltimore, Alex Brown & Sons, 1994.

13. American Medical Association: Managed Care Strategies for Physicians. Chicago, American Medical Association, 1993.

14. Palmer AR: Economics of Participation in Preferred Provider Organizations. Santa Monica, CA, Rand Corporation, 1985.

15. Oxford to use specialists as care coordinators. Health Care Capitation and Risk Contracting 3:1–2, 1997.

MELINDA B. EVERETT, AB, MS, APR

8

Using the Media to Promote Your Practice

When famous stick-up artist Willie Sutton was asked why he robbed banks, he replied tersely, "Because that's where the money is." Similar logic dictates why it is important for physicians to work with the media: because the media offer the best access to prospective patients. Medical and fitness news holds an abiding fascination for the American public, and most major newspapers, talk shows, and newscasts are replete with medical information. The media need experts to interview for such stories, and one of those experts could be you. This chapter outlines simple, effective "how to's" for tapping into media—and prospective patient—interest.

First and foremost, keep the target audience(s) firmly in mind as you seek media representatives with whom to foster a rapport. By selecting media that put you in front of your target audience, you maximize your chances of attracting future patients. For example, if you are a pediatrician, taking the opportunity to speak to a Parent-Teacher Association meeting about childhood immunizations may net more patients than a stint on a more esoteric lecture circuit or even on a national television program.

Also, remember that while you are a medical authority, media producers and reporters are the final authorities in determining what their audience will ultimately read, hear, or see. The media have the last word on how your message is packaged and presented. Medical experts frequently decry the media's preference for 10-second soundbites and easily digested—some would say oversimplified—information. Although this admittedly is not the ideal way to dispense health information, it is what the media dictate. Fortunately, the technique of speaking in soundbites and coming rapidly and powerfully to the point *can* be mastered with a little practice.

ADVERTISING AND PUBLIC RELATIONS

Advertising and public relations are two basic and important tools to use in promoting your practice. Keep in mind the two key differences between advertising and public relations, which are a major consideration in determining which media strategy you will want to use in any given instance. **Advertising** is paid for and, therefore, within certain guidelines can be controlled, whereas **public relations** is not paid for and, because it is free, cannot be controlled or produce guaranteed results.

Two examples illustrate the differences between advertising and public relations in action. You want an ad to announce that your practice recently opened on Main Street in Anytown, U.S.A. You call the advertising representative at the local newspaper, provide relevant details (e.g., office hours, phone number), and agree to look at a mock-up of the ad before it runs. You decide which days and perhaps even in which section of the newspaper you want it to appear. Then you pay for the ad, and it appears as ordered.

The public relations scenario may work this way: the public relations director of the hospital with which you are affiliated calls and says, "I've got a reporter from the *Anytown Times* who's interested in interviewing an expert on bicycle safety tips. As a pediatrician, you're a perfect choice for the interview." You agree to do the interview and to call the reporter at the paper at 3 PM on Tuesday. You check several journals, gather relevant statistics, and follow through on your commitment to talk with the reporter.

The interview goes smoothly, and you wait for the article to appear in the *Times* Health Section next Monday. Monday arrives, you check the newspaper and—nothing. You debate about calling the reporter and asking what happened and why he wasted your time. Fortunately, the reporter calls first and explains that the story was "pulled" because the local nursing home just bought a huge ad to announce the opening of its new recreation room. "Next week," the reporter promises. Next week, something else causes the article to be pulled.

Finally, after three weeks of disappointment, the article runs. Because it was "free" (except for wear-and-tear on you), you obviously had no control over when or where the story appeared. The **element of control** is the most important difference between advertising and public relations.

Before you decide that public relations results are too unpredictable and not worth the effort, consider the significant advantage of public relations over most advertising: public relations is viewed as "real news" and is, therefore, inherently more believable than advertising, which is "bought." For example, an ad for aspirin may run repeatedly on television with little result. However, a cardiologist interviewed on television cites the benefits of aspirin for poststroke patients, and there is a run on aspirin in local supermarkets.

Granted, there are numerous times when a simple, tasteful ad—for example, announcing a new staff member or new office location—is all that you need to get your message across. However, there may be many other times when it is vastly more effective if you can harness the power of public relations to build your practice.

Fortunately, tapping into public relations resources is not difficult in today's health care environment. Virtually every health care facility, from community hospitals to urban medical centers, has one or more public relations practitioners on staff or as consultants. That expert or team of experts is also available to help you. Even if you are in solo practice and have not been exposed to the ins and outs of public relations, consultants are available to help you at a relatively moderate cost. Even implementing your own public relations program is not overly difficult (more about that later). But, first, consider in-house public relations teams.

Public relations practitioners often wear many different hats, bear many different titles, and interface with numerous other health care facility departments, such as marketing, development, human resources, and strategic planning. Some public relations experts also serve as government affairs officials, working with lobbyists, legislators, and the institution's constituencies to ensure that the facility is perceived favorably. Public relations offices also may be responsible for community benefit and educational outreach activities, such as health fairs and screenings.

You are looking for the public relations professional charged with arranging media interviews and securing favorable press for the institution. Depending on the size of the facility, that person probably will have a title such as media relations director, coordinator, or manager. If you are not sure which person to contact, there is nothing wrong with calling the department directly and asking to speak to the person in charge of media relations. Most public relations departments will welcome your interest.

It is always to your advantage to work yourself into the media relations director's plans rather than the other way around. The media relations director is responsible for all staff interactions with the media and is usually the institution's designated spokesperson. The director knows which representatives of the media are the most reliable, which are interested in specific subjects, and how best to present news and feature ideas. The director also can plug you into the institution's speaker's bureau, grand rounds, and other lecture circuit opportunities. By working with the media relations department, you are a hero. Try going around the department, and you are a loose cannon—or worse.

But what if you are in private practice, not affiliated with a hospital, health maintenance organization, academic medical center, or other health care facility? Your two basic options are to go it alone or to hire a public relations consultant or agency. Before you decide, consider the various media outlets, their respective rewards and pitfalls, strategies for accessing each outlet, and the amount of work required to implement a successful public relations plan for your practice.

MEDIA OUTLETS AND HOW TO ACCESS THEM

Today there are more media outlets than ever before, and health care is one of the hottest of hot topics. To position yourself as a sought-after interview subject, it is important to find the medium that is best suited to your message, your style of presentation, and your target audience(s).

To unearth and assess the media outlets, head for the humanities reference section of any large public library. In the Boston area, for instance, the Boston Public Library provides access to *The Boston University Media Guide*, which contains information about virtually every media outlet in New England, complete with producers' and reporters' names and relevant phone numbers. The *Standard Rate and Data Service* is also a good source of information about magazines and other periodicals. The effectiveness of these reference materials, of course, is greatly enhanced if you spend some time studying the programs and periodicals to get the flavor of each medium. Armed with this information, you are ready to dig in.

NEWSPAPERS

For a society supposedly on its way to becoming paperless, Americans are still surprisingly devoted to their newspapers. Newspapers also have pass-along value—a person reading the paper may pass along an interesting article to friends, family members, or coworkers. Thus one interview in a small, local weekly may generate many times the weekly's actual circulation in pass-along readership. This is good news because smaller papers, such as weeklies and "shoppers" (free newspapers supported by ad revenue), are usually much easier to interest in doing local interviews than large daily papers, which have their own usually well-developed sources.

Review several copies of the paper in which you are interested in appearing. Many would-be interviewees overlook this simple step, and reporters have a keen sense of when they are being conned. Determine whether the target publication has a regular health section and, if so, whether a particular reporter is assigned to the health/medical beat. If no particular reporter is listed, ask to speak to the assignment editor, who will give you the name of the reporter with whom you should talk or tell you that the idea probably is of no interest at that time. If so, do not argue. Bide your time, and come up with a different suggestion later.

Decide the topic about which you want to be interviewed. Think about interviews in terms of what the paper's readership will be interested in hearing about. For example, as a pediatrician, you know that seat belts save lives, but that is not news. However, many parents probably are not aware of seat belt "dos and don'ts" and how seat belt safety requirements change for infants, toddlers, and children. Present your story this way, and you are thinking like a reporter.

Next, call the reporter. The first words you utter after, "Hi, I'm Dr. Yourname," should be "Are you on deadline? Or do you have a quick minute to listen to a story idea?" If the reporter indicates that he or she can talk for a minute, make it just that. Pitch your story quickly and vividly. (See tips under "How to Get Your Foot in the Media Door.") Then arrange for an interview time and follow through.

CABLE TELEVISION

Most cities and towns have cable television stations that feature news and local programming. And, although many programs are done by professional producers and newscasters, some programs, particularly local access programming, are often produced by trained volunteers.

To decide whether cable television is the medium for you, spend an hour or so watching the local station. If you decide that the results are suitably professional, local access programming may be a good starting point. Even if you decide not to work with the local access programmers, you may be able to arrange for an interview with the station's professional news and features team.

To do so, call the station and ask to speak to the news or features producer. Mention that you have watched the station (be specific) and wonder whether they may need a medical professional from time to time. Then *briefly* offer one or two story suggestions, such as, "I know this is prom season, and I thought you might like to talk about how alcohol affects teenagers and about some common misconceptions about drinking and sobering up." Make your topics *timely* and *intriguing*. In most instances, the smaller the station, the better your chances of getting a placement. And even small stations can be popular with your target audience(s).

LOCAL TELEVISION

Local or regional television is produced in most major cities across the country in affiliation with national networks such as ABC, NBC, and CBS. Your best hope of securing appearances on local or national television is through your hospital's media relations department or by hiring a media or public relations professional. Most television news teams are routinely inundated with requests for their time and, unless you are a recognized medical guru, prefer to work with their own contacts and sources. By keeping your target audience(s) in mind and working assiduously with media outlets to which you have good access, you will not need the difficult-to-attract "big" television stations.

NETWORK TELEVISION

The above comments go double for national network television. However, if you are able to work with a network through media relations at a hospital or other health care facility, by all means consider network television in your media repertoire.

TRADE AND PROFESSIONAL JOURNALS

Writing articles for professional journals can be time-consuming, but there can also be benefits—if you follow the first rule of public relations, never do good silently. In other words, once you have an article published, display copies in your waiting room. Send a small, tasteful announcement to your local newspaper: "Dr. Yourname recently had an article published in *Name of Professional Publication*. Dr. Yourname, who is in practice at Youraddress, discussed infant safety." Provide your patients with photocopies or reprints, if appropriate, and use a copy of the article to accompany your next pitch letter or to follow up on a call to a radio or television program director. The point is to maximize your media success and use it to build future successes.

REGIONAL AND NATIONAL RADIO

Even in major cities, local radio stations are often more accessible than newspapers and, certainly, than television. Furthermore, radio program directors are generally more accessible than television producers and program directors. Better yet, radio stations do not have to schedule cameras and film crews, making their interview times more flexible than television's.

To find a radio station that has talk shows suitable for a guest interview, check your local station listings in the newspaper, or simply check the phone book listings and call each station's program director. (Stations are usually listed in the business pages under "radio.") Of course, it is best to listen to a program before you call to pitch yourself. (Tip: Look in the library's media guide for radio stations that broadcast on 50,000 watts; they have a much wider reach and listening audience.)

ADVICE COLUMNS AND ADVERTORIALS

An extremely useful, cost-effective media strategy is the medical advice column, placed in your local newspaper. In the past, doctors, depending on their specialties, were often invited to guest-author such columns—but not any more (or, at least, rarely). The columns are now "advertorials," paid advertising that presents messages for the public good (while also promoting the person or organization sponsoring the message).

The advantage of tastefully done advertorials is that you control the message and frequency of appearance. The disadvantage is that you need to write the copy and pay for the ads. However, if you are going it alone, without benefit of an institution's media relations director or a paid consultant, weekly advertorials are a strategy worth pursuing.

To gauge the success of an advertorial campaign, you should be prepared to run the column weekly for at least three months. Then decide whether the benefits—new patients, requests for interviews, good will—outweigh the costs of time and money.

PRO BONO CAUSES

As the saying goes, it is often possible to do well by doing good, especially when supporting popular public causes to gain media attention. For example, you might volunteer to serve on the board of Mothers Against Drunk Driving, the local chapter of the American Heart Association, or any number of worthy health- and safety-related organizations. By helping such groups, you also may become their medical spokesperson (working with their media relations professional, if they have one). You help the organization, develop your media skills, and gain access to interested media at the same time.

HOSPITAL AND HEALTH CARE FACILITY PUBLICATIONS

If you are affiliated with a local hospital or similar health care facility (e.g., nursing home, rehabilitation center), many opportunities may be available to publicize your practice. Most health care facilities have an active mailing list and send their publications to former patients, business and civic leaders, and targeted families within their service areas. The facility's public relations or public affairs director is the person to approach about including you in institutional publications. Although many directors and/or publications editors who determine content have special themes and topics for the various publications, they are usually receptive to good suggestions and may use them in future issues. Be helpful but never pushy, and you may be on their list of favorite contacts.

INTERNET

There is plenty of interest in using the Internet to attract interest in one's service or product. However, a poorly designed web site or one that is eternally "under construction" is far worse than no web site at all. If the institution with which you are affiliated has a web site, introduce yourself to the web master and public relations director and see whether you can use the web as a media vehicle.

If you are on your own, however, the benefits of building and maintaining a web site probably are far outweighed by the time and effort demanded, especially if you are looking for rapid payback with minimal problems. A compromise strategy, if you specialize in the treatment of rare diseases or disorders, is to contact the national or local chapter for that particular condition and ask to be listed on their web site.

At the same time, always remember your target audience(s). Are they likely to be web savvy? You can grow old and frustrated waiting for your audience to climb the learning curve into web world.

SUPPORT AND DISCUSSION GROUPS

If you are affiliated with a health care organization, you may already be working with a patient and family support group. You can organize a support group of your own, depending on your office facilities and time constraints. For example, if you are a pediatrician, you may give a talk about schoolyard safety in the fall. Or, if you are a geriatrician, you may hold a series of talks about topics of interest to senior citizens. (Should I continue to drive? How do I talk with my children about my health concerns?) Remember to take scheduling and accommodations into careful consideration. Do not schedule programs in the evening for seniors who have trouble driving in the dark, and do not hold the talk in a hall that is shabby or too small.

Support and discussion groups also need to be fully publicized. Consider the time involved in sending flyers to your patients, displaying posters in public buildings, and sending calendar listings to local newspapers and radio stations. Is this a productive use of your time?

PERSONAL APPEARANCES: THE LECTURE CIRCUIT

Physicians, especially those newly in practice, are usually too busy for any circuit, except perhaps the drive to the office. However, if you have been asked to speak at a symposium or forum, take advantage of the media opportunity that you have been handed. Provide your local newspaper with a brief, tasteful announcement of the fact that you will be speaking. Being available to local civic groups is also an important way to make your presence known in the community and to build awareness and good will.

MAGAZINES

As with the Internet, it is usually difficult and time-consuming to build a practice via magazine articles. If you are fortunate enough to be affiliated with an institution with a national reputation, your chances are much improved. Your best approach is to work with the institution's media relations director and to let the director arrange interviews. Do not be discouraged if the interviews sometimes do not pan out. Many magazine articles are written by freelancers who have an entire country—sometimes the world—of interview sources from which to choose.

If you want to try writing and submitting an article yourself, *Writer's Market* (available in most bookstores and libraries) lists hundreds of possible markets.

Consider the competition, and, if you truly want to write, consider purchasing advertorial space in a publication in your own backyard. (Remember what Willie Sutton said.)

PHOTOCOPIES

Photocopies are an excellent, inexpensive way to make your media successes do double duty. Make sure that the copies are professional-looking. A local copier service will handle the process for a small charge. Have the copies available in your waiting room, and see how your practice grows.

HOW TO GET YOUR FOOT IN THE MEDIA DOOR

Now that you are aware of the myriad of media outlets, here is how to get your foot in the media door.

Your chances of media access will be enhanced greatly if you never contact any medium unless you have done your homework and can deliver your story pitch in no more than five concise sentences. (The entire Gettysburg Address was only 14 minutes, after all.) Reporters, editors, producers, and program directors are busy people. They are short on time, short on energy, and sometimes short on patience. Do not waste their time—and your opportunity— with a poorly thought-out, unfocused pitch.

Here is an example of a well-planned and well-presented pitch: "Hello, Mr. Smith, this Dr. Yourname. Are you on deadline? No? Great. It's prom season, and I thought your [readers, listeners, or viewers] might want to have some common drinking and driving myths explored. For instance, if you drink three cups of coffee, you'll sober up. Instead, coffee can really do a job on your system."

Use two or three vivid examples, and you will have the reporter hooked because the pitch is timely, relevant, interesting, easy to understand, and professionally delivered. (Tip: practice, practice, practice. Set a kitchen timer to two minutes, and start practicing your delivery. Or try the pitch on your toughest critics—your children.)

SELECTING A MEDIA CONSULTANT

If you are not affiliated with an institution and are not comfortable with developing media possibilities on your own, your best option is to hire a media relations consultant. Your problem, however, is not a lack of consultants—it is access to too many. Although many senior-level public relations practitioners are "accredited" by the Public Relations Society of America (PRSA) after passing a lengthy written examination, there is no licensure requirement for public relations counselors. As usual, the buyer must beware.

In selecting a public or media relations consultant, your two best sources are word of mouth (ask colleagues for their recommendations) and the telephone book. Look under public relations counselors, agencies, marketing communications, and related categories. You may decide to steer away from large public relations agencies that may eat up your budget and are geared to servicing national clients.

Your best resource may be a solo practitioner or a small agency. Talk with the local chamber of commerce, local health care reporters, and—most importantly—the consultant you plan to hire. Ask for samples and references, and check them out carefully. You are looking for someone to handle your most precious commodity: your reputation.

Expect to pay hourly rates of $25–75, although many counselors are receptive to per-project pricing. Do not be afraid to negotiate, but be realistic and fair. Run a mile from any practitioner who promises what you cannot realistically expect to be delivered. (Remember: advertising can be controlled; public relations cannot.) It is reasonable to ask a prospective public relations consultant to suggest several ways to build your practice—it is not reasonable to expect him or her to present an entire plan.

A basic plan may include such elements as a weekly advertorial in the local paper (perhaps ghost-written by the consultant), three bimonthly talks to the chamber of commerce, two bimonthly talks to the Parent-Teacher Association, and a guest interview on at least one major radio station. You do not need the *New York Times*; you want the audience in your own backyard.

CONCLUSION

As you go about working with the media to build your practice, make sure that your practice—your "product"—is a good one and that your expert opinions and interactions with reporters attract favorable media interest and keep the reporters coming back for more.

Once you have created demand for your product—*you*—continue to be accessible and responsive to the media. Establish clear guidelines with your staff as to how and when to reach you with media inquiries. When the media come calling, it is never to your advantage if reporters cannot reach you. Nothing turns a reporter off faster than voice mail (except perhaps "no comment").

Certainly, patient care must come first, but if you need to reschedule a media interview, make sure that the reporter is informed and that an alternative time is selected. Both print and electronic media have become increasingly competitive as television, radio, and newspapers battle fiercely for audiences, ad dollars, and ratings. A reporter whose source falls through may even lose his or her job. Reporters cherish sources that they can rely on, and they never forget a source who has stood them up. Your responsibility is to make every reasonable effort to be available for the scheduled interview and to prepare for it as you would for any important presentation.

Then sit back and enjoy your media success and your new patients.

BIBLIOGRAPHY

Look on any bookshelf—make that bookshelves because there are dozens of them—in any good-sized bookstore, and you will find plenty of publications to help you with every facet of writing. Believe it or not, there are guides to everyday life in the 1800s (for writers of historical fiction and/or time travel), books on writing erotica, and guides to poisons, weapons, wounds, and forensics. Perhaps surprisingly, however, there are few guides to medical writing for a lay/consumer audience.

To aid in attracting the media and writing for a general audience, your best bet is probably to purchase a few books or magazines that provide lists of consumer and special interest publications that may want to receive a submission—or at least a query letter—from you. I have listed several below. You do not need all of them, but each is helpful and informative, depending on your specific needs.

The Writer's Digest (magazine)
"Your Monthly Guide to Getting Published"
$2.99
Subscription Service
PO Box 2123
Harlan, IA 51593

The Writer (magazine)
$2.50
The Writer, Inc.
120 Boylston St.
Boston, MA 02116-4615
Note: Offers a special subscription rate to new subscribers of 5 issues for $10.

The Complete Guide to Magazine Article Writing (hardcover)
John M. Wilson
$17.99
Published by Writer's Digest Books
F&W Publications, Inc.
1507 Dana Ave.
Cincinnati, OH 45207

Writer's Guide to Magazine Editors & Publishers (paperback)
Judy Mandell
$23
Prima Publishing
PO Box 1260 BK
Rocklin, CA 95677

1998 Writer's Market (paperback)
"Where & How to Sell What You Write"
Edited by Kristen Holm
$27.99
Writer's Digest Books
F&W Publications, Inc.
1507 Dana Ave.
Cincinnati, OH 45207
Note: The granddaddy of how-to books for all aspiring writers. It is updated every year, with
hundreds of new markets. There is even a CD-ROM version for about $45. If you are
serious about getting published, do not sit in front of your computer without it.

WENDY W. FINK, BA

BARRY BEDER, MSW

ROBERT NAPARSTEK, MD

BARRY S. TAYLOR, ND

9

Practicing the Art of Medicine

Practicing the art of medicine is a fascinating and compelling topic. It provides opportunities to bring our knowledge and experience into practice and to fine-tune our technical and human interactive skills. It can be, for each health care provider, a source of fulfillment that enables us to be happier and more productive in our work and in our lives. The art of practicing medicine is a broad topic. For this chapter, however, art is defined as managing the powerful relationship between physician and patient, including activities, attitudes, and interpersonal skills that make effective and empathetic doctors.

The art of medicine allows us to bring our clinical skills to each patient in ways that dramatically and positively optimize the potential outcome. Without the art, we are technicians. With the art, we become healers.

This chapter is the result of collaboration among four authors who represent a variety of approaches to healing. It is different from most other chapters in this book and different from most texts that you read in medical school. We want to share our collective experience of many decades of assisting people in the healing process. We want to do so in ways that are comfortable and, hopefully, inspiring to our readers. We want to raise the flag for the importance of interpersonal skills—skills that we think are woefully under-emphasized in the training of most health care professionals—and invite readers to think seriously about the humanistic aspects and rewards of the physician–patient relationship.

We have interviewed dozens of patients and asked what the art of medicine means to them. We asked them to describe their best and worst experiences with health care providers. Invariably, they responded that the art had to do with the way their physician interacted with them. Typically, they would say, " I know my doctor knows his [her] stuff. My doctor is a well-educated person." Often they would add, "But my doctor's communication skills aren't so hot," or

"But I find it really difficult to talk with my doctor," or "My doctor seems too busy to talk, so I just don't ask. I don't want to waste his [her] time."

Our goal is to help you focus on (1) the importance of the physician–patient relationship and (2) specific skills and approaches that can be integrated into your practice.

Although you bring exceptional technical skills to each situation, it is important to be aware that your diagnosis and treatment plans are significantly affected by the quality of your interactions with your patients. Most ultimate outcomes of life, death, health, and morbidity are *not* a direct result of your specific acts. Rather, they are the result of the choices and acts of your patients. You can help your patients realize this fact. In so doing, you give them power. You can then guide this new-found power to help the patient arrive at healthy outcomes. Managing the quality of the doctor–patient relationship will help you and your patients make effective treatment plans that the patient will implement because of the bond between you.

The art of medicine provides skill sets that enable you to be a more effective healer. In addition, the techniques involved in the art of medicine have been shown to be the most important factors in the prevention of malpractice suits.

Doctors who talk with and listen to their patients have fewer malpractice suits. Research has clearly shown that *nice doctors do not get sued!* A study reported in *Lancet* in 1994 consistently pointed to "lack of caring" as the number one reason why doctors are sued.[15] Other factors and behaviors include inaccessibility of the physician, lack of information, aloofness of the caregiver, and reluctance to apologize. More than 30% of patients and relatives included in the *Lancet* study said that they would not have sued if they had received an explanation or an apology from their physician.

THE ART OF MEDICINE MAKES US MORE EFFECTIVE HEALERS

The art of medicine regulates the heartbeat of the healing process. Unlike the science of medicine, which is specific, concrete, and quantifiable, the art of medicine cannot be measured in clinical or tangible units. It involves many intangibles such as communication, leadership, empathy, and bonding, all of which are orchestrated (along with many other intangibles) by you in your interaction with each patient. The *Microsoft Word* thesaurus lists the following synonyms for art: "aptitude, artfulness, skill, adroitness, ability, inventiveness, expertise, imagination and dexterity." All of these factors can come into play when you meet with your patients.

As we explore the depths of the art of medicine, however, our definition goes beyond the *Microsoft Word* thesaurus. Our art is separate from our clinical skill and expertise. It has more to do with our mood, tone, and being than the skills on which we focused in our training. This art is not derived from science but complements science with its own vulnerable truth. This truth is what the relationship with the patient yearns to achieve. The art communicates and provides our service to others as they seek their own truth about their medical status and prognosis.

In his classic book, *The Lost Art of Healing*, Bernard Lown, M.D., suggests that our health care system is suffering because the patient is not considered to be central to the healing process.[10] We have become more concerned with technology, pharmacology, financial pressures, and malpractice than with involving the patient as the number one member of his or her health care team. Lown recounts vignettes from his remarkable 40-year practice as a cardiologist and professor at the Harvard School of Public Health and cofounder of International Physicians for the Prevention of Nuclear War, on whose behalf he accepted the Nobel Peace Prize in 1985. He proposes a new paradigm of medicine built on our shared humanity, one in which the art of healing is as valued as the mastery of medical techniques.

THE PHYSICIAN–PATIENT RELATIONSHIP— AN ENDANGERED SPECIES?

The patient–physician relationship should be part of every treatment plan because so much responsibility for a successful outcome rests with the patient and the choices that he or she makes after leaving your office. The relationship between some physicians and their patients has become increasingly compromised over the past several decades in direct relationship to the exponential increase in the number of technical and pharmacologic advances.

Dr. Herbert Benson, Director of the Mind/Body Clinic at Beth Israel/Deaconess Hospital in Boston, suggests that the practice of health care can be illustrated by a three-legged stool.[2] According to Benson, one leg is pharmacology, one is surgery, and one is behavioral interventions. The art of practicing medicine is part of the third leg of the stool.

Many factors have resulted in the breakdown of the doctor–patient relationship, including physician specialization, astounding advances in the science of medicine, the need for continuing education to maintain competency, marked increase in paperwork, and the demands of managed care protocols. As physicians have become more and more preoccupied with all of these factors, their attention to the human interactions between caregiver and patient has taken a secondary role. The art is becoming lost in the shuffle. This loss is tragic.

Patients play an important role in the phenomenon as well. Most patients are not educated to be conscious about their role as consumers of medical care. More resources are available to guide them in the purchase of a car than to help them select a physician.

In some instances, society has placed the medical profession on a pedestal, and this idealization has created a sense that the doctor's time is too valuable to "waste" with uneducated questions. In our culture, we also have been socialized to believe that no matter what we do to ourselves, someone else (the doctor) can make us better. Our society is only now beginning to become aware of the fact that each and every one of us is our own ultimate caregiver.

Another barrier to the powerful doctor–patient relationship is that we have not learned to speak intimately with one another. We may be effective at exchanging information and data, but we have not learned to communicate fears, expectations, respect, and guilt to each other. Communication is much more than information exchange. It involves "communing."

It is time to honor the importance of the human connection—the bond—between patient and physician. This bond makes the difference in supporting each patient's choice to participate fully in the recovery process by understanding and actively participating in the creation and implementation of the treatment plan. Attention to the art of medicine is a crucial step.

ARTFUL PRACTICES

The art of medicine requires that you see yourself as an educator in addition to a diagnostician and clinician. The skills outlined in this section help to create a context that supports the patient education process.

COMMUNICATION

One of your most challenging tasks is to engage in meaningful communication with your patients. Most physicians have not had much instruction about what constitutes good communication. What can we learn from communication specialists that can be applied to the patient–physician relationship?

An important rule of effective communication is to be a conscientious **listener**. This is not an easy task for any of us, and you, when pressed by your sense of lack of time and a waiting room full of other patients, may find it an especially difficult challenge. There are short cuts, however, that can help. You can learn to listen with your ears, with your eyes, and—most importantly—with your heart. What is really going on with the patient who presents with the cough that has lingered for five weeks? Is he having marital problems? Has his teenager been caught with marijuana in her backpack? Is his aged father nearing death?

You need to do **investigative listening** that gets beyond the cough, which is the chief presenting complaint. Often all it takes is a single question to bring the real problem to the surface. That question may be, "Is anything else going on in your life?" or "Is there anything else you want to tell me?"

The focus on the art of medicine means that you set different objectives for each patient's visit. Each visit focuses not only on a symptomatic, systematic review but also on an inventory of issues on a human level. To be a more effective practitioner of the art of medicine, you must have objectives in addition to those you bring from basic medical training.

The success of this dynamic rests in the importance of (1) being focused enough on the patient to be truly listening and (2) not interrupting or anticipating the words that you will say back. These two suggestions may seem trite, but they address a communication problem that is endemic in our culture. Almost everybody interrupts others. Almost everybody acts as if what they have to say next is more important than what the other person in the conversation is saying. These bad habits seriously interfere with effective communication.

The use of **eye contact** is critical to clear communication. Poets, philosophers, and healers throughout time have called the eyes the windows of the soul. When we look into each other's eyes as we speak, the power of our words is enhanced many times. The human connection becomes stronger. The feeling of being heard and understood is enhanced. Reflect on the different effect of (1) establishing eye contact or (2) looking at the medical record for the majority of time you are with a patient. Although it is important not to give a patient more eye contact than she or he can take (the patient will automatically look away when she or he needs a rest), eye contact is an important way truly to "see" our patients.

Another technique that speaks volumes is **body language**. One of the authors recalls a graphic example when her mother was in day surgery. The patient had just had arthroscopic surgery on her knee and was sharing a recovery room with a woman who had just had a colonoscopy. When the surgeon visited the other patient, she spent about 5 or 6 minutes with the patient. Although this was probably long enough to determine that the patient was recovering satisfactorily from the procedure and to answer a few questions, the doctor spent the entire time standing perpendicular to the bottom of the bed and facing the door. It was obvious that she could not wait to get out of the room.

Then the other surgeon came into the room and went to the side of his patient's bed. He gently took her hand and asked how she was feeling. The patient responded that she had more pain than she had expected. He asked her to describe the pain—was it constant or stabbing? It was constant. He said that he would increase the dosage of her pain medication for the next 24 hours. She should call him to let him know how she was doing. (His office called the next morning to check.) He also spent time telling the patient and her family what he had found during the procedure. The prognosis was excellent. There were no complications. He talked with the family and told them how good it was to have them there, even though the procedure was simple. He also had been in the room for 5 or 6 minutes.

This scenario raises the question of **touch**. Is it appropriate for a physician to do this kind of connecting and bonding? Many doctors do not feel that they have permission to touch their patients. We believe, however, that a simple touch offers an incredible opportunity to establish trust with patients. For example, when a patient comes into the office, a doctor might shake the patient's hand, place his other hand on top of their joined hands, and look the patient in the eye. This gesture can be an extraordinary moment of bonding. Touching a patient in appropriate ways—a hand on the shoulder, shaking a hand, touching a hand—can be a highly effective way of delivering your art.

Another important communication skill is **validation**, which consists simply of feeding back to the patient what you heard him or her say: "So, I hear you saying that your cough started about the time you realized that your father was critically ill." Validation is not the same as agreement. You are recreating the scenario that the patient has described to be certain that you understand what has been said. It is a highly technical, surgical-like communication that lets the patient know that you heard exactly what she or he said. It does not mean that you are agreeing with what was said. Validation allows the patient to feel seen and heard. You have brought the patient into the diagnostic process. And having clearly heard the patient's statement, you can guide the discussion to build on his or her understanding or to correct it if necessary. The critical process, however, is to discover the patient's interpretation of what is going on.

AN OPEN ATTITUDE

You will improve significantly the quality of your relationships with your patients if you examine your own attitudes about the relationship and what happens within it. As you begin to value good communication, empathy, and connectedness as part of your work, part of the business of being a doctor, you will begin to see your patients respond in amazing ways. Your attitude needs to value the humanistic aspects of medicine as part of your work. You need to hold the attitude that the dynamics of the patient–physician interaction are every bit as important as the patient's history and chief complaint. The art of medicine is how you are *being*, not just what you are *doing*.

It is also important to acknowledge that your patients usually know more about themselves than you do. You need to embrace them as the number one member of their own health care team because they know the truth of their own experience—far more than you could possibly discover in a routine history and a few office visits.

TIME

Managing time is one of the most difficult challenges faced by physicians. Patients are typically scheduled at regular intervals, depending on the practice and whether the patient is presenting for the first time. But patients' needs do not fit into prescribed time slots.

If your objectives for the session are strictly clinical, the visit is all about data collection and analysis. If your objectives are also to practice the art of medicine, you will need to redefine what you do with the time you have. Redefinition does not necessarily mean that you need more or less time. You are looking at the objectives of what you want to accomplish when you are with the patient. The real question is, "What do I do with the time that I have?" What is the quality of the time that you spend with your patients? The skills of practicing the art of medicine allow you to make the most of it.

One possibility is to tell your patients that you wish you had more time to be with them and that you appreciate their understanding of your time constraints. But also tell them that, no matter what the schedule says, you want to be with them long enough to understand the problem and that you have time to work together to decide what can be done about it. The visit, in fact, may still be completed in the allotted time, but the quality of the patient–physician interaction will have been significantly enhanced.

Sometimes it is absolutely necessary to spend a lengthy time with a patient. If a breakthrough is about to occur in which a patient will finally divulge a closely guarded secret or finally fathom an important connection that has affected his or her health, time must stand still. This moment is so vitally important that any premature ending will forever rupture trust. These are times when other patients simply must wait. You, meanwhile, are working hard and maintaining the highest standard of professional integrity.

The management of time also can be affected by your attitude. If you can adopt the philosophy that "what needs to get done gets done," you may feel more relaxed as you go through your busy day.

BEING FULLY PRESENT

Being fully present means that you must leave everything outside the examining room door each time you meet another patient. You must knock and then walk through the door with complete focus on the patient who waits for you. You must walk through the hospital room door having let go of the interactions that you just had with another patient or caregiver. You must take your entire intellectual, emotional, spiritual, and physical energies to the patient who waits, leaving all else behind. This task is not easy, but it becomes easier with conscious practice.

Being in the present moment is an amazing experience. This skill is not highly practiced in Western civilization. But it is incredibly powerful because it allows you to create an environment for the patient–physician exchange that is special—even sacred. The trick is to be conscious that you must be fully present to have an effective interaction with each patient. One physician consciously

Assurance of Confidentiality. Confidentiality needs to be brought out of the closet of assumed beliefs at the beginning of every new patient interaction and at any time when a privacy issue may be of concern. When you make confidentiality explicit, you create an opening for trust in the partnership. Even the appearance of a breach of confidentiality can generate ultimate mistrust in a patient. Mistrust makes the doctor–patient relationship worthless.

Compassionate Care. The practice of the art of medicine requires that you embrace the concept of compassionate care. You must be able to feel something of the patient's own experience of illness and the patient's perception of his or her own quality of life.

The feature film, *The Doctor*, presents a compelling story about the need for compassionate care and about how undervalued it is in our medical delivery system. The main character is a surgeon who is diagnosed with cancer of the larynx. We follow him through the stressful experience of having a magnetic resonance scan, radiation treatment, and, eventually, surgery. We see him "fire" the hospital's noted otolaryngologist because she does not provide compassionate care.

We share his experiences of learning from other patients with cancer what the system—his profession—typically lacks in terms of humanistic response (the art of medicine). We watch his transformation from a highly efficient, competent, but aloof surgeon into the weaker state of powerless patient (the hospital system does not recognize his status as an attending physician when he sits in a patient's chair) and his eventual metamorphosis into a compassionate human and physician.

Inspiration. Your patients need to hear success stories from you. They need you to convey your belief that they can recover—if not complete health and balance—at least some sense of control over their lives.

You become your patients' standard bearer. You lead them into their battle. You reveal to them their own power and abilities to do battle and to create their own states of health and balance. Then you become the presenter of their medal of valor—that is, you proclaim them cured or not. Even if patients are not cured, you validate a sense that their suffering has meaning.

THE PATIENT'S PERSPECTIVE

The patient comes to you for help in varying degrees of anxiety, depending on her or his perception of the problem. You may diagnose a "cold," but the presenting symptom may be a reminder that Uncle Don's fatal pneumonia started with a runny nose. It is critical to remember that the patients who come to your office for anything other than routine physicals may not have expected to be spending this time with you. They have lives to live, things to do, deadlines to meet. Most patients do not make medical care the center of their personal lives. Therefore, when they have to seek medical help, they are looking for understanding and empathy as well as a cure.

Patients come to you in fear. They come with a sense that something is wrong, that there is an imbalance in their life. They are confused, and they bring a sense of unworthiness based in the societal imbalance of power created by the system that empowers physicians and devalues the patient's role in healing. Patients often translate these feelings of imbalance to "My problem isn't worthy of your time."

However, patients also come to you with many positive qualities, such as their knowledge of themselves, their attitudes and beliefs, and their expectations. All of these are part of the human experience that you can use as you practice the art of medicine.

A MODEL PROCESS FOR PRACTICING THE ART OF MEDICINE

How, then, do you pull together all of these intangibles (and those that each individual patient brings by virtue of his or her uniqueness) to practice the art of medicine? We suggest a six-step approach:

1. Establish control. Your leadership role requires that you help the patient to feel in control. Trauma and disease often create a sense of loss of control. Your assurance that control is possible will help the patient to regroup. In a sense, patients borrow a sense of control from you. As long as people feel taken care of by someone stronger than themselves, psychologic and biologic systems seem to be protected against becoming overwhelmed. When you provide education, support, sharing of information, specific behavioral recommendations, identification of additional resources and support, and assistance in navigating the health care system, you are helping the patient to regain control.

2. Encourage communication. Communication is one of the most important elements of the patient–physician relationship. People need time and space to tell their stories. Your response, shared thoughts, and feelings help to provide a balanced dialog. Communication itself can be a therapeutic process. The openness or invitation for shared feelings creates the foundation for a therapeutic relationship.

3. Reduce guilt and alienation. Guilt and feelings of alienation are common when patients find their world disturbed by trauma or illness. You can reduce such feelings with acceptance, assurance, and support. Validation is important. Patients often blame themselves for what has gone wrong. They are embarrassed and feel less than whole because they are sick. Telling your patients that these feelings are normal will help.

4. Educate. Educating your patients is an ongoing process. You may want to provide some practical information such as, "It's important to take good care of yourself for the next few weeks. Get good sleep, eat well, drink a lot of water. Avoid alcohol while you're taking this medication." Basic information is an expression of caring. It is vitally important than you see yourself as educator as well as clinician.

5. Codevelop a treatment plan. Talk to the patient about what is and is not possible for him or her to do over the course of recovery. The treatment plan will be more likely to be carried out and more effective if the patient "owns" it. The best way to create ownership is to invite the patient into its design. You must take time to explore what a patient is both able and willing to do and to ascertain the patient's level of support in terms of human and financial resources. You create a partnership by suggesting a therapeutic course of action instead of taking charge and telling the person what he or she must do.

6. Identify resources and involve family and significant others. Your profession is richly endowed with resources that have been organized to support patient education and healing, ranging from pamphlets supplied by volunteer agencies to thousands of 800 telephone numbers and resources on the Internet. Your patients have access to more information and support than they (or you) can imagine. The trick is helping them to navigate their way through these resources so that they can choose those that will be most helpful. You provide an immeasurable service for your patients when you study the resources within your speciality and provide a list of important materials and programs for your patients' use.

You also are helped by understanding the nature of each patient's relationships with his or her family, friends, and significant others. These relationships can provide important support for the patient's quest for health. They also can provide little or no support. These possibilities require special attention in developing a treatment plan.

THE NEW PATIENT–PHYSICIAN RELATIONSHIP

The basis for the new patient–physician relationship outlined by Lown will be supported by many factors. One of them is our **shared humanity**. Doctors have problems and human frailties just as patients do. We know stories about the doctor whose wife is battling breast cancer and another physician who has rheumatoid arthritis and has had to give up his surgical practice. Still another physician is having serious behavioral problems with a teenage daughter. The realities of your own life should help you to be empathetic with your patients. We are not suggesting that you share the details of your life with your patients (unless you want to do so). We are suggesting that you can acknowledge your shared humanity in an empathetic way.

You can try to be in your patient's shoes through **empathy**. You can think about how your life would be affected if you had the patient's disease and/or disability. You can also ask patients to be in your shoes. You do so when you tell them that you wish you could spend more time talking with them. You can also ask them to come to their next visit with a list of questions so that together you can focus on their concerns in the precious time that you do have.

Another factor that comes into the equation is **shared responsibility**. The wellness movement has brought health promotion and disease prevention programs to virtually every major corporation and many small businesses. These programs have broadcast the message that more than 70% of the disabilities and premature deaths in the United States are directly related to behavioral lifestyle. You now have incredible support for helping your patients understand that you are not God and that you cannot magically repair the damage done by their own life habits. You can clearly help your patients to understand the role of their lifestyle practices in their own health and well-being. Most patients will be willing, even eager, to become actively involved in their pursuit of optimal health.

You can learn to speak more authentically by taking time to listen to your own feelings. These feelings are the expression of your heart and soul. Sometimes your heart will tell you to give the patient a hug. Admittedly, this is a sensitive issue, but you receive highly accurate information from your heart and soul when you listen to them. Some patients will welcome a hug or a warm handshake; others will not. Their body language and your own internal messages will help you to identify clearly who needs what. Your office should be sterile. You do no have to be.

Patient follow-up traditionally has been in the clinical setting. Nevertheless, the new paradigm for patient–physician interaction is greatly enhanced when you call a patient at home. Doing so makes the patient feel cared for, and the call provides useful feedback. An extra bonus for you is that it contributes to your sense of well-being and love of your work.

ACKNOWLEDGE PROGRESS

You can celebrate success with your patients, even when small successes are achieved. For example, a celebratory phone call when a new baby arrives or at the end of a chemotherapy series speaks volumes about the fact that you think of your patients even when they are not in your office. Celebration can also be appropriate when treatment plans are complete, when a behavioral goal (such as being smoke-free for 6 months) has been achieved, or when a patient completes physical therapy. The symbol does not have to be big—a card, a single flower, a balloon—to express your compassion and humanity. Recognition of what works and what has been accomplished in an office session is as important as continued exploration to correct imbalances.

All of these factors—the artful practices of medicine—are your best insurance against malpractice. They also will help to protect you against burn-out and exhaustion. We know that giving is more rewarding than receiving. To give of ourselves is the most important blessing that we can receive.

WISDOM FROM THE PAST

In his commencement address at Johns Hopkins Medical School in 1906, William Osler listed three qualities that help to make a good doctor.[12] They summarize the art of medicine:

1. Thoroughness, including attention to detail and doing things that we do not like to do. If you think of it, you should check it out. Thoroughness comes from broad-based education, getting to know the patient and his or her own environment and educating the patient at every possible opportunity.

2. Humility to realize that the outcomes are not the result of the physician's work alone. In fact, they are more likely related to the choices that the patient makes after leaving our sphere of influence.

3. Equanimity, which comes from confidence and the ability to weather any storm. Equanimity speaks of an inner peace that provides a trust that the proper outcome will be reached.

Through your work, you can elevate yourself to an improved state of personal, healthy equilibrium. When you are allowed to reveal yourself as a fellow human and sufferer, you can stop the myth that the doctor knows it all and has all of the answers.

You need the patient as much as the patient needs you. Together you become more conscious and caring people. That, after all, is practicing the art of medicine for yourself and your patients.

SUGGESTED READINGS

1. Benson H, Stuart E: The Wellness Book. New York, Simon & Schuster, 1992.
2. Benson H, Friedman R: The three-legged stool. Mind/Body Med 1:1–2, 1995.
3. Carlson R, Shield B: Healers on Healing. Los Angeles, Tarcher, 1989.
4. Cousins N: Anatomy of an Illness (As Perceived by the Patient). New York, W.W. Norton, 1979.
5. Frankl V: Man's Search for Meaning. New York, Simon & Schuster, 1984.
6. Hamilton A: Exploring the Dangerous Trades. Beverly, MA, OEM Press, 1995.
7. Kabat-Zinn J: Wherever You Go There You Are. New York, Hyperion, 1994.
8. Kazantzakis N: The Saviors of God. New York, Simon & Schuster, 1960.
9. Koop CE: Koop: The Memoirs of America's Family Doctor. New York, Random House, 1991.
10. Lown B: The Lost Art of Healing. New York, Houghton-Mifflin, 1996.
11. Mann T: Death in Venice. New York, Modern Library, 1970.
12. Osler W: Aequanimitas: With Other Addresses to Medical Students, Nurses and Practitioners of Medicine, 3rd ed. New York, McGraw-Hill, 1932.
13. Peck MS: A World Waiting to Be Born: Civility Rediscovered. New York, Bantam, 1993.
14. Pollen I: Medical Crisis Counseling: Short-term Therapy for Long-term Illness. New York, Norton, 1995.
15. Vincent C, Young M, Phillips A: Why do people sue doctors? A study of patients and relatives taking legal actions. Lancet 243:1609–1617, 1994.
16. Zukov G: The Seat of the Soul. New York, Simon & Schuster, 1989.

10

Successful Medical Marketing for Practice Survival

> In the past two decades or so health care has become commercialized as never before, and professionalism in medicine seems to be giving way to entrepreneurialism. The health-care system is now widely regarded as an industry, and medical practice as a competitive business.
>
> Arnold S. Relman, M.D.
> *Atlantic Monthly*, March 1992

Beginning a medical practice has never been easy. Today, however, it is more difficult than ever, largely because of the many changes in the nature of physicians' practices. The percentage of solo private practitioners has decreased significantly, and salaried physicians who work for industry, hospitals, or managed care organizations are now in the majority.

This chapter discusses techniques to market yourself and your practice. I assume that you have already made a decision about certain fundamental issues, such as being a self-employed clinician in a solo or group practice. I also assume that your success in this "business venture" will enrich your life and influence your financial security, personal reputation, and standing in the medical and social community.

Another basic assumption is that you endured the ordeal of medical training because you deeply care about people and are committed to improving their health and well-being. Financial remuneration was not your primary motive for becoming a physician. Some of the decisions that I made throughout my career may apply to choices that you make or, in some cases, avoid.

My role model for a successful physician was my father, who, as a clinical allergist and immunologist, was also involved academically at the medical school, was chief of a busy clinic at the medical center, and had a private practice. He enjoyed the practice of medicine, and it enriched his life. He was proud to be a physician and shared that pride with his family. I looked forward to visiting his office, occasionally making rounds or house calls with him and observing the mutually gratifying and fulfilling relationships that he shared with his patients. They looked forward to his visits. He was their ally and advocate; they felt better as a result of his assistance. The bond between my father and his patients was based on respect, trust, and confidence in his integrity. He, in turn, always attempted to convey to his patients that it was his privilege to be their physician. The relationship was not with a health care "provider" but with a physician, educator, and healer.

Role models play a major part in our choice of careers. I was fascinated by the study of human behavior as an undergraduate. In medical school, neurology and psychiatry were my favorite rotations. In my fourth year elective with a professor of pediatric endocrinology I found my calling: to pursue a career in adolescent medicine. I planned to combine training in psychiatry and pediatrics. While in my psychiatric residency at the Harvard Medical School's McLean Hospital, I took my electives in neurology at Massachusetts General Hospital. While I was there, several experiences influenced my decision to change career paths. First was the realization that patients with chronic pain presented a challenge to conventional medicine and that most physicians did not enjoy having such patients in their practice. I also recognized that all too often people with chronic pain fell through the cracks in the health care system. Medical patients with neurologic, orthopedic, and other disorders frequently had significant emotional problems contributing to or resulting from their pain. These issues complicated treatment and added to their debilitation, chronicity, and disability. The process fascinated me. I then took fellowship training in psychosomatic and consultation–liaison psychiatry. It was my good fortune to meet Dr. Nat Hollister, neurosurgeon, psychiatrist, and founder of the first multidisciplinary pain center (MPC) in New England. He became my mentor in the study of pain.

The field, which later was to become known as pain medicine, had not yet developed; I believed that I could participate in its maturation. Laying the foundation, I began supplementing training experience with work experience, which meant learning from the experts. I participated in every major organization related to my field, became involved in clinical research, served on committees, and presented papers at medical meetings.

Point: Initially present posters or abstracts of your work. Refine your presentations, and ask the organizing committee to let you give a plenary lecture or participate in a workshop. Medical organizations welcome enthusiastic physicians, especially those who are dedicated and willing to work. For me, the path meant working on committees, then chairing them, and participating in elections for board of directors, executive committee, and finally president.

Point: Directly and indirectly, as you develop relationships with your peers, you are also marketing yourself. Whether you are entering an emerging field or one that is well established, develop your area of expertise and let people know of your interest. Each of us will do so in our own way.

In 1983 I was invited to become a founding member of what later was to become the American Academy of Pain Medicine. By now I was chairing the American Pain Society Committee on Pain Centers. I became vocal in the many clinical and political issues affecting my field.

Point: Take a position in which you believe and about which you feel passionately. Become known for your position, but be able to support and defend it.

Pain was inadequately treated in the United States. Based on the pioneering work of others, it became clear to me that complex chronic pain syndromes required a multidisciplinary and interdisciplinary team approach for optimal management. In addition, I became concerned about what appeared to be a "disability epidemic," related less to pathophysiology and more to psychosocial and sociopolitical issues, changes in the work ethic, and changes in medical–legal relationships, with increasingly litigious patients suffering personal or work injuries. I believed that the disability epidemic could be reversed or prevented and began writing and lecturing about this belief. It became clear that conventional treatments, which restricted and limited patients vocationally and recreationally, often contributed to iatrogenic disability. The increasing trend toward the medicalization of suffering not only was a disservice to patients, creating states of learned helplessness and encouraging passive dependency, but also threatened to cripple society. I advocated comprehensive rehabilitation as an alternative to further medical/surgical treatment and to disability. I believed in those principles then and continue to believe in them today. I took further training in disability medicine and forensic medicine.

Point: As you develop expertise in your area of specialization, you also develop views about the best way to practice medicine within your particular patient population. Each of us is unique. Give thought to your unique qualities—cultivate and nourish them. Make your uniqueness part of your practice, but also make it part of what you stand for professionally.

Decide which medical organizations are important for your career and which are important for your soul and well-being (ideally some are both). You may choose to join the major organization of your board certification as well as county, state, or national societies as a way to enhance referrals or to demonstrate that you are in the mainstream of medical practice. Other organizations may allow you to express who you are in a way that is extremely fulfilling. Such medical groups will encourage your professional and personal growth.

I was extremely fortunate in the evolution of my career to have had a talented support staff of physicians, nurses, therapists, and other pain center personnel, without whom my career successes would have been more difficult—and perhaps would not have occurred.

Point: Select a competent and dedicated staff. Do not forget to thank the people who help you look good. Share your successes and triumphs. When people feel appreciated, they work harder, and your practice is more likely to thrive.

Do not overlook the importance of your secretary, receptionist, or office manager. From a marketing perspective they are vital to your success (or can contribute to your failure). They are often the first point of contact with prospective patients. If they are not courteous, helpful, empathic, and encouraging, you will lose patients. The same rule holds for contacts with your current patients. Patients call your office for appointments because they need help. In one way or another they are not feeling well. Your scheduling secretary should have a policy to deal with routine appointments as well as emergencies. There should be a policy about prescription refills. When you are unavailable, your staff should know who is on call for medical coverage. On a given day you may not be on schedule for your appointments. It is essential that your office staff explain the problem to your patient (or other scheduled appointment). People recognize and can accept that physicians have emergencies and cannot always be on schedule. They cannot and will not accept the lack of courtesy in being forced to wait for a prolonged time without an explanation.

Early in my career, when I thought I knew a great deal about coordinating an inpatient medical unit, I was fortunate to have had a charge nurse/supervisor who was mature enough to recognize my need to take charge and make important clinical decisions while she and I were making daily rounds. She was supportive and secure enough that she had no difficulty as I implemented most of her suggestions.

Point: You and your office staff are a team. You may be the team leader—or perhaps not. The issue is not who gets credit with the correct answer but whether your patients are treated well and improve. Every one of your office personnel has an important role to play and provides an important service to you or your patients. If they do not, they should be replaced or are superfluous.

As our team concept for the treatment of difficult chronic pain syndromes developed, it became a model for pain centers nationally and internationally. Physicians wanted to tour our facility, to spend time training with us, and to pattern new programs after the Boston Pain Center. The 1980s were the golden era for pain centers and for medicine generally. In the early 1990s the clinical success of our pain program continued, but health care was changing. Insurers were demanding more in terms of justifying the cost of health care. We published outcome studies and continued our clinical research. We were proactive. We met with insurers, case managers, claims adjusters, and medical directors of insurance companies—anyone who needed to know more about our treatment program so that they could pay for it. We justified it clinically and economically. Treatment in our pain program was cost-effective and could be justified. Patients felt better and functioned better; many returned to work. As mentioned earlier, patients with chronic pain are in general a difficult population with which to work. Increasingly we became a tertiary care center, and more than 25% of our patients came from outside the immediate catchment area, frequently from another state and occasionally from another country.

Patients with work-related or personal injuries are especially difficult because of complicating variables such as involvement in disability proceedings and the medical–legal system. In the early days of the pain center movement, outcomes were considered successful if they improved pain control, reduced suffering, and had a positive impact on the quality of life. This definition changed rapidly, especially for patients with work-related injuries. Increasingly pain programs emphasized functional restoration with specific goals of return to work. Clearly this change was a direct result of the third-party payors from workers' compensation programs who viewed return to work or maximum medical improvement (MMI) and claims closure as acceptable outcomes. This change in philosophy at times causes conflict with patients or their attorneys. Frequently this conflict has a negative impact on patient satisfaction. Doing well at a pain program for some patients represents a threat to their disability status and workers' compensation benefits and may mean returning to work at a job that perhaps was not satisfying even before the injury.

Such factors need to be recognized as we discuss marketing a practice because having an understanding of your consumer is vital to the survival of your practice. Our primary consumers are the patients we treat. As an attending physician you are their advocate. However, as their advocate, you may decide that rehabilitation is preferable to disability. They and their attorneys may disagree. Your treatment program may be unpopular with a subgroup of patients, and, although on many objectively measured parameters you and your treatment team believe that the patient achieved a successful outcome, the patient leaves treatment dissatisfied and unhappy. Patients may not share your enthusiasm about their "successful outcome" or appreciate your "assistance," and their vocal discontent will not help your marketing efforts. On the other hand, this treatment outcome may be viewed as successful in the eyes of the insurance carrier and employer, if the patient was successful in returning to work or if the insurance claim was closed. In this case, your other consumer, the payor, without whom your office would close, was pleased with the treatment outcome. Does this pose a conflict? It certainly may; however, it does not need to do so if you carefully define your treatment goals and explain them to all involved before undertaking treatment. The goals of pain treatment for a work-injured patient are to alleviate pain and suffering and to improve function so that the patient can return to work when appropriate, with or without restrictions. You cannot be all things to all people.

Point: Avoid conflicts of interest. There is an inherent conflict of interest in requiring the attending physician who functions in the role of patient advocate to make ratings of impairment for disability determinations. Frequently this conflict of interest will compromise your therapeutic relationship and, whenever possible, should be avoided.

Dr. Relman, the former editor in chief of *The New England Journal of Medicine*, has expressed his concern that medicine increasingly finds itself in an ethical quagmire. He takes issue with entrepreneurial medicine and finds that frequently financial and technologic pressures may have adverse consequences for patients and for society. The roots of the medical profession are based on the assumption that physicians' responsibility to their patients takes precedence over their own economic interests. Relman[1] reviews dilemmas faced by many physicians and discusses in detail the distinctions between what society has a right to expect of practicing physicians and what it expects of people in business:

> [P]atients depend on their physicians to be altruistic and committed in advising them on their health-care needs and providing necessary medical services. Most patients do not have the expertise to evaluate their own need for medical care. The quality of life and sometimes life itself are at stake, and price is of relatively little importance, not only because of the unique value of the services rendered but also because patients usually do not pay out of pocket for services at the time they are received. Although most physicians are paid (usually by the government or an insurance company) for each service they provide, the assumption is that they are acting in the best interests of patients rather than of themselves. A fact that underscores the centrality of the patient's interest is that advertising and marketing in medical practice were until very recently considered unethical.

This position is contrasted with commercial vendors, who, although obligated to produce a good product and not to advertise it deceptively, have no responsibility to consider the consumer's interests. Inherent in the contrast is the premise that when people are in the sick role, they frequently are incapable of making decisions about their health care without being guided by physicians. It is essential that the advice rendered not be motivated by economic self-interest. The American Medical Association (AMA) has modified its position as stated in the 1957 code of ethics with its many anticommercial recommendations to viewing advertising and marketing as acceptable if they are not deceptive. Relman noted that the AMA actually encourages competition, stating that "ethical medical practice thrives best under free market conditions when prospective patients have adequate information and opportunity to choose freely between and among competing physicians and alternate systems of medical care."

Throughout the growth years of the pain center, marketing took many forms. The hospital had a public relations representative who sent out press releases whenever I or another staff member did something noteworthy, such as an academic presentation or appointment, scientific article or book publication, election to a major office, or community service event. Each release was marketed to a different population, and each population was considered important to the marketing of the pain center (and to the hospital). For several years I wrote a regular column about pain in the health section of the local newspaper. Although at times these projects proved to be time-consuming, they were also gratifying and exposed the community to a little-known service.

Point: Use of the media to disseminate information and educate the public can provide an important public service while serving as a powerful marketing strategy.

One of the questions most frequently asked by patients has been why it took so long for anyone to refer them for treatment at the pain center. Education through local and national television, radio, newspapers, and magazines leads patients to request their physicians to refer them for evaluation.

Point: If you are going to use such marketing strategies, be well prepared and base your information on scientifically sound principles.

The media are often more interested in sensationalism than in sound science. An effective communicator learns to make the statements believed to be important, regardless of the questions asked by the interviewer. You are a professional. Some of the people listening to you may be in a vulnerable position as a result of health problems. You will not be a target for criticism if you adhere to the same principle that guides your clinical practice of medicine: "Above all do no harm." In my experience, using the media for marketing, with national exposure on syndicated television and radio shows, is a good strategy, improves your visibility, and enlightens the viewing audience. However, in the days after your presentation, the office switchboard will be constantly busy and secretaries overburdened, but few calls will result in new patients. Most of the calls will be patient-specific questions about the caller's pain and resources available in their geographic regions. Local media appearances, on the other hand, are significantly better for marketing to prospective patients and may result in more new patients.

Point: Do not get involved in activities that compromise your credibility or that of your practice.

In the late 1980s I was approached by several business groups to develop a chain of pain centers as part of a joint venture. I developed a business plan and corporate name—Pain Centers of America. After much discussion with colleagues I decided not to partner with business for several reasons. The most important was related to a basic philosophical difference. My main concern was to develop centers of excellence for the management of chronic pain. The investors were concerned primarily with profit and secondarily with patient care. I did not want to turn a gourmet restaurant into a fast-food chain. What made our pain center unique was a culmination of the dedication and experience of our staff under my guidance. In retrospect, I believe that my decision was flawed. Carefully run, the venture could have been extremely lucrative without compromising patient care. We are not indispensable, and others can be trained to replicate our treatment program. Having said that, I add that several of my respected colleagues across the country attempted to establish chains of pain centers and were highly unsuccessful; the outcome was financially disastrous. Understand business trends and perform a market analysis before embarking on a new venture. Verify that you will be reimbursed adequately for your proposed treatment. In the 1970s and early to mid 1980s, comprehensive pain programs were generally hospital-based. Insurance carriers were familiar with the traditional medical model and reimbursed for it. Although it could be shown that for most patients comprehensive day treatment, at times coupled with housing in local hotels, was clinically as effective, more in keeping with a wellness model, and more cost-effective than in-hospital treatment, insurance carriers initially were inflexibly unwilling to reimburse for this "new" service.

Point: Philosophically you may have highly creative ideas. However, they may be thwarted by a system that is inflexible and may not be ready to implement them. Einstein once said, "Great spirits have always encountered violent opposition from mediocre minds." It probably is wise that I not expand on this point as it relates to our health care system.

MARKETING STRATEGY

The medical environment has never been more competitive than it is currently. Provision of health care increasingly is encumbered with many audiences, each with its own interests. It is critical that planning and marketing efforts incorporate an approach to each audience.

Although it is generally appropriate to consult with experts in marketing, do not delegate analysis of your marketing—check it for yourself. Verify the data that you have been given. No one can advocate for you as well as you can. As you attempt to establish your practice, expand it, or market it to new sources, you would be wise to follow certain fundamental principles.

In years past, physicians relied on word of mouth or relationships established during medical training as they opened an office and built their medical practice. Today, however, to be successful often requires becoming more marketing-oriented. The public has certain expectations of your practice that they take for granted. People assume that you are well trained, stay current with technologic advances in your field, and have convenient hours and that you and your staff will treat them courteously. To distinguish your practice from others and to give prospective patients a reason to contact you may require marketing efforts. Many of the recommendations in a recent article about business marketing[2] can be adapted to marketing a medical practice. Once you have evaluated your practice and identified growth opportunities, the following five steps can guide you to success.

Step 1: Establish your goals. For successful marketing you must make certain decisions about where you want your practice to go. Schlarb[2] emphasizes that specific, written, action-oriented goals are the goals most often achieved. An example of such a goal may be that over the next six months you will increase the number of your new patient evaluations from 15 to 20 per week. Goals may be short-term or long-term and focus on any aspect of your practice. It is important that goals be articulated well and shared with your staff so that they understand your priorities. If you have multiple goals, prioritize them. Goals should be:

- **Payoff-oriented.** Know the expenditures and resources necessary to accomplish each of your goals, and then prioritize them. I find that this exercise is important and frequently may modify the priority of certain goals because of the costs and efforts involved in implementation.
- **Realistic.** Review your goals with appropriate key personnel to assess the likelihood that they can be achieved.
- **Observable.** When you implement your action plan, you should be able to monitor the change in your practice.

Step 2: Define your target market. Your market may be defined demographically or geographically, but you should know who and what you want to target. What is this population most concerned about? Your marketing efforts may be different for existing and prospective patients. Schlarb[2] emphasizes the following points:

> In planning a promotion with a specific goal, you might look to your existing patients first as this should yield better results. After all, they already have a relationship with you and are familiar with your practice and services. You have credibility with them that you have not yet established with consumers outside your practice.

You also should be aware of whether and to what extent your competition is marketing to the same patients. Before deciding on the venue for your marketing, attempt to learn when your competition last utilized the same source. Saturation is an important factor. You do not want to spend your resources advertising a free evening lecture about a medical topic that was recently covered.

Step 3: Develop your marketing program. Schlarb's mnemonic[2] for the marketing program is **SMART**:

- **S**imple, specific, and easy to understand
- **M**easurable, so that progress toward your goal can be easily tracked
- **A**ttainable, providing your target market with what they want or need
- **R**ewarding—for the target market, you, your practice, staff, and suppliers
- **T**imely, creating a call to action within the target market and a sense of urgency within the practice

The promotional tools that we currently use at the Mid-Atlantic Center for Pain Medicine or have used at the Boston Pain Center include:

- A professionally designed marketing packet with biographies and specialty credentials for each physician in the practice as well as detailed discussion of each treatment program offered with the practices. Included is detailed discussion of insurance issues with our offer of assistance in clarifying issues that patients find confusing. In addition, the fact that we were one of a relatively small number of pain centers accredited by the Commission on Accreditation of Rehabilitation Facilities (CARF) was prominently displayed in our marketing information.

- A brochure entitled *A Patient's Guide to Pain Medicine* was purchased in bulk from the American Academy of Pain Medicine (AAPM). On the cover is space for each physician to put his or her name and mailing address. The brochure addresses many of the more commonly asked questions about chronic pain and, along with the marketing packet described above, is given to patients during registration on the day of the appointment. It is an opportunity for them to learn about the physician whom they will be seeing and the practice itself.
- Holiday cards
- Bulletin board prominently displaying recent honors or awards of physicians and other staff (e.g., recent lectures, books or articles published).
- Focus groups. Annually we meet with insurance carriers, case managers, rehabilitation nurses, and other key personnel involved with our patient population in an attempt to understand better how well we are meeting their needs, how well we are accomplishing our treatment goals, and how we can improve our "product." On occasion we get together with physician referral sources. More often, however, the interaction is either by phone or in the medical staff lounge. **Point:** Do not underestimate the importance of casual interactions with colleagues. In my experience this is one of best marketing tools available. I highly recommend that periodically you have your meals in the medical staff dining room and attend your medical staff meetings.
- Open houses—whenever you open an office, expand your practice, take in a new colleague, or have something newsworthy to report.
- Flexible hours, including the availability of early or late hours on request.

Although it is estimated that 4–5% of the gross practice revenues should be committed to marketing, Schlarb[2] notes that you will need to spend more if you wish to do aggressive marketing and if you depend on external sources. You may be able to spend less if your marketing efforts come from within your office.

Step 4: Implement your program. Barring unforeseen events, a carefully developed, realistic, and well-implemented marketing plan should bring successful results. However, success may come gradually, and progress must be carefully monitored with periodic adjustments as necessary. Both marketing and advertising have cumulative effects. Abandoning your effort prematurely without repeating your message often enough is a common marketing mistake.

Step 5: Analyze your results. Did you achieve your goal? If so, use what you learned to work toward your next goal. If not, based on what you learned, make the necessary modifications in your next marketing plan. It may involve changing some of the individuals, strategies, or media types that you utilized.

Make sure that you have adequate ways to track what worked and what did not. Schlarb[2] concludes with sound advice:

> Always analyze your return on investment [ROI]. How did the revenues, expenses, and profits track to your plan? ROI analysis gives you a basis to compare one marketing plan against another. It also helps you understand where practice growth is coming from.

CONCLUSION

This chapter has emphasized that although medical training prepares most physicians to be good clinicians and some to be good healers, rarely does it train us to be successful at marketing ourselves or our practices. Marketing can be done ethically or deceptively. You worked hard to become a physician. Being deceptive jeopardizes that prized status. Marketing must be done carefully and with much planning. Find your niche. In what way are you providing a service different from and better than your competition? Medicine today is more competitive than ever before. To survive, physicians make increasing use of marketing strategies to attract more patients and to improve the profitability of their practice.

REFERENCES

1. Relman AS: Atlantic Monthly, March 1992.
2. Schlarb S: Marketing for the Professional: Five Steps to a Healthier Bottom Line. Varilux Practice Report No. 8, 1995.

11

Running the Office without a Glitch

Running the business office of a medical practice smoothly, efficiently, and cost-effectively—in other words, without a glitch—has always been the goal of the medical practice manager (the general term applied to practice administrators, managing physicians, and office managers). But in an increasingly hostile health care environment, the glitch-free office is imperative because of the forces at work to reduce payments for medical services and, at the same time, to increase demands on practices for greater compliance with more rules and regulations, higher levels of patient satisfaction, and tighter control of overhead costs. The list of complicating factors goes on.

Be aware of the most important factor: managed care. Managed care changes the way in which physicians practice. Most physicians already have managed care contracts; they have learned through experience that it is vital to reengineer the office to flourish under the new conditions generated by managed care. It is best to perform the tasks demanded by managed care in the way that managed care organizations (MCOs) need and want them to be performed. If you have no managed care contracts, be aware that some experts predict that all health care eventually will be managed care. Physicians who do not contract with MCOs may find it impossible to do so later, when most patients have already left fee-for-service medicine to join health plans and the health plans have signed all of the physicians that they want and need for their panels.

Physicians must cope effectively with MCOs and their impact on physician practices. You may need to downsize, add associates, merge your practice, add offered services, drop services, affiliate, open new offices, close old offices, revamp your business systems, or computerize if you have not already done so. Even if your office already is computerized (and most are), you may need to upgrade your information system to compete even more effectively in an increasingly managed care environment.

In the jargon of the business establishment, the bottom line is that practices must redouble their efforts to run a glitch-free office if they are to flourish. Furthermore, it is the responsibility of everyone in the practice—physicians; clinical, clerical, administrative staff; and ancillary personnel—to work toward this end. When the practice thrives, everyone in it also thrives. When the practice falters—by failing to maintain a high level of patient satisfaction and losing patients and enrollees, by failing to capture all possible payments, by inviting a fraud audit through sloppy or misguided billing and coding, or by various other failings—the practice may struggle, downsize, be sold to an entity that dismantles it, or just close its doors.

RESPONSIBILITIES

Thus, it is a matter of enlightened self interest for each employee and owner of a medical practice to understand that it is his or her own personal goal to strive for practice excellence and to find the necessary motivation from within to do the work assigned to the best of his or her ability. But even more is involved. Everyone needs to look beyond the scope of his or her own position, to be aware of the extra things that he or she can do to help, to pitch in as needed, and generally to work as though the practice depends on each individual. It does.

The secret to success is two-fold. First, everyone in the practice must adopt the above philosophy and practice it, or those who do will be taken advantage of by those who do not. Second, it is management's duty to encourage adoption of this philosophy, to reward those who practice it, and, if necessary, to replace those who do not.

MANAGEMENT RESPONSIBILITIES

In most practices, the practice manager is not *solely* but *primarily* responsible for practice success. Practice size and organization influence the role of the physician in the management of a medical practice. Some physicians are directly involved in practice management; others delegate hands-on responsibilities of staff employees to others who, in turn, are directly responsible to them; others simply establish goals and parameters for a practice administrator; and some physicians even find themselves taking instructions and directions.

Your particular situation may be more complex, but, in general, if you are:
- the owner of a solo practice, the primary responsibility for practice success is squarely on your shoulders.
- the coowner of a small or medium-sized practice, you and your coowners must work together to develop a consensus on each matter vital to practice success and express these.

- the coowner of a practice large enough to have a practice administrator, you and your coowners may well perform no direct day-to-day practice management functions, but you still must establish the parameters within which your practice administrator manages the practice.
- an associate physician or physician employee, you must do whatever is necessary to achieve practice success and use whatever means are available to you—even if you are limited to using the corporate suggestion box—to influence practice management positively.

Staff members also are responsible for practice success at the most basic level, because they do all of the work that is not directly associated with the practice of medicine. But practice management and ownership must understand that, to a large extent, staff are only as good as management *permits* them to be. Remember three basic tenets of management:

1. Those at the top stand to gain the most when the practice flourishes or to lose the most if it fails.

2. Tone and tenor are established at the top; management can encourage and reward staff members or discourage and denigrate them.

3. Management sets the rules and regulations by which the staff live.

As practice manager or owner/coowner, you must work proactively to establish practice rules, regulations, and goals; to build a plan to achieve practice goals and objectives; and to make it as easy as possible for others to do the same. Make sure that everything is spelled out and written down to avoid misunderstandings. Maintain discipline, but also be quick with praise. Reward good work and achievement when it counts, at employee review time, with appropriate salary raises. And when things fall apart, have the sense to recognize the problems and the courage to make the necessary adjustments.

STAFF RESPONSIBILITIES

Staff members take their instructions from the practice management. They must understand that the practice counts on them, in large part, for its success. No matter how skillful and charismatic the physicians are, one poor staff member—for example, a surly receptionist, a finagling coding expert, an arrogant secretary, an obnoxious medical technician, or a slovenly computer expert—can damage a practice. Help your staff members understand that your patients count on them, you count on them, and they must rise to the occasion and take pride in their work. Furthermore, you should gently emphasize that the practice pays everybody's bills.

Effectively communicate to each member of the staff that his or her personal success is vitally linked with the success of the practice. Make it understood that, whatever your function is within the practice, *it is your job*. If you make the best of it, you will be rewarded; if you do not, you may be out of a job. Also emphasize that the job includes pointing out problems, especially, if possible, before they develop.

Then prove it. Be a careful, patient listener. Actually consider what your staff members tell you. Investigate potential problems thoroughly. Take required actions, rather than allowing problems to fester. Remain objective, even-handed, and fair. If you are unreasonable, if you show that you do not care, if you play favorites, or if you manage your practice with fire one day and ice the next, your staff will become confused at best. At worst they will develop a poor attitude about their jobs and either leave, which will make it difficult for you to maintain staff cohesion, or remain, which may be worse.

MANAGED CARE RESPONSIBILITIES

Most practices are in transition from a 100% fee-for-service population to a managed care basis; your practice probably has a mix of self-pay, discounted fee-for-service (e.g., Medicare), and managed care patients.

Expect changes. For example, if you have added one discounted fee-for-service contract and two capitation contracts within the past 6 months, you may be experiencing cash flow problems. If so, you simply may not have enough people in your billing department to do the work. Furthermore, your employees may be struggling with the new system(s), and your patients may need someone in your office to explain benefits, formulary restrictions, and rules and regulations. To compensate, you must:

- determine what tasks you need to have done;
- have the people on board you need to do those tasks; and
- make sure they are properly trained and motivated.

Talk with your personnel. Find out if any tasks that must be done are being neglected, who is doing which tasks, how well each employee is performing within those parameters, and whether everyone is properly motivated. Assess workloads, tasks, attitude, motivation, and skills.

Survey your patients and referring/referral physicians to ascertain their impressions of your practice and staff. Talk with representatives of your health plans. Most make it absolutely clear what they need and want from participating practices; make sure that you fully understand what is needed from you and provide it.

Then review your findings. Ask yourself direct questions and develop honest answers. Consider these possible areas to investigate:

1. Is your staffing on target?
- Do you need more people?
- Are your employees doing the right tasks?
- Are they motivated?
- Do they need more training?
- Will your managed care partners train your personnel?

2. Should you upgrade your information system?
- What do you need? Consider, for example, electronic systems for:
  Claims processing
  Claims posting
  Checking of capitated lists
  Generation of the reports you need to manage effectively
  Cost analysis
  Managed care contract analysis and comparison
- Will the HMOs and insurance companies provide the software you need to send and receive data packages?
- Does your computer vendor have a managed care software module?
- Do you need a computer expert?

3. Is your telephone system able to meet your practice's current and growing needs?

4. What other areas need your attention?

PLAN FOR SUCCESS

Having completed your basic research, draw up a mission statement to establish the guiding principles of your business plan. Include your managed care strategic plan in your comprehensive business plan, but make sure that your business plan drives your strategic plan. MCOs want to do business with physician practices that help the MCOs to achieve their own corporate goals. Successful medical practice businesses are highly desirable to MCOs as managed care partners.

Thus, your business plan should address all areas of practice improvement. It is, in a sense, your road map for business success. If you do not have a business plan, develop one. Be sure to write down every part of your plan. Distribute copies throughout the office. Establish deadlines for goal achievement and assign responsibilities. Involve everyone. Establish your strategies based on partner consensus. Keep them few in number, realistic, and doable. Assign personnel to accomplish implementation; assign responsibilities. Allocate the necessary resources. Include financial "how-to" sections.

Most medical practices in the United States are small, service-oriented businesses. The typical business plan for a small service oriented business includes five steps:

1. Establish your practice goals.
2. Analyze your practice and its environment.
3. Develop your business plan.
4. Implement the plan.
5. Monitor and adjust the plan.

ESTABLISH YOUR GOALS

If you have practice partners, meet with them and develop a consensus on every issue. Start with developing a consensus list of the most important issues. This task may best be done on retreat, and you may want to consider enlisting the assistance of a business consultant to act as facilitator. Regardless of what method you choose, you and your practice partners need to give the issues your full attention and consideration.

Establish each physician owner's personal and practice goals. Focus on the development of the practice first, and then address personal needs and wants. Be aware that this step tends to be the toughest part of the process for some groups, especially if some physicians refuse to put the group first. You may be faced with difficult decisions. If consensus is impossible to achieve, perhaps it is time to reorganize the practice.

Above all, make your goals attainable. Write them down. Make each of your goals succinct and absolutely clear. How will you know if your plan is working if your goals are vague or ambiguous? For example, consider a practice that must control its accounts receivable. Consider these goals, established at the end of the calendar year, by a hypothetical practice:

1. Make the reduction of accounts receivable our number one priority.

2. Reduce accounts receivable significantly.

3. Eliminate all accounts receivable by the end of the year.

4. Reduce accounts receivable by 10% within 60 days, by a total of 20% by the end of the second quarter, and by a total of 30% by the end of the year.

The first goal means nothing. It cannot be measured in terms that can be quantified. The second goal is a bit better, but what does *significantly* mean? Is 5% within a week significant? Perhaps, but if your staff starts off like gang-busters and achieves that reduction in the first week of January but has accomplished little else through December, what is the true impact? If that 5% represents the only receivables that you can hope to collect, the result is wonderful. However, if 5% makes only a dent in your receivables, you have accomplished nothing at all. The third goal is on the right track, but can you eliminate *all* your receivables, and should you not check your progress well before 12 months have passed? The fourth goal is excellently presented. It is doable; it recognizes that the easiest-to-collect receivables will be the first goal that your staff will accomplish and that things will become increasingly more difficult thereafter; and it gives you reasonable checkpoint dates.

ANALYZE YOUR PRACTICE AND ENVIRONMENT

Begin your analysis with an objective assessment of practice management. Focus on function, structure, and hierarchy. Know how decisions are made and whether you are proactive or reactive. If necessary, revise your decision-making process. Resolve to become proactive. Assign responsibilities.

Next analyze your business. Who are your patients? What are their demographics, in terms of medical needs (range and intensity), geographic coverage, and payment (self-pay, health plan, traditional insurance, Medicare, Medicaid)? What are your referral sources? What is your payor mix? Does one health plan dominate? If so, how strong are your ties to it, and what will happen if the plan goes bankrupt? What is your reputation among your patients, other physicians, managed care partners, health plan purchasers, and the general public?

Examine your finances. Analyze your revenue streams and costs. Are you offering only money-making medical services? Use a proven activity-based costing (ABC) method to perform an objective analysis. Make sure you do not offer MCOs services that cost you money. Control your costs.

Assess your market. What is your market share? Should it be higher? How can you improve it? Must you merge your practice, hire more physicians and/or staff, or downsize and find a niche? Is affiliation with a network in your future? What are your competitors doing? Why? Can you should you— merge with them, step up your competition, or ignore them?

Which MCOs are offering contracts in your area? What terms are they offering? If they are dealing only with practices of eight or more physicians and your group has only five, what are your options? Managed care tends to upset traditional alliances as former friends become competitors and former competitors become allies or partners.

Use patient and physician questionnaires to augment your self-analysis process. Determine your strengths, weaknesses, opportunities, and threats so that you can better determine your optimal responses and take the appropriate actions.

Strategic Plan. Weave your managed care strategic plan into your comprehensive business plan at this stage. Eventually, it will behoove virtually every physician who wants to remain successful to have managed care contracts. Your managed care goals are to obtain and retain favorable managed care contracts. That is the essence of the basic managed care strategic plan: get what you need and want from MCOs by providing MCOs with what they need and want. From MCOs, you need and want:

- Optimal market share (high enough to keep a steady stream of income flowing into your practice, but not so high that you are unable to handle the load)
- Good payment rates
- The highest possible level of input into the MCO's decision-making process (understand that this level is typically far lower than the level you enjoy in fee-for-service practice)
- Good contract terms (e.g., no indemnification clause, but a clause that will allow you to vacate the contract without cause if conditions become intolerable)
- A hassle-free working relationship

MCOs are in continual competition with other MCOs and with fee-for-service practices; they compete for "covered lives" (patients and potential patients) by selling their health plans to purchasers, usually employers in the private sector, government, and academia. MCOs do not practice medicine; only physicians do. Thus, MCOs must market their plans to purchasers through the physicians with whom they contract to provide services. Physicians who fail to measure up can be excluded from provider panels or deselected (MCO euphemism for "fired"). From physicians, MCOs typically need and want:

- Specific geographic coverage
- A specific range of services
- Low costs
- Low utilization
- Good outcomes
- Physicians with good reputations and proper credentials (e.g., board certification)
- The right attitude toward managed care in general and the MCO in particular

The particulars vary from practice to practice and MCO to MCO. Thus, it is difficult to be any more specific in terms of MCO and physician needs and wants, negotiations, tradeoffs, contract review, and the like.

Generally, you should draw up a weighted list of what you want and need and determine what you are willing to trade off. Give yourself an information advantage by obtaining copies of contracts that the MCOs in your area (those seeking to contract with physicians) have negotiated with similar practices and discuss with impaneled physicians their negotiating and practice experiences with each MCO.

Thereafter, incorporate your managed care objectives—what you must do to win managed care contracts (e.g., add new associates, redesign your practice floor plan, merge your practice, upgrade your computer system, or paint, paper, and carpet your office)—into your comprehensive business plan. Plan point by point and include funding options and deadlines. Be certain that these points make good business sense and do not conflict with your "pure" (i.e., not part of your managed care business plan) business plan items. In summary, make sure that your business plan drives your strategic plan.

DEVELOP YOUR PLAN

Think of your medical practice's business plan as a road map. Use it to plot the optimal course from point A, where your practice is now, to point B, where you want your practice to be. Feel free to compare your plan with plans suggested by others, but remember that medical practices are unique. Your goals and situation, on the surface, may appear to be the same as those of some other practice, but the differences are probably significant.

Consider two hypothetical practices. Each appears to be a mirror image of the other. They are both at point A and headed for point B. But one practice has a deep pool of capital reserves, whereas the other must borrow and save investment capital. Thus, the timelines and financing options of the two plans are significantly different, and they may need to take different routes to their mutual destination. The practice with the deep capital reserves may take the superhighway toll road and step on the accelerator, whereas the other practice may need to take a few back roads and conserve fuel.

Whatever you decide to do, cover all your bases. Must you hasten or delay plan elements? Do you have enough reserve capital to take the new risk(s) you must consider? How much money do you have available for investment? Do you need to plan your practice improvements in stages? Should you start a capital improvement account? Do you need to borrow money? How good is your credit? How can you remain financially independent? Draw up an implementation timeline that considers your goals, the actions that you must take to achieve your goals, and the funding necessary to accomplish the necessary actions.

IMPLEMENT YOUR PLAN

Once you have established your goals, made your analyses, and developed your written plan, it is time to implement your business plan. Consider posting copies on the walls and entering salient points on your paper and electronic calendars. Refer to them often.

The worst thing that you can do with a business plan is to stick it in a desk drawer or computer file and forget about it. A business plan may fail because its goals are unreasonable or out of focus. It may fail because of incompetent analysis or lack of development. But usually when a plan fails, it is because it was not implemented in the first place. The second most common reason for failure: it was not written down. No one can remember the details or perhaps even the main points, or memories conflict. Consider the following hypothetical conversation:

Dr. A: Did we want to add two new physicians over the course of three years or three new physicians over the course of two years?

Dr B: Wasn't it supposed to be two new physicians this year and a nurse practitioner the following year?

Dr. C: I remember distinctly that it was supposed to be a nurse practitioner this year and then two new physicians over the course of the following two years.

Dr A: Of course, that's it! Now, does anybody remember what we did with the money we were going to set aside to pay those salaries?

(Long pause, for memory jogging)

Dr. C: I think we decided to expand the reception area and upgrade the computers instead.

(General agreement—more or less)

Dr. D: Weren't we supposed to do that in year 4?

Avoid the above conversation or anything resembling it. Write down your plan. Implement what you wrote down.

MONITOR YOUR PLAN

The worst thing that you can do with your business plan once you have implemented it is to follow it blindly. Is your plan working? Are you sure? Monitor your plan from the day you implement it and continue to evaluate it to make sure it is working. If it is *not* working, measure the plan's performance against points 1–4, analyze the discrepancies, and make the necessary adjustments.

What can go wrong? One or more of your goals may be unreasonable or out of focus. Reconsider them. Your initial practice or environmental analysis may contain one or more miscalculations. Correct them; hire an analyst if necessary. Does your plan lack funding parameters? Is your timeline faulty? Did you implement the plan? Has your situation changed since you implemented the plan? If your practice has changed considerably, factor in the changes. Consider: if your plan calls for adding three new physicians over the course of two years, it will be a significantly different practice at the end of 24 months. Have your revenues increased? Decreased? Is your new computerized billing system in place? Did you decide to delay hiring because no candidate was right for the position you must fill?

Monitor your current and potential future competitors and allies. Is there a major shift in allegiances or in power? Are multiple MCOs starting to compete for market share in your area? Are you in or out of the plans of either or both MCOs? Can you determine which will be successful and join it? Are MCOs competing for your participation? If so, consider joining one now rather than two years from now, as your plan initially recommended. Is competition for market share much more intense than you anticipated that it would be at this point? Consider making your move now. Downsize into a niche practice, if you must. If the new MCO in town wants to deal only with groups of 10 or more physicians, merge *now* with those four other practices to create your 12-physician practice rather than wait four years. Is it time to join a powerhouse network?

Perhaps the problem lies elsewhere. If, for example, you intended to install a new computerized business system within two months but have not done so three months after plan implementation, it may be because vital components were back-ordered, because you had to wait for the financing, or because your key vendor had to handle a crisis situation and could not juggle personnel. If computer upgrade was the focal point of expanding your practice by adding a new physician and a few new staff members, these plan points also may be delayed for a valid reason.

FOCUS ON PERSONNEL

Your employees make the first impressions for your practice. They take telephone calls, make patient appointments, and deal with vendors, managed care plan representatives and referral/referring physicians before they reach you. They help your patients with insurance and health plan forms, escort patients to examination rooms, perform your billing, collections, and coding, take care of your computers, perform clinical functions, and in short do everything except practice medicine. Your employees can and will make or break your practice. You must be certain that:

- You hire the best possible personnel.
- They are doing the tasks that you need to have done.
- They are performing at an appropriate level.
- They are well motivated.

USE RELEVANT JOB DESCRIPTIONS

Job descriptions are necessary to your hiring and employee evaluation processes. In addition, you can use them to make sure that everyone on your staff is doing the right job, which means doing all tasks that are necessary for practice success and not tasks that may have been important two years ago but are no longer necessary.

The sample job descriptions in Tables 1 and 2 are for nonexistent general medical practices. Your job descriptions should reflect the unique needs of your own practice. The ideal job description is generated from established practice needs, implemented at hiring, reviewed at employee evaluation, and updated as the practice changes. It reduces to writing the tasks that are necessary to the practice, that each employee must perform. Develop all job descriptions comprehensively. Coordinate each position so that it meshes with all others. Your objective is to see that all tasks are covered without redundancy. Naturally, if you need two billing clerks, for example, each will be doing the same tasks without redundant effort.

Review your job descriptions at least once a year and immediately before you hire anyone. Talk with the people doing the work to detect problems, to determine the causes, and to develop a solution. Talk with department heads, supervisors, and physicians. Consider all recommendations, but also consult your own employee performance files.

Revise your job descriptions, if necessary. For example, if your registered nurse is escorting patients to examination rooms, taking patient histories, and cleaning up, you can save money by having your medical assistant, who probably earns several dollars less per hour, do such work. In turn, your nurse is freed to perform higher-level functions, which can save time and improve efficiency.

TABLE 1. Sample Job Description: Receptionist

General definition: Position requiring the ability to interact well with clients and staff members and to remain calm under stress. Immediate Supervisor: Office Manager.

Typical examples of work: (Note: this job description may not include all of the duties required and may not include examples of the tasks that may be required.)

- Operates Isoetec Telephone Terminal and answers incoming telephone calls
- Greets visitors
- Keeps daily log of physicians' in/out schedules
- Records incoming payments and distributes to billing, etc.
- Assists with special projects, as necessary

Necessary occupational traits:

- Pleasant telephone manner
- Organization skills
- Communication skills
- Ability to follow written and oral instructions
- Ability to exercise good judgment and tact in dealing with clients
- Knowledge of general office procedures
- Skill in typing

Minimum education, training, and experience required:

- High school degree
- Office experience helpful

Full-time staff position (35 hours)
Regular hours of work:

Monday	Tuesday	Wednesday	Thursday	Friday	Saturday
8 a.m.–4 p.m.	8 a.m.–4 p.m.	1–9 p.m.	7–11 a.m.	7 a.m.–3 p.m.	9 a.m.-noon
1-hour lunch	1-hour lunch	1-hour lunch		1-hour lunch	

Reviewed and discussed with: _____ _____

                                                                                            Date

Employee's signature: _____ _____

                                                                                            Date

---

HIRE THE RIGHT HELP

The main reason to have job descriptions is for your hiring process. When you need a new employee, your job description is your hiring blueprint. But it is only part of the process. Successful hiring starts with your help-wanted ad. Design it to attract attention. Word it to attract multiple candidates with the right qualifications, and place it in the most appropriate location(s). Make sure not to mislead potential candidates. You do not want to waste time with under- or overqualified candidates, or candidates not in your salary range.

Consider the following sample help-wanted advertisements for a hypothetical medical practice in Figure 1. Obviously, the second ad is more likely to attract the specific type of candidate that you want to interview for your specific position and also to discourage under- and overqualified applicants.

Review the qualification briefs that you receive; compare them against your job descriptions. Interview the top candidates. If the response to your ad indicates fewer than 10 qualified candidates, reconsider your ad and/or its

---

TABLE 2. Sample Job Description: Business Manager

Reports to managing doctor with special reporting, as indicated, from time to time.

RESPONSIBILITIES

1. Office Coordination
   a. Attend doctors' meetings; record decisions from discussions; implement ideas arising from these meetings; investigate alternatives; report results to doctors.
   b. Coordinate activities among physicians on a day-to-day basis.
   c. Work with managing doctor on projects requiring administrative support.

2. Financial
   a. Assist with proposed annual budget.
   b. Approve all expenditures.
   c. Prepare, review, and analyze monthly statements.
   d. Prepare all studies, reports, etc. requested by doctors, or as necessary.
   e. Liaison with accountants, attorneys and other advisors.
   f. Monitor pension and profit-sharing funds, including seeking various investment vehicles. Keep records for each participant's account balances.
   g. Monitor all practice savings and checking accounts.

3. Personnel
   a. Recruit, hire, and fire office personnel.
   b. Supervise employees, including salary review and proposed adjustments.
   c. Maintain control and records of vacations, sick leave, etc.
   d. Organize regular office meetings and set agendas.
   e. Determine and change personnel assignments and job descriptions as needed.

4. Business systems
   a. Institute any new business systems as may be appropriate (scheduling, filing, billing); investigate alternatives and work with physicians and staff to assure that systems are implemented.
   b. Keep current on new laws and regulations that affect the business systems of the practice.

5. Collections
   a. Institute a system to handle delinquent account follow-up, including telephone and preprinted letter.
   b. Use Small Claims Court to handle accounts not paying.

6. Audit controls
   a. Review and supervise internal systems for handling cash, recording mail receipts, writing checks, etc., in both offices.
   b. Follow-up audit control systems devised by accountants.

7. Office facilities
   a. Assure proper maintenance of present offices; order new equipment; obtain supplies and services; including comparison price shopping.
   b. Be responsible for all aspects of office maintenance and coordination with landlord.

8. Personal for doctors
   a. Act as business agent for doctors personally in all areas where their time can be saved for medical work.
   b. Carry out assignments for doctors as may be required of their civic, medical, or other committee positions.

---

placement. Use your job description to generate interview questions. Include input from your physicians and staff, particularly those who will be working with the new employee. Consider consulting with your attorney before you interview to make sure that you do not ask questions that may violate, for example, the Americans with Disabilities Act or that may be perceived as biased.

1. Secretary/Medical Office.
   Typing experience necessary.
   Call Rita, 555-1234.

2.
   SECRETARY/MEDICAL OFFICE

   Growing medical practice located near suburban hospital needs experienced person to transcribe dictation tapes, compose letters for physicians, etc. Some familiarity with word processing, medical terminology helpful. Will also act as secretary for all non-patient activities. This is a fast-paced, 35-hour per week position. Salary open; benefits.

   Call Rita at 555-1234.

FIGURE 1. Sample help wanted ads.

Revise your candidates list to include the top two or three, and reinterview these candidates before making your selection. Consider having your candidates talk with selected current staff members. Check references, employment background, and education points. Rely on your gut feelings.

To avoid paying overtime and minimize your turnover rate, consider exercising nonstandard personnel measures. Many talented people are looking for part-time employment. Perhaps former employees reentering your location or the job force are seeking just a few hours per week. Part-timers may be highly trained and motivated, and they may not care about obtaining benefits (especially if they have a primary full-time job or are covered by a spouse's benefits package).

You also may consider the job-sharing option, in which two employees share the position, set their own hours, and function as a single employee. Communication is the key to making this option work, and you may need to halt the experiment if one employee dominates the position or one fades out of the picture or if coordination fails.

Another option is flex-time, which may be perfect if you need to remain open to accommodate patients during lunch time, evenings, weekends, and vacations. Retirees and people in multiple-income families may have nontraditional scheduling needs that match your practice needs.

PAY OPTIMAL SALARIES AND BENEFITS

Certainly you must pay a competitive salary and provide necessary benefits to attract and keep good help, but be sure to remain within established industry norms. It is imperative to control your costs. To get an idea of whether you are paying optimal staff salaries, compare your salaries with industry standards (this comparison helps you to assess fair wages for each employee). Establish a salary range for every practice position, based on the responsibilities and demands of the job and industry norms. Compare your practice's staff salaries against those listed in Table 3.

Be careful with fringe benefits, which can get out of hand. If you are in a highly competitive situation, you may want to consider offering such unorthodox benefits as paid or subsidized parking, tuition reimbursement, or assistance

TABLE 3. Selected Staff Salaries*

Position	< 2 Years' Service			2–5 Years' Service			5+ Years' Service		
	Low	Avg.	High	Low	Avg.	High	Low	Avg.	High
Executive Director	$26,000 annually	$56,165 annually	$95,000 annually	$30,000 annually	$56,930 annually	$140,005 annually	$24,000 annually	$55,728 annually	$140,000 annually
Office Manager	$15,000 annually	$29,724 annually	$50,000 annually	$18,200 annually	$32,742 annually	$52,000 annually	$15,600 annually	$35,006 annually	$65,000 annually
Billing Coord.	$6.50 per hr	$11.47 per hr	$19.01 per hr	$6.50 per hr	$12.28 per hr	$22.00 per hr	$8.10 per hr	$13.35 per hr	$34.84 per hr
Book-keeper	$6.50 per hr	$10.84 per hr	$17.75 per hr	$8.65 per hr	$12.41 per hr	$20.00 per hr	$7.95 per hr	$14.70 per hr	$25.16 per hr
Nurse Pract'ner	$15.14 per hr	$24.98 per hr	$44.56 per hr	$18.20 per hr	$27.37 per hr	$40.87 per hr	$16.40 per hr	$24.16 per hr	$36.05 per hr
File Clerk	$4.00 per hr	$6.73 per hr	$12.00 per hr	$5.15 per hr	$7.81 per hr	$11.40 per hr	$6.34 per hr	$9.43 per hr	$14.75 per hr
Lab Tech	$7.50 per hr	$11.72 per hr	$20.00 per hr	$7.50 per hr	$12.82 per hr	$21.60 per hr	$8.46 per hr	$13.70 per hr	$20.55 per hr
Medical Assistant	$4.50 per hr	$9.17 per hr	$17.42 per hr	$6.25 per hr	$9.81 per hr	$22.00 per hr	$6.75 per hr	$11.41 per hr	$25.88 per hr
Physician Assistant	$16.82 per hr	$25.19 per hr	$40.87 per hr	$15.86 per hr	$26.88 per hr	$48.44 per hr	$15.00 per hr	$25.74 per hr	$39.90 per hr
Reception	$5.10 per hr	$8.69 per hr	$17.50 per hr	$5.25 per hr	$9.27 per hr	$16.63 per hr	$5.70 per hr	$10.72 per hr	$20.19 per hr
Regist. Nurse	$8.00 per hr	$14.65 per hr	$25.00 per hr	$9.00 per hr	$15.13 per hr	$33.00 per hr	$9.00 per hr	$16.28 per hr	$27.00 per hr
X-ray Tech	$8.00 per hr	$12.31 per hr	$19.80 per hr	$8.25 per hr	$13.17 per hr	$23.01 per hr	$11.00 per hr	$15.21 per hr	$22.88 per hr

* This information is from the 1997 Staff Salary Survey, which is published annually by The Health Care Group. The averages are national; figures may vary significantly by region.

with child care. Also avoid extensive largess at the holidays. Throw a party if you can afford one, but not if you must use funds earmarked for employee raises. Also try not to be too lavish. A secretary with an annual salary of $22,000 may be aghast, angry, and insulted enough to quit if you throw a holiday party that costs what you pay her for six months of hard work. Instead, consider a small, catered luncheon at which your employees can relax and feel appreciated. This may be an excellent opportunity to make achievement awards and even to disburse bonuses or cash gifts, again if you can afford it and if it does not affect raises. Consult with your attorney about tax laws if you do.

EVALUATE YOUR EMPLOYEES OBJECTIVELY

Have and use a standard employee evaluation system. We have already addressed using job descriptions as the basis of employee evaluation. You also must maintain employee performance files in which you note each employee's accomplishments and shortcomings throughout the year.

Keep your personnel files current and record relevant data for each employee based on the employee's job description. Your regular staff meeting will supply you with basic data. Other relevant data will be obvious at the time it is generated. Record relevant incidents in your personnel files. For example, if an employee makes a major mistake or performs an outstanding accomplishment that may be beyond the scope of his or her standard duties and responsibilities, praise the employee's progress or point out any problems or shortcomings, as appropriate. Suggest corrective measures and actions and establish performance goals. Provide training, if necessary. Make a note in the appropriate file. Your employees, department supervisors, referring physicians, patients, and others also may provide you on an ad hoc basis with information that should enter these files.

Evaluate every employee under your direct supervision on a regular basis. Be evenhanded in your evaluations. Stick to objective indicators of job performance, and avoid emotional input.

New Employees.　For new employees, perform the first evaluation at the end of a 90-day probationary period. It takes about three months for most new employees to become acclimated, learn your system, and show positive signs that they will be good contributors to your practice. After 90 days, either welcome the new employee into your practice or release him or her at a formal exit interview, explaining that things just did not work out as expected. Remain cordial, but stick with your decision.

If you can—and if he or she is willing to listen—make recommendations. Perhaps you may genuinely be able to suggest a different line of work or to direct your former employee to another practice or entity that is more suited to his or her capabilities and in need of another employee. If not, sincerely wish the person well and end the interview. Be sure to have the employee return keys, passes, and badges, and change computer passwords.

In some cases, particularly if the position is intrinsically difficult to master or if, for some reason that is no fault of the new employee, adjustment to the job or to the practice has been unusually difficult, consider extending the probationary period. If you choose to do so, make the extension a short one; 30 days is probably best. Explain to the employee that you believe he or she shows promise but must show obvious improvement to keep the job. Establish quantifiable goals. Use the probationary period extension sparingly and make only one extension per case, unless extenuating circumstances are extremely compelling. The speediest possible resolution to the hiring situation is best for all:

- You need to return your full attention to seeing patients or to start the hiring process over again.
- Your staff needs to have a new member in place and producing at an appropriate level.

- The new employee needs to know whether to settle into the new position or recirculate his or her qualifications brief.

At every employee evaluation, refer to a standard employee evaluation form. Prepare it in advance, and after each review put a copy in each employee's personnel file so that you can track progress. You may use the sample employee evaluation form in Figure 2 as a template.

GIVE PAY RAISES WISELY

If the employee remains with the practice, formally welcome him or her aboard and explain that your practice reviews all employee performance annually on the same date (or, if you have many employees, dates) each year.

Base raises on performance, and avoid across-the-board raises. If everyone in a hypothetical practice receives the same 4% raise, slackers conclude that they need not improve performance to receive the highest (only) raise, and the best people conclude that, no matter what they do, they will receive the same reward as their slower, less motivated, less talented coworkers.

Budget your raises each year; set the needed money aside. At review time, if you have more money to add and feel so inclined, do so, but avoid shunting funds out of this pool. Determine the average raise percentage, if you were to give everyone the same amount; then weight raises based on performance. For example, if the average raise is 4%, give that amount to people who are making average improvement. Give the best people higher raises, perhaps 6–8% or 10% to reward outstanding progress and initiative. Give your poor performers less, perhaps 2–3%.

At each review, make sure that each employee knows why he or she earned the raise and exactly what he or she must do to reach the next level of compensation. Set goals and deadlines. Allow your employees to speak their minds and clear the air. Investigate any potential problems you discover. For example, if you learn that an employee is unable to do his or her work to expectations because of the recurring need to cover for a coworker who is undertrained or undermotivated or has a problem, monitor the situation, find out exactly what is happening, and make adjustments. In general, you want to stick to your plan and keep your stated pay raises; however, if you need to increase the first employee's raise the following year, do so.

ESTABLISH A FAVORABLE WORKING ENVIRONMENT

Some offices that seem to have all of the components in place to ensure the best possible performance from their personnel still have serious problems. They use excellent, updated job descriptions, know how to hire good personnel, pay them well without breaking the budget, maintain discipline, and should reap the rewards—but do not.

THE HEALTH CARE GROUP, INC.

EMPLOYEE EVALUATION FORM

Employee Name _____ Position _____

Supervisor Name _____ Date _____

Rating Period from _____ to _____ Date of Last Raise: _____ Amount $_____ Pr. _____

This Raise Effective _____ Amount $_____ Pr. _____

RATING VALUES:
O = Outstanding; E = Exceeds Requirements; M = Meets Requirements;
N = Needs Improvement; U = Unsatisfactory

Check as Appropriate					Outstanding	Exceeds Requirements	Meets Requirements	Needs Improvement	Unsatisfactory
O	E	M	N	U					
1. Job Knowledge									
					Broad knowledge of the position and its relationship to others in the practice.	Good knowledge of position and its relationship to others in the practice.	Enough knowledge to perform routine aspects of job. Sometimes must seek advice of others.	Often requires advice from others to perform even routine aspects of position.	Cannot perform even the most routine tasks.
2. Quality of Work									
					Produces exceptional, precise, well organized quality of work.	Produces high quality work.	Produces acceptable quality of work.	Work quality is below acceptable standards.	Work falls considerably short of acceptable standards.
3. Patient Interaction									
					Displays exceptional skill in communicating with patients and managing difficult situations.	Communicates well with patients and displays tact in handling difficult situations.	Satisfactory skill in communicating with patients and managing difficult situations.	Skill in communicating with patients and managing difficult situations is below acceptable standards.	Unsatisfactory level of skill in communicating with patients and managing difficult situations.
4. Punctuality and Attendance									
					Always punctual and has few absences.	Employee is punctual with good attendance record.	Employee meets attendance and tardiness requirement.	Employee is below attendance and tardiness requirement.	Employee is considerably below attendance/tardiness requirement.
5. Cooperation									
					Exceptionally willing employee. Always works well with others.	Willing employee. Works well with others.	Cooperation of employee is at satisfactory level.	Cooperation level is in need of improvement.	Cooperation level well below acceptable standards.
6. Relationships									
					Maintains outstanding relationships with employees, physicians and/or patients.	Maintains very good relationships with employees, physicians and/or patients.	Maintains satisfactory relationships with employees, physicians and/or patients.	Relationships with employees, physicians and/or patients need improvement.	Relationships with others are far below acceptable standards.

FIGURE 2. Sample employee evaluation sheet. *(Continued on following page.)*

EVALUATION FORM (Continued)					
Check as Appropriate	**Outstanding**	**Exceeds Requirements**	**Meets Requirements**	**Needs Improvement**	**Unsatisfactory**

O	E	M	N	U					
					7. Attitude				
					Displays outstanding level of enthusiasm and interest about the job and practice.	Usually displays enthusiasm and interest towards job and practice	Displays satisfactory level of enthusiasm and interest.	Level of enthusiasm and interest needs improvement.	Level of enthusiasm and interest far below acceptable standards.
					8. Initiative				
					Displays outstanding level of initiative with little or no supervision	Displays very good level of initiative with little or no supervision.	Displays satisfactory level of initiative with little or no supervision.	Level of initiative needs improvement.	Level of initiative far below acceptable standards.
					9. Communication				
					Exceptionally effective in all phases of communication.	Good communication skills.	Communicates at a satisfactory level.	Communication skills are below standards.	Communication skills are far below standards.
					10. Dependability in Decision-making				
					Extremely reliable and consistent in making sound decisions.	Very reliable and consistent in making sound decisions.	Reliability and consistency in making sound decisions at satisfactory level.	Reliability and consistency in making decisions needs improvement.	Reliability and consistency in making decisions is far below acceptable standards.
					11. Planning and Organization				
					Assigns priorities exceptionally well. Anticipates problems.	Assigns priorities well. Usually meets goals on time.	Plans and organizes at a satisfactory level.	Planning and organization ability needs improvement.	Planning and organization ability far below acceptable level.
					12. Awareness of Practice Philosophy and Patient Services				
					Exceptional. Often makes suggestions to improve patient relations and services. Demonstrates a thorough understanding of practice philosophy in patient care.	Good awareness of practice philosophy and patient services.	Satisfactory awareness of practice philosophy and patient services.	Awareness of practice philosophy and patient services needs improvement.	Awareness of practice philosophy and patient services is below acceptable level.

Evaluator's Comments

Areas where improvement is needed _____

Specific goals for upcoming year _____

_____

Other _____

_____

Prepared by: _____

Employee's Comments

_____

_____

Date: _____ Signature: _____

Historically, the fifth level of motivation has been difficult to accomplish in smaller practices because there are few levels of responsibility. However, in larger practices, where there are more opportunities for promotion, the fifth level is an important consideration.

Emphasize that if everyone in the practice takes pride in his or her work, operates efficiently with little or no supervision, knows what to do and how to do it, and supports everybody else's efforts in the best way possible, the practice and all of its people will be rewarded. It is necessary to involve the entire practice in this process. If everyone buys into it, working toward common goals that are commonly accepted will be the rule rather than the exception.

Hire employees who are self-motivated, and establish an environment that fosters self-motivation, interdependence, pride in one's work, and pride in self. By focusing on each employee's hierarchy of needs, keeping the lines of communication open, and helping each employee become self-motivated, you can foster practice-wide motivation from within.

USE DISCIPLINE AND FIRING WHEN NECESSARY

Distinguish between discipline and firing. Establish a written code, make sure that everyone has a copy, and enforce it. Refrain from discipline by reducing salary. Usually, issuing a warning, establishing a cure period, and monitoring the employee for progress can accomplish behavior modification. If the unacceptable behavior persists, consider dismissal. Have documentation of previous offenses and prior failed attempts to modify unacceptable behavior or of the employee's inability to perform the job satisfactorily.

FOCUS ON YOUR SYSTEMS

As your practice transitions to managed care, it will be necessary to develop your business systems. Most medical practices already are computerized, and the few that are not probably will be so soon. MCOs are universally computerized, and some MCOs that acquire medical practices offer to install or improve the acquired practice's information systems as added inducement to join. In part, this is necessary for many MCOs that require direct claims reporting and other computer functions.

Because computer technology is expanding extremely rapidly, increasingly more medical office functions are being computerized. Computer systems are relatively expensive; a good-quality information system for a small practice may cost as much as a luxury automobile. Other similarities to a luxury car include the fact that they tend to become obsolete in a short period and may require substantial maintenance and repair efforts.

For all these reasons, focusing on systems means, first and foremost, focusing on computerized information systems—usually in terms of upgrading existing systems.

UPGRADING YOUR INFORMATION SYSTEM

Early computers required a degree of user programming. Now most programs are commercially available. You still may need a computer expert in house, especially if you have a local network or are part of a more extensive network. These complex systems often require full-time attention.

Virtually every information system now in use can help your practice with its billing, insurance, and collections. Chances are that you need a system that will also help to manage your practice. There are certain things that you can and should expect of your computer system. Your practice should review its operations monthly to detect potential problems. A good computer system should track practice expenditures and revenue streams, accounts receivable, and insurance figures.

A good computer system also generates patient flow statistics and tracks correlations with particular physicians or health plans. It should detect excessive delay between the time that a patient calls to make an appointment and the actual appointment date and spot any trends in reception-room waiting time. Your system should be able to help you collate and analyze patient and referring/referral physician survey results. It also should be able to give you pertinent patient demographics and referral information.

A good information system quantifies patient outcomes, tracks procedure frequency by CPT or ICD code, monitors and categorizes services provided in terms of physician, health plan, or payor, and runs numeric relations of all sorts, including RVUs (relative value units; most payors use Medicare's resource-based relative value units), visits, and referrals per patient.

If your computer system is not able to report the number of hospital admissions and length of stay per patient, prescriptions per patient, and average wholesale price of the drugs you have prescribed, consider making changes. Your system should be able to track your charges-to-collections ratio, denial rates, and write-offs, categorized by payor.

If your practice is even partly capitated, your computer should be able to tell the cost to the practice of providing each service, your total costs of providing services, and your capitation profitability for each managed care contractor (expressed by RVU). It should allow you to compare all of your capitated managed care contracts not only against one another but also with your discounted fee-for-service contracts and against your usual and customary fee-for-service rates. A good computer system compares your business numbers from month to month, from year to year, and by month and year. It should make all numbers available on a practice-wide basis and by physician.

Larger MCOs and computer software vendors should be able to provide physician practices with direct links to MCOs for claims processing and posting and also to give practices immediate information about enrollee eligibility, allowable services, and required copayments. A good information system helps the practice to secure fast approval for referrals, which, in turn, reduces paperwork and improves collections.

A good computer system automatically generates letters to patients requesting payment of accounts in arrears and otherwise dealing with delinquent accounts. It can send out letters reminding patients of appointments. It can track physician and staff salaries, benefits, and overhead costs. A superior system also can perform paperless office functions, such as generating and updating medical charts and diagnostic images. Some systems also offer hands-free voice-recognition dictation.

Most vendors also offer managed care modules or packages of programs, which can help with quality assurance and utilization review as well as assess compliance with the rules and regulations of health plans, state and federal laws, and the Health Plan Employer Data and Information Set (HEDIS).

HEDIS is the assessment tool developed by the National Committee for Quality Assurance (NCQA). NCQA started as a collaboration of health plans and large employers (the main purchasers of health plans) to develop a way to compare certain aspects of health plans in common terms. It was originally offered to HMOs as a way to see how they measured up, and compliance was voluntary. However, many large employers are now demanding that health plans demonstrate HEDIS compliance. In turn, health plans are holding their impaneled physicians responsible for meeting the requisite standards.

The implication for medical practices is clear: managed care is taking over one health care market after another, and some experts predict a 100% managed care environment in a decade or two. If you have no managed care contracts now, you probably will need some shortly. Health plans live by HEDIS compliance and demand the same of the physicians with whom they contract. You need to be in HEDIS compliance—sooner rather than later. If you have a top-notch computer information system, you can track all of the necessary HEDIS statistics (e.g., contracting, managed care, revenue stream, overhead cost).

For a copy of the latest HEDIS document, version 3.0, contact the NCQA. The document is large and seemingly daunting but also self-explanatory and relatively easy to use. It contains a mechanism to evaluate your score, and the NCQA also offers assistance.

DO NOT FORGET THE TELEPHONE

Although computerization is perhaps the most important business system for many practices, remember your telephone system. It is at least your second most valuable business system, and if you are not yet computerized, its importance increases. To flourish in an increasingly competitive marketplace, you will need to expand your market share, which means adding more patients, most of whom probably will be health plan enrollees, as more and more people join such plans each year. Most of your practice business will be arranged by telephone, starting with patient appointments and continuing with referrals, vendor contacts, and managed care business calls. Your staff probably will grow, especially if you merge or add physician associates. Staff members use your phones, too.

Do you have a fax machine? You probably should. Are you linked with another site by telephone modem? Are you "on line" from the office? If so, your practice requires even more telephone service, to accommodate your access to the Internet, which is also probably by telephone modem. Many regions around the country are subdividing in terms of adding new area codes to handle all the burgeoning telephone traffic.

Make sure that your practice can handle all of its phone traffic. Have enough lines and enough personnel to answer all calls promptly as well as to manage a dedicated fax line and a dedicated computer modem line. Peak hours may be problematic; thus, you should consider using an automated attendant. Make sure that you use the attendant to field calls during busy times, not to evade them. The referral you miss costs income. So does the patient whose business you lose when you put her on hold, keep her there for long minutes at a time, and then lose her when someone pushes the wrong telephone button. Make sure that all employees are fully trained in the use of the system.

Have an emergency option on your system. Consider announcing that option first. Experience indicates that if you structure the caller's choices correctly, they will use the system properly. People tend to use the emergency option indiscriminately most often when the choice that they seek is not there. Also include an option for the operator to handle miscellaneous calls.

Hire a competent answering service. Make sure to check your service personally. Call and try to make an appointment. See how long you wait to speak with someone, how long you are on hold, whether the person answering the call is pleasant and efficient, and whether the person can cope with you effectively if you pretend to be difficult and impatient, as you should.

Install a voice-mail system for personal calls to your office when your staff members are busy and for nonemergency calls from vendors, other physicians, and pharmacies. You may even tie in your voice-mail system with your automated teller to handle nonemergency patient calls.

Triage all calls from patients. As the health care delivery system transitions away from fee-for-service and toward capitation, it is important for staff to schedule office visits only for patients whom you really must see. Perhaps even more importantly, they must know what to tell callers in emergency situations. Ideally, a registered nurse should triage all calls; if that is not possible, a licensed practical nurse is the best option. Of course, you should expect to receive patient calls—even emergency ones—when neither your RN nor your LPN is available. In such cases, another member of your staff will need to take the calls.

Develop a triage protocol for your practice, and write it down; put together a formal manual. Use standard guidelines. Your physicians (assuming that you are in a group practice) need to get together and reach a consensus about how to handle each situation. After all, staff members must be able to use your manual efficiently and effectively; you cannot ask them to leaf through several different pages or sections with an anxious patient on the phone, looking for a specific doctor's instructions. That wastes time, and time is vital, especially in an emergency.

Ideally, all of your physicians, nurses, and owners should participate in the development of the manual, remembering that your staff people will be the ones who use it. Consider laying out the information not only by condition but also by body part (alphabetically). Include specific scheduling instructions for emergency situations, patient visits that must be scheduled immediately, patient visits that may be delayed, and patients who need not visit but rather may receive a return phone call from the doctor. Also include questions and answers that your triage personnel can use to help them decide how to handle each caller.

Post your emergency instructions near each telephone, and make sure a copy of your written triage protocol manual remains at each telephone station. Also, do not always expect to "go by the book." Some questions are not easily categorized or expected; a doctor should become involved if there is any question at all. Also be aware that some people simply will not talk to anyone but the doctor. They will stay on line, call back, and wait until the physician answers. If you can identify such people in advance, simply give them what they want. Why lose a patient?

Under no circumstances should nonclinical personnel give medical advice or answer a patient's questions in terms of "what the doctor usually does." Your triage nurse may answer some of these questions; others should be handled by a mid-level practitioner or physician.

If you or your practice maintains a presence on the Internet, if you are "on line," especially if you have a page or site on the world wide web, your patients will find you. So will others. Beware making any medical recommendations on line; they may be forwarded inappropriately, and you may be held responsible. If you are on line, consider listing your address, hours of operation, health plans and insurance accepted, and telephone number. Also post an emergency option directing patients with immediate problems to call or connect with your emergency number, hospital, or ambulance by telephone or e-mail.

FOCUS ON SATISFACTION

To keep your medical practice successful, you must keep your market share high. Focus on satisfaction. Just as you must keep employee morale high, you also must work to keep your customers satisfied. Who are your customers? Your patients, referring physicians, and managed care partners.

KEEP PATIENT SATISFACTION HIGH

Patient satisfaction is vital to your practice for a number of reasons. First, if you have fee-for-service patients, you must keep them satisfied to keep them in your practice. Second, MCOs must sell their health plans to employers. To do so, they must show that the physicians on their provider panels maintain a high level of patient satisfaction. Thus, you must prove the same to your MCOs. Third, purchasers of health plans are increasingly using HEDIS compliance to help determine whether to remain with the health plans they have or to contract with new MCOs. In turn, MCOs are holding their plan physicians accountable for HEDIS compliance. HEDIS rates patient satisfaction high on its list of priorities.

In effect, patient satisfaction is a major driving force of managed care. As discussed earlier, staff members who are well trained, pleasant, efficient, and motivated improve patient satisfaction. So does having great outcomes. What else should you be doing? It never hurts to address patient-oriented scheduling again, not only from the perspective of telephone efficiency, but in terms of wasting their time in other ways. Consider the following pointers:

1. Start on time. Schedule your first patients of the day to arrive at the office 15 minutes early so that they are escorted to the appropriate rooms, prepared, and waiting for you when you start.

2. Keep scheduled appointments. If you have a patient scheduled for 10:30, see that patient at 10:30 or as close to that time as possible. If you are delayed at the hospital or called away on an emergency, have your secretary or receptionist tell your patients, and give them your estimated time of arrival. If they cannot stay, offer to reschedule them and give them preferred appointment times. If it is late in the day, offer new appointments to patients who cannot stay and see those who can. Stay as late as you must. And make sure to give every patient at least as much of your time as is "normal." A few moments more is better. Never rush a patient after making him or her wait for you.

3. Deal with walk-ins. If you can schedule a time for walk-ins, do so. If not, discourage the practice. If a patient has an emergency, try to squeeze him or her in as long as the visit does not unduly delay your seeing other patients. If the emergency is imminent and critical, send an ambulance. If a patient without an emergency walks in, see your scheduled patients first, and make sure the walk-in understands that he or she will have to wait.

4. Be open when patients need you. If you find that your patients need you on evenings and weekends but your Tuesday, Wednesday, and Thursday mornings are slow, close the office on those mornings and open it on evenings. Stay open Saturdays and close Mondays. If you can see patients earlier than your usual starting time twice a week, make those hours available and measure the response. If patients like those hours, keep them. If necessary, add hours rather than switching them. If you already are working a 60- or 70-hour week, consider hiring an associate physician or a physician extender.

5. Keep track of the seasons. Maintain a lighter schedule of regular appointments when you expect heavy seasonal "sick visit" traffic. For example, know when flu season begins and, especially for Mondays during flu season, leave room to accommodate unscheduled patients who truly need your services. Make similar plans for vacation season and back-to-school physical examination time.

Extend the concept of convenience for patients beyond telephone triage and extra hours. Consider payment methods. Many families live on a budget. Many people hate to carry cash. What can you do about it? Accept payment by credit and/or debit card. For patients who are not in health plans or on Medicare or Medicaid, consider arranging payment by schedule. Accept payment by check with caution.

Some medical practices are located in areas with substantial populations of non–English-speaking people. Having an employee on your staff who can converse with such people in their native language and who understands the culture and its customs can substantially boost patient satisfaction and draw such patients and enrollees to your practice.

Catering to your patients is always a good idea. Is there a school for hearing-impaired students in your area? Perhaps someone on your staff—even one of the physicians—can learn sign language and offer this value-added service.

Although it is not widespread, some MCOs are starting to pay for certain alternate therapies. Find out which ones your MCO will reimburse. If there is enough demand from your fee-for-service patients for alternative medicine, consider adding those services. You also must consider what it will cost you to acquire the necessary skills and discipline or to hire a physician who already is versed in such practices.

Make your practice accessible to and friendly toward people with disabilities. Have ramps installed. Have your doorways widened. Consider your restroom facilities.

If your practice has young children as patients or if adult visitors to your office tend to bring young children into your reception area, consider adding changing tables in the restrooms. Parents and other caregivers will appreciate the convenience.

Pay attention to your reception area. Provide comfortable seating, adequate soft lighting, reading lamps, and a wide range of current reading material. For children, have coloring books and crayons (with parental permission), reading books, activity books, games, and puzzles. Provide water, juice, and coffee. Have soft music playing on the radio. Consider making a television available (*you* should control the settings at all times). Give visitors access to a telephone for free local calls.

Make sure your examination rooms are secure, private, and as comfortable as possible. Provide security escort to your parking lot on request. Make sure that your business sign is as large as local zoning ordinances allow and visible from a block away.

Provide patient education; consider adding a tape player to your television set for education films. Supply brochures, which are available free of charge or at reduced cost from many medical societies and vendors.

KEEP REFERRING PHYSICIAN SATISFACTION HIGH

If you are a specialist or subspecialist, referring physicians are also your customers. Generally, they want you to be able to schedule their patients when they need you. Again, make sure your telephone system is superior. Also find out what type of reporting each of your referral physicians prefers. Some like to be advised at every step of the way. Some only want to know when you become involved, what your course of action is, and the final result. Some want details, whereas others want only summaries. All referring physicians want you to provide excellent outcomes and respond to their needs promptly. Find out what each wants and provide it.

SURVEYS

Survey patient and referring physician satisfaction using a standard form with well thought-out questions. Analyze the results. Make appropriate changes based on the feedback. Focus on doing the work you can most easily afford first, and delay more costly projects. Notify your patients of changes you have made and changes to expect in a letter. Include survey results, improvements you have made, and pending improvement. Thank your survey participants. Leave copies in your office for your patients. Consider a similar letter for your referring physicians. Send copies of each letter to your managed care partners.

Alternatively, consider starting a practice newsletter, which you can also use for more general purposes. Your computer system should be able to accommodate a modestly priced desktop publishing program.

In general, turn patient complaints into patient compliments and turn patient compliments into successful practice marketing. You may use the sample patient and referring physician satisfaction survey questionnaires in Figures 3, 4, and 5.

MANAGED CARE PARTNERS

There is no need to survey managed care partners or partners-to-be. If your physicians are seeking managed care contracts, find out what the MCOs that offer contracts in your area want and gear your practice to provide it. Focus on

---

Your Practice's Name

Today's date: _____

Which doctor did you see? _____

How many days did you have to wait to schedule an appointment?
☐ 1 to 2 days   ☐ 3 to 5 days   ☐ 6 to 10 days   ☐ 10 to 15 days   ☐ more than 15 days

How did you get to our office?
☐ Car   ☐ Public transportation

How many miles did you travel to get to our office?
☐ Under 1 mile   ☐ 1 to 3 miles   ☐ 3 to 5 miles   ☐ 5 to 10 miles   ☐ Over 10 miles

Which of the following influenced your decision to use our office? (Check all that apply)
☐ Referred by another patient   Name: _____
☐ Referred by a doctor   Name: _____
☐ Referred by a friend or family mamber
☐ Physician referral service   Name: _____
☐ Doctor participates in your HMO
☐ Telephone listing
☐ Close to home or office
☐ Other   Specify: _____

What health insurance do you have?
☐ Medicare   ☐ HMO 3
☐ Blue Cross/Blue Shield   ☐ HMO 4
☐ Medicaid   ☐ HMO other: _____
☐ HMO 1   ☐ Cash
☐ HMO 2

Are you satisfied with your insurance? (Circle one)
Yes, very   1   2   3   4   5   No

How long did you wait to be seen by the physician?
☐ under 15 min   ☐ 15 to 30 min   ☐ 30 to 45 min   ☐ 45 min to 1 hr   ☐ over 1 hr

Please rate us	excellent	good	fair	below avg.	poor
Courtesy and helpfulness of our receptionist when you called to make your appointment	☐	☐	☐	☐	☐
Ability to get a timely appointment	☐	☐	☐	☐	☐
Office location	☐	☐	☐	☐	☐
Parking availability	☐	☐	☐	☐	☐
Convenience	☐	☐	☐	☐	☐
Reception area	☐	☐	☐	☐	☐
Appearance and quality of our staff	☐	☐	☐	☐	☐
Courtesy and knowledge of our staff	☐	☐	☐	☐	☐
Appearance and professionalism	☐	☐	☐	☐	☐
Waiting time after you arrived	☐	☐	☐	☐	☐
Courtesy of doctor	☐	☐	☐	☐	☐
Doctor's patience and interest in your problem	☐	☐	☐	☐	☐
Time our professionals spent with you	☐	☐	☐	☐	☐
Doctor's explanation and treatment	☐	☐	☐	☐	☐

FIGURE 3. Sample patient satisfaction survey questionnaire. *(Continued on following page.)*

Please rate us *(Continued)*	excellent	good	fair	below avg.	poor
General quality of medical care you received	☐	☐	☐	☐	☐
Explanation of billing	☐	☐	☐	☐	☐
Other: _____	☐	☐	☐	☐	☐
Other: _____	☐	☐	☐	☐	☐

Tell us the best times for you to make appointments:

	Mon.	Tues.	Wed.	Thurs.	Fri.	Sat.	Sun.
Morning							
Afternoon			XXX				XXX
Evening						XXX	XXX

Personal: Your answers are helpful, but the following are optional.

Age: _____   Home Zip code: _____

Thank you for participating in our survey. We will use your responses to help improve our practice and our service to you.

(Signature) _____

FIGURE 3.   Sample patient satisfaction survey questionnaire *(Continued)*.

Your Letterhead

Date

Physician Practice Name
Address
_____
_____

Dear _____:

We at (your practice's name) are making a special effort to be sure that we are providing the quality and types of services that are important to our patients and to our referring physicians.

You are a valued referrer, and we want to know what you think about us. We would appreciate your taking a few minutes to complete the enclosed questionnaire and return it to our consulting firm, (consulting firm's name), in the enclosed envelope. It is important to us that you be completely open and honest so that we will be able to make changes to the benefit of our mutual patients.

We want to be sure that you are properly informed about the care we are providing to our mutual patients. Please be sure to let us know how well we report back to you as well as how you may prefer to be kept informed during the time we are involved in the patient's care.

We know your time is valuable. It is important to us, however; therefore, we look forward to receiving your comments. Thank you very much for your help. If you prefer not to identify yourself or your practice, that certainly would be acceptable to us.

Sincerely,

(Your practice's name)

Enclosures

FIGURE 4.   Sample cover letter for referring physician satisfaction questionnaire.

Was your patient able to schedule an appointment in a timely manner?
☐ Yes,   ☐ No (specify problem below)
Problems:

Was your hospital consultant seen promptly?
☐ Yes   ☐ No (specify problem below)
Problems:

Did your patient report any problems?
☐ Yes   ☐ No (specify problem below)
Problems:

Do you prefer a phone call as soon as the patient is seen and prior to written report?
☐ Yes   ☐ No

Do you usually receive the written consult report in a timely manner?
☐ Yes   ☐ No

Please rate us	excellent	good	fair	below avg.	poor
Physician availability	☐	☐	☐	☐	☐
Physician responsiveness	☐	☐	☐	☐	☐
Quality of care provided	☐	☐	☐	☐	☐
Clarity and breadth of consult report	☐	☐	☐	☐	☐
Our business office staff	☐	☐	☐	☐	☐
Our clinical office staff	☐	☐	☐	☐	☐
Other:	☐	☐	☐	☐	☐

Please tell us what you like about our practice:

Please tell us what you do not like about our practice:

Any other information you can give us about our practice, to improve it:

We appreciate your referrals. Thank you for taking the time to complete this questionnaire. Our goal is to improve our service to our mutual patients and to our referring physicians.

Your Practice Name: _____

FIGURE 5. Sample referring physician satisfaction questionnaire.

geographic area, patient demographics, range of services, payment rates, and expected utilization rates. Be aware that MCOs want to deal with physicians who keep costs low, provide excellent patient outcomes, are outstanding citizens of the community, are board-certified, and are in compliance with HEDIS guidelines and all state and federal laws. They want physicians who embrace the principles of managed care and will help them to market their health plans to employers and other purchasers.

If physicians are on health plan panels, MCOs will tell them exactly how well or poorly they are doing by issuing report cards designed to help physicians analyze their current practice status and to suggest strategies for practice improvement.

It will be up to you and your information system to measure outcomes, perform practice cost analyses, and generate the data your physicians need to prove practice excellence to MCOs.

CONTROL COSTS

As physician payments continue to shrink, practices must reexamine their practice costs with an eye toward controlling costs and improving efficiencies. Review your expenses line by line, and review your systems, human and electronic, to make sure that there is no waste. Trim wherever possible.

REDUCE PERSONNEL WITH CAUTION

Typically, the most costly component of doing business for any medical practice is personnel. Not counting physician compensation, staff salaries routinely account for the largest numbers on the debit side of the ledger. Thus, it may occur to you that firing or laying off employees may help you to control costs, but remember that your staff is your practice's most valuable asset as well as its largest operating expense. A good staff can make or break a practice.

Before you cut personnel, make sure you are *really* over-staffed. If you cut key personnel, you probably will disrupt operations and decrease practice efficiency. Furthermore, you may send a negative message to remaining staff members, who may consider themselves not only hard pressed to compensate for the work your employee(s) did but also probably next in line when you swing the ax again.

Lowering office morale will not help to achieve high levels of patient satisfaction. And if your remaining employees are distressed enough, they may decide to find new jobs, which will leave your practice coping with a high turnover rate. You may need to hire more employees, train them, and wait for them to adjust to your practice before they become efficient.

If you *must* restructure and/or restaff your practice, consider hiring a health care business consultant to assess your needs and current staff and recommend necessary changes. An external consultant most likely will be more objective than you can be, and your employees can focus their resentment on the consultant, not you. Furthermore, an experienced health care business consultant can also help you assess the rest of your practice for other cost control potentials. For example, review your malpractice insurance rates. Remember to assess *all* practice expenses and possible alternatives before you cut personnel to reduce your overhead costs.

Resources are available from many organizations to help you determine if your salary and benefits package is on target, including the *Staff Salary Survey*, cited above. The Medical Group Management Association and Society of Medical-Dental Management Consultants also have figures that you can use.

CAN YOU CUT COSTS BY ADDING PERSONNEL?

Consider controlling costs by adding personnel. Consider adding, for example, a physician's assistant, a medical assistant (who also can act as a practice chaperone and/or scribe), and a patient advocate. Although adding staff members will cost your practice money initially, staff additions may prove invaluable by improving practice efficiency and allowing you and other physicians in your practice to treat more patients.

CONSIDER ADDING A PHYSICIAN EXTENDER

A physician extender (PE) may allow you to control practice costs and also increase productivity. In addition, a PE may relieve you of some time-consuming and mundane tasks. Consider hiring a PE particularly if you are contemplating the addition of a new associate physician. Do you really have enough work to keep a new associate busy, or are you actually looking for help with peripheral tasks that cannot be performed by a secretary or receptionist but *can* be performed by a PE—typically a certified registered nurse practitioner (CRNP) or physician assistant (PA).

A PA can work in hospitals, clinics, agencies, and, in general, family, emergency, and most specialty practice situations, doing a wide range of work historically performed by physicians, including:

- Taking medical histories
- Assessing primary health problems
- Conducting routine check-ups
- Handling patient education and counseling
- Performing some diagnostic procedures
- Ordering laboratory tests for cultures
- Interpreting test results

CRNPs are registered nurses who have completed additional training. They perform in much the same way as PAs and provide services in a variety of settings. Bear in mind that diligent physician supervision is absolutely necessary. The physician is usually required to be on the premises or at least reachable by telephone and must review and countersign the patient's chart documentation. Many states require PAs and CRNPs to practice under written protocols.

The economic benefits are obvious. Compare the annual salary range of the typical physician extender—$45,000–50,000—with the starting salary range for a typical primary care associate—$70,000–90,000. Also note that future salary expectations of the typical physician extender are significantly lower than those of the typical physician. Also consider the comparison calculation in Table 4, which is based on the cost to a hypothetical medical practice of a comprehensive new patient encounter.

MCOs rate their panel providers on a number of factors, including cost-effectiveness and patient satisfaction; a good physician extender can improve

TABLE 4.   Hypothetical Comparison: Physician vs. Physician Assistant Costs

Personnel	Hourly Cost	Old Time Allocation	Old Unit Cost	New Time Allocation	New Unit Cost
Physician	$62.20	.75	$46.65	.4	$24.88
Registered nurse	$22.60	.3	$ 6.68	.3	$ 6.68
Medical assistant	$ 9.68	.5	$ 4.84	.5	$ 4.84
Physician assistant	$20.67	0	$ 0	.35	$ 7.23
			Total direct cost: $58.27		Total direct cost: $43.63
			Total indirect cost: $21.46		Total indirect cost: $21.46
			Total cost: $79.73		Total cost: $65.09

By having the physician assistant perform some of the preliminary work, the practice can save $14.64 on each CPT-4 #99203. It this hypothetical four-physician practice performs 40,000 patient encounters a year, and CPT-4 #99203 accounts for 25% of all encounters (10,000 per year), then having the physician assistant perform part of this work saves the practice $14,640 annually.

both. In addition, most payors—including Medicare—reimburse extenders' services if they work under the proper physician supervision. If used effectively, the typical physician extender can generate revenues equaling 120% of his or her salary.

CONSIDER ADDING A PATIENT ADVOCATE

In an environment of increasing managed care, a patient advocate on your staff may pay big dividends. The patient advocate's job is to educate patients about managed care and teach them that it is necessary to stay within the health plan to receive medical services. The patient advocate will teach your patients how to receive MCO-covered resources from the most appropriate providers. For example, a patient advocate will facilitate referrals, list which pharmacies patients should use to get their prescriptions filled, discuss any formulary restrictions, and tell your patients at which hospitals to seek services, such as radiographs and laboratory tests. In general, a patient advocate helps your patients to stay in the loop and to deal with physicians and other health care providers in the same loop. Thus, he or she helps your medical practice to eliminate unnecessary financial losses and to improve your relationships with MCOs.

Practices bearing substantial managed care risk lose money when patients go outside the health plan for services that they do not directly provide. Most MCOs penalize the practices in which patients generate such costs. By teaching patients what they need to know about managed care, health plans, and their restrictions, rules, and regulations, the advocate eliminates or at least controls these potential losses. Furthermore, by working closely with your patients, the advocate tends to improve patient satisfaction and helps to reestablish the vital

YOUR PRACTICE'S NAME

Patient Advocate's Managed Care Checklist   As of _____

Fin. Cls.	Insurance	Type	Reim.	Ambulatory Surgery	Hospital	DME	Pharmacy	Home Health	Mental Health	In House *See Attached Notes	Outside *See Attached Notes	Dental	Vision	Transp.	Notes**
1	Regional Health	Medicare Risk	3	Med. Ctr. All Saints	Med. Ctr., University	UrCo	Worthy's Eastern	InCare 111-2222	HCM 333-4444	MA IHRF *To MCO for auth.	MA-PRF Form 198	Enamel Net 999-9999 *Adult ref only; use ENet form; Y5 <20 see ref	User MA-IHF	Call Member Services	A, B, C, G, Q, R, W
2	PriCare	HMO Commercial	1	General	University, Med. Ctr., All Saints	Eastern 7th & Main	Worthy's U-Mart	ABC Home Health	PriCare Ref on Form 184A	IHS Form *Regarding In-house Specialists: Return pink copy to MCO, filled in	IHS Form	SEE ATTACHED NOTES <20 self ref >20 w/acute problems, use IHS Form	SEE ATTACHED NOTES	Call Member Services	C, E, G, H
3	The Blues HMO	Commercial	5	General	OmniSys, All Saints Med. Ctr.	AllStar 777-7777 DeltaCare 888-8888	Worthy's Eastern	InCare 111-2222	HHAC 444-5555	The Blues Short Form	The Blues PAR	N/A	Call The Blues Cust. Svcs. 232-3232	N/A	A, B, C, X, ZZ
4	Medicare Primary; ABC Secondary	Medicare Risk	3	PRIMARY CARE ONLY	University	PRIMARY CARE ONLY	University Greene's	PRIMARY CARE ONLY	PRIMARY CARE ONLY	IHS Form * In-house Specialists: (pink copy)	Form 201; Return to MCO				X
5	AllCare Neighbors Choice	Medicaid Risk	3	PRIMARY CARE ONLY	University	PRIMARY CARE ONLY	University Greene's	PRIMARY CARE ONLY	PRIMARY CARE ONLY	IHS FORM * In-house Specialists: (pink copy)	Form 201; Return to MCO	Use ENet Form	AAA PAR for Ophthalmic and Optical	Call Member Services	X
6	OmniSys	HMO Commercial	5	General	All Saints University	UrCo 666-7777	Clinic United Eastern Greene's	SNI UrCo	The Source 1-800-333-2211	MA-IHRF	MA-PRF Form 208	N/A	N/A	N/A	D, I, J, M, P
7	OurGroup	HMO Commercial	1	General	Med. Ctr., CCH, All Saints	AllStar 777-7777 UrCo 666-7777	Clinic Greene's Smith	UrCo 777-6666	HHAC	MA-IHRF	ICG Form	N/A	N/A	N/A	O
8	OurGroup Commercial	Medicare Risk	1	General	OmniSys, All Saints	AllStar 777-7777 UrCo 666-7777	Clinic Greene's Smith	ABC Home Health	HHAC	IHS Form * In-house Specialists: (pink copy)	ICG Form	N/A	N/A	Call Easy-Ride 1-800-111-2345	R, S, X

This matrix is a fictional representation, for illustration only

FIGURE 6. Hypothetical/sample patient advocate's managed care checklist.

relationship in which patients and physicians (and, by extension, physicians' practices) work together to determine the optimal health care regimen for each patient in each case. Managed care tends to threaten this relationship; your advocate can help to restore it.

The patient advocate must make sure that the health care providers outside your office (from whom your enrollees seek care) also understand all of the appropriate health plan parameters. He or she will find out all of the rules for all of your managed care plans, maintain the necessary contact with them, and stay current with their changes. Your advocate will work with the physician(s) to identify appropriate referral physicians and providers. He or she also will follow up to make sure the system is working.

Even if your practice is small, has few managed care patients, and bears little managed care risk, you should perform patient advocacy. Rather than hire an advocate, establish a patient advocacy *program*. Later, if and when your practice needs a dedicated employee to perform this work, the foundation will be established and your advocate will have a head start. Advocacy programs may include posting charts that show each plan's requirements, distributing printed managed care forms to patients, listing participating pharmacies on the back of prescriptions, assigning someone to keep track of changes and make the necessary updates, and having health plan information readily available for practice personnel and patients.

Consider the hypothetical patient advocate's checklist in Figure 6 as a blueprint for a similar checklist for your practice. Any such checklist must be tailored for your particular practice's needs.

CONSIDER ADDING A CHAPERONE/SCRIBE

Another type of employee who can have a significant impact on your practice in terms of cost control is a chaperone/scribe. As a chaperone, she can often protect a practice against frivolous legal action that patients may press against physicians by being present during examinations. As a scribe, she can increase your patient throughput by taking notes (e.g., vital signs) during examinations and ordering prescriptions afterward. In addition, physicians can focus more attention on patients' needs, which will improve patient satisfaction. As an added bonus, health plans will give your practice higher marks for both improved efficiency and higher patient satisfaction levels.

If using a scribe allows a physician to see an average of only four more patients per day at a fee of $30 per patient, over the course of 48 weeks, you will add $7,200 (4 patients × $30 a day × 5 days a week × 48 weeks a year = $7,200) to your income stream over the course of a year. In fact, most practices report that adding a scribe improves patient throughput by significantly higher than four patients daily. In some cases, a scribe can boost throughput by as much as an additional two patients an hour.

If you are going to hire a chaperone/scribe, consider hiring a medical assistant to do the job rather than using a PA. For each task, use the lowest-paid employee capable and qualified to do the job. Both PAs and CRNPs are trained at a higher level than is necessary to perform the duties of a scribe or chaperone, and each earns a considerably higher salary.

Referring to a chaperone as "she" is deliberate, simply because in most legal actions involving claims of sexual assault, harassment, or unprofessional behavior, the allegation is made by a female patient against a male practitioner. However, remember that it is *not* unheard of for a man to charge a female physician with sexual misconduct. If you determine that your practice needs a male scribe/chaperone, hire a man.

It may be the case that you can easily see the need for a practice scribe but question the need for a practice chaperone. Traditional physician-patient relationships are becoming increasingly rare. Years ago, physicians generally developed cordial relationships with their patients, and physicians often treated multiple generations of the same family. Today extended families are rare, and the likelihood of patients living in one geographic area their entire lives is less likely now than in the past. Moreover, managed care is growing, converting ever more patients into enrollees, further disrupting traditional patient-physician relationships. Many enrollees simply pick a physician's name off a list of impaneled physicians who currently accept their health plan.

Bottom line: often your patients do not know you, and you do not know your patients, many of whom are not really "patients" but enrollees. Some people play malpractice games to make money. One of those people could be among your unknown enrollees.

Having a chaperone (who is the same sex as the patient) present during an examination could save your professional life in this increasingly litigious society. Adding a medical assistant to your staff who can function as both a scribe and a chaperone can help to control costs, increase throughput, and keep you out of a frivolous lawsuit. Even if you win such a suit, your reputation may be lost in the process.

INVESTIGATE OTHER COST-CONTROL MEASURES

In comparison, other cost-saving/cost-control measures you can take—measures that do not involve hiring new personnel—may appear to represent small savings. But in this environment every dollar counts. Consider the following measures:

1. Avoid paying employees for overtime work by keeping your office hours on time and staggering staff work schedules.

2. Consider the costs of professional services, such as payroll and laboratory. Will it cost your practice less to have these services provided in house or by an outside agency?

3. Review your physical plant. Can you redesign your floor plan for greater efficiency? If you need more space, can you negotiate a better lease with your current landlord? Look at your lease carefully, even if you do not need more space. Can you obtain better terms? Can you leverage new paint and carpeting? Can you schedule office hours so that each exam room is used for as many sessions as possible? If so, you can avoid underutilization. If you have excessive office space, can you sublet? Consider subletting during times when your practice is not in operation.

4. Consider your supplies and equipment. If you do not already do so, consider negotiating for all supplies that you will need for a year, and bid prices competitively. Send out new bids annually. "Panic ordering" is wasteful; use a perpetual inventory system to avoid it. Plan your purchases as part of your annual budget process. Purchase nonmedical minor supplies (e.g., pens, pencils, paper, transcription tapes, mouse pads, light bulbs) from discount suppliers; consider mail-order houses, which are typically less expensive for generic items. Before you simply buy them, determine if you really need maintenance contracts on fairly simple equipment. Negotiate price and terms whenever you buy; consider leasing options.

5. Review your staff's fringe benefits. Eliminate benefits that are not really important to your employees. Be careful to know what is and is not important. Once you provide a fringe benefit, it is difficult to take it back without causing employee dissatisfaction. Consider providing a cafeteria (which include dependent care plans and medical expense reimbursement plans, to name a few) and 401(k) retirement plans, which can save you money and improve employee satisfaction at the same time.

6. Review your physician-level perks. Eliminate duplicate subscriptions to the same journals, if you can. Also eliminate duplicate book orders. Assign one person to oversee journals and books. Carefully choose which professional meetings to attend. If your practice needs a "practice car," distinguish between which features you need and which you want. Cost counts.

7. Crack down on "nonbenefits," which usually are defined as the ignoring of the unauthorized use of practice resources, such as paper and other hard supplies, faxes, long-distance phone calls, and Internet service. If you can afford to allow your employees to avail themselves of these items, make sure that they know that such items are nonbenefits, and monitor their usage. If necessary, establish limits, especially on long-distance calls, which can become expensive, and Internet usage, which can become virtually addictive. Your people should be working, not chatting in cyberspace or playing computer games.

CONCLUSION

If you are the person who is primarily responsible for running your medical practice office without a glitch, remember the basics. Focus first on your personnel and then on your systems. If your staff members are doing the right jobs and doing their jobs right, you have the advantage. If your people are paid well and well motivated, you can accomplish what appear to be miracles.

Have a well–thought-out plan for practice development, and follow it. Make sure that your business systems are performing all the functions that you need them to perform. Focus on upgrading your computer system and getting all the use you can out of your telephone system. Fight to make sure that your business tools are at least adequate for the job you must do.

Remember that satisfaction is your business. If you can keep customers— patients/enrollees, referring physicians, and managed care partners—satisfied with your practice, you will maintain a steady stream of income into your practice. Now more than ever patient satisfaction is the key to practice success.

Cut your costs, wherever possible, but be careful about dismissing key personnel, which disrupts the office, reduces efficiency, and damages practice morale. All of these effects can lead to poor patient satisfaction. Consider cutting costs by adding personnel, such as a physician extender, patient advocate, or chaperone/scribe. Do not forget the other costs you can address, such as buying generic supplies in bulk. Remember: every dollar counts.

Whatever you do, remember that your medical practice is unique. Always remain focused on what *you* must do to keep *your* office running without a glitch.

PHYSICIAN RESOURCES

Medical Group Management Association, 104 Inverness Terrace East, Englewood, CO 80112-5306; telephone: (303) 799-1111; fax: (303) 397-1874; on-line: http://www.mgma.com.

National Committee for Quality Assurance, 2000 L Street, NW, Suite 500, Washington, DC 20036; telephone: (202) 955-3500; fax (202) 955-3599; on-line: http://www.ncqa.org.

Society of Medical-Dental Management Consultants, 3646 E. Ray Road, B16-45, Phoenix, AZ 85044; telephone: 800-826-2264.

The Health Care Group, 140 West Germantown Pike, Suite 200, Plymouth Meeting, PA 19462; telephone: 800-473-0032; fax: (610) 828-3658; e-mail: hcghcc@aol.com.

12

Monitoring the Financial Vital Signs of Your Medical Practice

Just as heart rate, temperature, respiration, and blood pressure can give a quick assessment of a patient's health, you can monitor business vital signs to assess the health of your medical practice. Regularly checking vitals such as patient volume, bread-and-butter services, revenue production, billing, and collections helps to ensure that your practice is as profitable as it ought to be. It also can make you aware of potential problems that need attention. Appendix I provides a glossary of relevant terms, and Appendix II lists sources of assistance.

Currently, most good computer systems used for practice accounting provide the raw data to calculate these vital signs. It is not necessary to spend megabucks on megabytes or custom software to produce a report for your practice like the example in this chapter. Any office manager should be able to duplicate the fundamental calculations using spreadsheet programs such as Excel or Lotus.

To keep track of how your practice is doing, consider a simple monthly report that displays the essentials on just two pages. In the accompanying example of a hypothetical four-doctor primary care practice (Table 1), three charts are involved: financial measurements, accounts receivable management, and procedural services. The format is roughly the same for each. Totals and monthly averages for the prior year of practice come first, serving as a benchmark.

Next are record tallies for each month, followed by a monthly average for the current year. Set up properly, the spreadsheet should be able to calculate automatically new averages, totals, ratios, and percentages each time the monthly data are entered.

TABLE 1. **Associates in Internal Medicine Monthly Practice Management Summary (Calendar Year 1996)** *(Continued)*

	Prior Year Totals	Average	Jan	Feb	March	April
Inpatient Services						
Consults, Hospital	302	25	25	36	10	32
Admissions	652	54	55	53	32	58
Follow-up Visits	5,725	477	418	641	192	568
Discharges	609	51	45	59	35	49
Observations	142	12	11	2	3	15
Total Hospital Encounters	7,430	619	554	791	272	722
EKG Interpretations	6,125	510	698	486	245	0
Stress Tests/DCG Interp.	87	7	13	12	6	9
Echos	138	12	6	12	9	24
Nursing Facilities						
New Patient Evaluations	298	25	25	60	16	14
Established Patient Visits	3,327	277	211	226	280	250
Total NF Encounters	3,625	302	236	286	296	264

A TELLTALE REPORT CARD

With a monthly report, you can track major procedures, assess your business manager's effectiveness, determine whether a special effort is needed to clear up aging accounts, evaluate the use of billing codes, and periodically answer the question, "How well is my practice doing?" Quite a few practices get an A+ when we look at this information. Such cases indicate a rock-solid administrator or office manager, whereas deficiencies usually mean weaknesses in office management. In addition, this information sometimes helps to add thousands of dollars to the bottom line. Even if the report does not result in a windfall, it will help you to understand where you are and where you are going.

The financial measurements section of the monthly report gives a good idea of what is happening on the revenue side of the practice and helps to monitor overall accounts receivable (A/R). Updating such information monthly helps to spot troubling trends or changes and hopefully nips problems in the bud. The object is to track trends in production, insurance write-offs, and collections. For example, if gross charges are increasing but collections are not, more attention ought to be devoted to obtaining full payment from third parties and patients.

Listed first in Table 1 under financial management are charges, which represent the gross fees charged at standard rates before adjustments are subtracted for insurance write-offs and contractual discounts for Medicare, Blue Cross/Blue Shield, and managed care plans. Isolating third-party write-offs also helps to monitor the impact of managed care. Some amounts are written off as bad debts or uncollectible accounts, such as charity and professional courtesy.

Table 1. *(Columns Continued)*

May	June	July	Aug	Sept	Oct	Nov	Dec	YTD Totals	Monthly Average
30	35	36	20	18	21	31	26	320	27
65	62	58	50	56	44	55	60	648	54
525	538	541	355	418	449	363	433	5,441	453
30	39	56	39	56	43	54	56	561	47
14	13	15	14	10	18	24	11	150	13
664	687	706	478	558	575	527	586	7,120	593
1,170	309	1,636	50	511	137	538	578	6,358	530
7	8	6	5	12	9	6	2	95	8
15	18	2	9	12	15	12	15	149	12
11	13	23	39	27	32	34	24	318	27
266	263	275	268	297	379	381	334	3,430	286
277	276	298	307	324	411	415	358	3,748	312

After subtracting adjustments from gross charges, you have the adjusted charges or collectible charges. These are the amounts that the practice can realistically collect. It is crucial to know what percentage of the adjusted charges the practice brings in. If it is 90%, there are some clear deficiencies. If it is 98%, the practice is doing a great job.

Next come gross collections or actual revenue to the practice. Subtract refunds to patients or insurance companies, and the result is net collections. Although at one time it was enough simply to record gross collections, today it is more instructive to look separately at fee-for-service receipts vs. the newer concept of capitation, by which doctors receive a monthly fixed fee per patient (similar to a budget) regardless of whether services are delivered.

Under capitation, the group is obliged to provide specified services when patients need them, and if the actual cost of providing care is less than the fixed fee, both the practice and the health plan profit.

TRACKING CAPITATION REVENUE

For physicians it is important to monitor how capitation revenue compares with charges that would have been billed under the traditional fee-for-service arrangement. At the end of the year, this calculation also may include return of capitated withholding amounts applied by the health plan as a hedge against potential losses. For example, if the physician is capitated at $10 per member per month and has a 10% withhold, the plan would pay the provider $9 per month per member. The other $1 would be held in a retention pool or charges significantly, some reduction in the net collection percentage should be expected early on. But it should not languish for months in the low 90s. The net collection ratio for our hypothetical group exceeded 100% in a few months. They not only captured all of their current adjusted charges but also collected on some old accounts.

ACCOUNTS RECEIVABLE MANAGEMENT

A look at the aging of receivables during the year can also give sharp insights into the health of your practice. Pay close attention to the amount and percentage of receivables aged beyond 90 days. Medicare is good at paying promptly within 17–25 days of receiving a claim. Some commercial companies and managed care plans lag quite a bit, and it is not uncommon to see some insurance companies taking 60–90 days to pay claims. By 90 days, however, providers should have collected a majority of what they can from the third-party payors as well as patient copayments and deductibles.

Acceptable levels, as a percentage of the total, vary from one specialty to the next. In primary care, typically 25–35% of accounts may be outstanding for 90 days or longer. However, for many surgical specialties, the number is significantly lower—20% or 25%. Table 3 provides examples of the typical percentage of total accounts received aged greater than 90 days for selected specialties.

Insurance pending is another area to watch in this section of the report. A subset of accounts receivable, insurance pending represents insurance claims that the practice has submitted but have not yet been paid by the insurance companies. This number varies widely—from as low as 50% in some practices to as high as 80% or 90% in others. This percentage gives a strong clue as to whether unpaid claims are really delinquent and aged. Because this is a fairly

---

TABLE 3.   Accounts Receivable (Aged > 90 Days)*

Specialty	%
Family practice	31.11
Internal Medicine	29.60
Pediatrics	23.59
Obstetrics/gynecology	21.89
Neurology	26.02
General surgery	26.94
Orthopedic surgery	31.85
Otorhinolaryngology	30.80

* 1997 MGMA Cost Survey, reprinted with permission from the Medical Group Management Association, 104 Inverness Terrace East, Englewood, Colorado 80112-5306; 303-799-1111. Copyright 1997.

new pulse point, the range that we have established is quite wide. As more practices record such information, we will be able to narrow the target range. At this juncture, something less than 60–70% is usually acceptable.

As payments on these gross billings are posted, your business office writes off part of the charge as a contractual adjustment, bills the patient for the balance, if necessary, then clears the claim from pending status in the computer system.

IS IT TIME FOR AN ACCOUNTS RECEIVABLE BLITZ?

Working with an internal medicine practice that the doctors thought was well managed, we discovered that 50% of receivables were more than 90 days old. We also were surprised to find that insurance pending represented 95% of gross charges for a full year. The computer system showed nearly $800,000 in pending claims that had actually been paid and should have been cleared. Furthermore, the net collection ratio was 89%. Clearly, there was a lot of room for improvement, because eight percentage points in the net collection ratio translated into $100,000 for the group.

Although failure to post insurance payments (and clear the insurance pending category) is a bookkeeping detail, it may mean that the patient has not received a statement for the balance due. Practice accounting systems often do not release a patient statement until the insurance claim has been cleared. In this case, we suspected that many patients had not been billed.

Our recommendation for the practice was to coordinate an accounts receivable blitz. Basically, this involves pulling out all stops to analyze every account outstanding for 90 days or more, then deciding on a specific course of action: initiate special calls or letters, write off the accounts, or turn them over to a collection agency. The blitz can be done after hours, during evenings and weekends, with overtime paid to participating staff members (business office employees who are familiar with insurance processing, delinquent accounts, setting up installment payments, and the like). Without exception, we have found that this is money well spent; claims that have been tied up with insurance companies and patients for months are paid en masse.

Do not be too alarmed if receivables older than 90 days occasionally swell beyond 50%. It happens even in the best-managed groups, requiring special attention every two or three years to purge old accounts. In other words, think of it as a reminder that it is time for an accounts receivable blitz.

Another statistic to monitor is the A/R ratio, or total accounts receivable divided by an average month's gross charges. If a group has $1 million of outstanding accounts and has averaged $400,000 in charges per month for the year that just ended, the A/R ratio is 2.5. In other words, there are 2.5 months of gross charges in accounts receivable. The A/R ratio varies from specialty to evaluation and management service levels 1–5 and to assign numbers to those that correspond to the last digit of the CPT code number. The key services used in every practice are office consultations, new patient office visits, and established patient office visits. On the hospital side are admissions, hospital follow-up services, and clinical consultations. Appendix III contains the AMA guidelines on how to determine the appropriate level of patient evaluation and management services for billing purposes.

In analyzing a practice, we look for an array of the use of these service codings, which should be prepared at least on a semiannual or quarterly basis. It is impossible to define a perfect distribution, but a classic bell curve is most likely appropriate. It is important to do an array not only for the group as a whole but also by individual physician. This approach enables the practice to determine whether the group as a whole is on target and to identify any outliers or individual doctors falling outside the normal distribution. If you can identify an outlier, you can work with the physician on his or her documentation to identify deficiencies and to improve code selection. Improving code selection can have a profound financial impact. Various Medicare, Blue Shield, and other major commercial carriers with managed care plans have created what they consider to be appropriate distributions.

An example of the difference that proper coding can make involved three hard-working internists who were concerned about their group's financial performance and how they might bolster profitability. We looked at each doctor's billing habits for new patient encounters, established patients, and follow-up services. Having audited a representative number of records, we found that they were undercoding about 40% of their services. After completing the study, we met with the doctors and showed them how they could make simple changes in documentation to qualify for higher levels of service. We then reviewed with them definitions of each level of service. They put the information to use immediately and increased their profitability by 5–8% without working harder.

MORE PROCEDURAL WRINKLES

If you put together a monthly report such as the example in Table 1, you also should take a close look at the line for preventive medicine services. Annual physical exams should be included in this line. For years, insurance policies covered only the treatment of acute or chronic illness; therefore, doctors tried to find diagnostic problems to report and to qualify these exams as acute or chronic care visits. Many physicians continue to bill in this manner. For example, a doctor will list "mild hypertension" as the problem, then try to collect a $95 feel for a level 4 established patient visit. But the diagnosis does not justify a 30-minute encounter, and third parties reject or down-code it. Thus many doctors deny themselves revenue to which to they are entitled.

Managed care has helped to solve the problem of getting proper reimbursement for preventive medical care. Many health plans today pay well for an annual physical—as much as $100–130. But you need to use the correct codes. On the other hand, if the patient's insurer does not pay for the exam, there is nothing wrong with asking the patient to pay the fee out of pocket.

To round out the patient services picture, you want to list a handful of procedures in your analysis. Most specialists can identify a half dozen key procedures that enable them to keep a good pulse on what is going on. In primary care, these may be office ancillaries such as laboratory tests, radiographic studies, electrocardiograms, and flexible sigmoidoscopies, which our hypothetical doctors performed at the hospital. Radiographic studies may apply to medical and surgical practices, and they are key procedures, of course, in orthopedic and radiologic practices. Surgical practices should keep track of major and minor operations. In orthopedics, examples include hip and knee replacements, exploratory arthroscopies, fracture treatment, and cast applications. In general surgery, they may include appendectomies and other abdominal surgery. Thoracic and cardiovascular surgeons should tally coronary artery bypass grafts and valve replacements, among others. The important point is to zero in on the key procedures that generate 75% of your revenue.

Under inpatient services, there are five categories to track—hospital consultations, admissions, follow-up visits or services, procedures performed, and discharges. Table 5 presents benchmark data for selected specialties.

TABLE 5. Procedural Service Activity*

Type of Service Percentile	Ambulatory Encounters[†]		Hospital Encounters[‡]		Surgical Cases[§]	
	50th	75th	50th	75th	50th	75th
Family practice (without obstetrics/gynecology)	4390	5514	298	561	236	453
Internal medicine	3275	4046	620	1077	120	303
Pediatrics	4671	5738	294	514	67	134
Obstetrics/gynecology	2988	3777	171	353	352	548
Neurology	2172	2975	712	1300	37	100
General surgery	1543	2083	439	766	615	844
Orthopedic surgery	3111	3995	131	276	381	601
Otorhinolaryngology	3403	3912	70	162	556	847

* 1997 Physician Compensation and Production Survey, reprinted with permission from the Medical Group Management Association, 104 Inverness Terrace East, Englewood, Colorado 80112-5306; 303-799-1111. Copyright 1997. (The Physician Compensation and Production Survey is available at $200 for members, $300 for nonmembers, order #4986.)
† Ambulatory encounters are defined as an identifiable contract between a patient and provider where advice, a procedure, service, or treatment is provided. Encounters attributable to physician extenders are excluded.
‡ Hospital encounters are those that take place in a hospital.
§ Surgical cases are those performed on an inpatient or outpatient basis.

TABLE 7. Staffing Ratios

	MGMA*	NAHC/SMD/PMG†
Family practice	4.77	4.24
Internal medicine	4.00	3.39
Pediatrics	3.40	3.91
Obstetrics/gynecology	4.20	3.82
Neurology	3.34	2.81
General surgery	2.50	2.34
Orthopedic surgery	4.56	4.02
Otorhinolaryngology	5.20	3.91

* 1997 MGMA Cost Survey, reprinted with permission from the Medical Group Management Association, 104 Inverness Terrace East, Englewood, Colorado 80112-5306; 303-799-1111. Copyright 1997.
† 1997 Medical and Dental Income and Expense Averages, jointly compiled by the National Association of Health Care Consultants (NAHC), the Society of Medical-Dental Management Consultants (SMD), and the PM Group (PMG). Reprinted with permission.

the office manager, the business manager, or someone that he or she designates handles inputting of information. This fairly routine task can be delegated to an administrative assistant.

Items that should be checked monthly include a count of key procedures performed, office encounters, and hospital encounters. In addition, each quarter the practice should do an array of levels of care and the distribution of levels of care by each physician in the practice. Once a year, the practice should take a critical look at the overall financial picture, including charges, revenues, expenses and profitability, and staffing ratios.

Keeping track of the vital signs of your practice provides key information so that you can monitor and fortify the business side of your medical practice.

ACKNOWLEDGMENT   This chapter is an updated and substantially expanded version of an article published in *Medical Economics*, March 11, 1996, p 135.

APPENDIX I

GLOSSARY OF TERMS

Accounts receivable ratio: the number of months of gross fee-for service charges in total accounts receivable.

Adjusted fee-for-service collection percentage: the percentage of fee-for-service adjusted charges collected. The percentage is calculated by dividing net fee-for-service charges.

Adjusted fee-for-service charges (collectible charges): gross fee-for-service charges less third-party (insurance) contractual charge adjustments and other adjustments to charges, e.g., charitable, professional courtesy, bad debts, and uncollectible charges. In other words, the value of services performed for which payment is expected.

Aged accounts receivable: unpaid fee-for-service charges by the number of days outstanding since the date the service was provided.

Capitated services/fee-for-service equivalent charges: a measure of undiscounted fees (rates) of professional services activity on patients covered by at-risk, capitation contracts. In other words, services extended to capitation patients are recorded as equivalent charges using the standard fee-for-service rate.

Capitation revenue: income derived from per member per month payments made to a practice by managed-care plans to pay for all goods and services due to the patient under the terms of at-risk capitated contracts.

Gross fee-for-service collection percentage: the percentage of fee-for-service gross charges collected. The percentage is calculated by dividing net fee-for-service collections by gross fee-for-service charges.

Gross fee-for-service charges: a measure of full value, at the practice's standard, undiscounted fees (rates), of all services provided to fee-for-service, discounted fee-for-service, and noncapitated (at-risk plan) patients.

Net fee-for-service collections: a measure of practice revenue (collected from patients and third-party payors for services provided to fee-for service, discounted fee-for-service, and noncapitated patients) remaining after patient refunds and returned checks.

Staffing ratio: the number of full-time equivalent (FTE) support staff to FTE physician.

TABLE A.   Categories and Subcategories of Service *(Continued)*

Category/Subcategory	Code Numbers
Prolonged services	
With direct patient contact	99355-99357
Without direct patient contact	99358-99359
Standby services	99360
Case management services	
Team conferences	99361-99362
Telephone calls	99371-99373
Care plan oversight services	99375-99376
Preventive medicine services	
New patient	99381-99387
Established patient	99391-99397
Individual counseling	99401-99404
Group counseling	00411-99412
Other	99420-99429
Newborn care	99431-99440
Special E/M services	99450-99456
Other E/M services	99499

3. Review the level of E/M service descriptors and examples in the selected category or subcategory.

The descriptors for the levels of E/M services recognize seven components, six of which are used in defining the levels of E/M services. These components are:

- History
- Examination
- Medical decision making
- Counseling
- Coordination of care
- Nature of presenting problem
- Time

The first three of these components (i.e., history, examination, and medical decision making) should be considered the **key** components in selecting the level of E/M services. An exception to this rule is the case of visits that consist predominantly of counseling or coordination of care.

The nature of the presenting problem and time are provided in some levels to assist the physician in determining the appropriate level of E/M service.

4. Determine the extent of history obtained.

The extent of the history depends on clinical judgment and on the nature of the presenting problem(s). The levels of E/M services recognize four types of history defined as follows:

Problem-focused: chief complaint; brief history of present illness or problem.

Expanded problem-focused: chief complaint; brief history of present illness; problem pertinent system review.

Detailed: chief complaint; extended history of present illness; problem pertinent system review extended to include a review of a limited number of additional systems; pertinent past, family, and/or social history directly related to the patient's problems.

Comprehensive: chief complaint; extended history of present illness; review of systems which is directly related to the problem(s) identified in the history of the present illness plus a review of all additional body systems; complete past, family, and social history.

The comprehensive history obtained as part of the preventive medicine evaluation and management service is not problem-oriented and does not involve a chief complaint or present illness. It does, however, include a comprehensive system review and comprehensive or interval past, family, and social history as well as a comprehensive assessment/history of pertinent risk factors.

4. **Determine the extent of examination performed.**
   The extent of the examination performed depends on clinical judgment and on the nature of the presenting problem(s). The levels of E/M services recognize four types of examination that are defined as follows:

   Problem-focused: a limited examination of the affected body area or organ system.

   Expanded problem-focused: a limited examination of the affected body area or organ system and other systematic or related organ system(s).

   Detailed: an extended examination of the affected body area(s) and other symptomatic or related organ system(s).

   Comprehensive: a general multisystem examination or a complete examination of a single organ system. *Note:* The comprehensive examination performed as part of the preventive medicine evaluation and management service is multisystem, but its extent is based on age and risk factors identified.

   For the purposes of these CPT definitions, the following body areas are recognized:

   - Head, including the face
   - Neck
   - Chest, including breasts and axilla
   - Abdomen
   - Genitalia, groin, buttocks
   - Back
   - Each extremity

   For the purposes of these CPT definitions, the following organ systems are recognized:

   - Eyes
   - Ears, nose, mouth, and throat
   - Cardiovascular
   - Respiratory
   - Gastrointestinal
   - Genitourinary
   - Musculoskeletal
   - Skin
   - Neurologic
   - Psychiatric
   - Hematologic/lymphatic/ immunologic

6. **Determine the complexity of medical decision making.**
   Medical decision making refers to the complexity of establishing a diagnosis and/or selecting a management option as measured by:
   - The number of possible diagnoses and/or the number of management options that must be considered;
   - The amount and/or complexity of medical records, diagnostic tests, and/or other information that must be obtained, reviewed, and analyzed; and

Table B. Complexity of Medical Decision Making

Number of Diagnoses or Management Options	Amount and/or Complexity of Data to be Reviewed	Risk of Complications and/or Morbidity or Mortality	Type of Decision Making
Minimal	Minimal or more	Minimal	Straightforward
Limited	Limited	Low	Low complexity
Multiple	Moderate	Moderate	Moderate complexity
Extensive	Extensive	High	High complexity

- The risk of significant complications, morbidity, and/or mortality, as well as co-morbidities, associated with the patient's presenting problem(s), the diagnostic procedure(s) and/or the possible management options.

Four types of medical decision making are recognized: straightforward; low complexity; moderate complexity; and high complexity. To qualify for a given type of decision making, two of the three elements in Table B must be met.

Comorbidities/underlying diseases, in and of themselves, are not considered in selecting a level of E/M services unless their presence significantly increases the complexity of the medical decision making.

7. **Select the appropriate level of E/M services based on the following:**
   1. For the following categories/subcategories, **all of the key components** (history, examination, and medical decision making) must meet or exceed the stated requirements to quality for a particular level of E/M service: office, new patient; hospital observation services; initial hospital care; office consultations; initial in-patient consultations; confirmatory consultations; emergency department services; comprehensive nursing facility assessments; domiciliary care; new patient; and home, new patient.
   2. For the following categories/subcategories, **two of the three key components** (history, examination, and medical decision making) must meet or exceed the stated requirements to qualify for a particular level of E/M services: office, established patient; subsequent hospital care; follow-up inpatient consultations; subsequent nursing facility care; domiciliary care, established patient; and home, established patient.
   3. In the case in which counseling and/or coordination of care dominates (more than 50% of) the physician/patient and/or family encounter (face-to-face time in the office or other outpatient setting or floor/unit time in the hospital or nursing facility), then time is considered the key or controlling factor to quality for a particular level of E/M services. The extent of counseling and/or coordination of care must be documented in the medical record.

---

* Reprinted by permission of the American Medical Association—CPT only. Copyright 1996 American Medical Association. All rights reserved.

SUNG J. LIAO, MD, DPH
LORENZ K. Y. NG, MD

13

Opportunities in Alternative and Complementary Medicine

The current resurgence of interest in acupuncture and other unconventional healing arts is evidenced by the cover story of a recent issue of *Life* magazine;[2] an article about alternative medicine, entitled "The Frontiers of Medicine," in a special issue of *Time* magazine;[4] and the cover story, "Acupuncture Boom," in the Health section of the *Washington Post*.[7] Eisenberg's survey of "Unconventional Medicine in the United States"[3] in 1990 found that 34% of respondents used at least one unconventional therapy, with an estimated expenditure in the United States of about $14 billion on such treatments. Three-fourths of the total was allegedly paid out of patients' own pockets. About 425 million visits were made by patients for alternative therapeutics—about 40 million more than the number of visits to their own physicians. Several years have passed since that survey and presumably, with the continued interest in alternative medicine, these numbers have increased. Perhaps the most troubling finding from the survey was that 72% of the patients using alternative therapies did not discuss them with their physicians. This finding suggests that the American public may not see their medical doctors as a helpful source of guidance for unconventional therapies. The February 1997 issue of *ACP Observer*, a monthly newsletter published by the American College of Physicians, reported that some members are adding alternative therapies to their practice "to get a piece of the action or risk losing business."[8] An increasing number of physicians believe that by adding alternative therapies to their mainstream practices they offer better health care to their patients.

Thirty-four American medical schools have departments or divisions of alternative medicine. Establishment by Congress of the Office of Alternative Medicine at the National Institutes of Health in 1992 and increasing coverage of alternative practices by health care insurers further suggest the need for physicians to understand these practices. Increasing interest in alternative medicine by mainstream physicians is evidenced by the increasing number who enroll in courses about alternative therapies.

As leading providers of primary and subspecialty health care, physicians must understand the potential benefits, risks, and other issues pertinent to increasingly prevalent alternative health practices. Armed with this information they can counsel their patients appropriately about the broad ranges of potentially helpful and harmful modalities to which they are increasingly exposed.

In spite of the tremendous number of new discoveries in many fields of medicine, such as genetic engineering, interventional radiology, and organ transplant surgery, the prevention and management of common problems, such as stroke, cancer, and heart disease, are still beyond the grasp of scientific Western medicine. Therefore, opportunities for research in alternative therapies, clinical and basic, abound.

CATEGORIES OF ALTERNATIVE AND COMPLEMENTARY MEDICINE

The following short list of alternative therapies illustrates the more commonly used varieties in the United States:

ACUPUNCTURE

Acupuncture is probably the most widely known and used as well as the best researched of all alternative therapeutics. It entails inserting a thin needle at strategic loci on the body to effect relief of a disease condition. Acupuncture dates back to several millennia B.C. Its therapeutic efficacy undoubtedly has kept it in existence through so many centuries. Scientific research in recent years has unraveled at least part of its mechanism of action. Basically the needle provides a stimulus to different levels of the central nervous system with release of endorphins, catecholamines, cortisol, and other neurochemicals.

The basic tenet of traditional Chinese medicine and acupuncture is that the universe is composed of two opposing forces, *yin* and *yang*, in equal parts. They resonate with each other and complement and supplement each other in harmonious balance. If one is in excess, the other is deficient. When imbalance occurs, disease is a result. Acupuncture is thought to restore the balance. The yin-yang concept allegedly led Leibnitz to devise the binary theory.

The ancients noticed the prevalence of certain diseases when one of the five orbiting planets appeared in the sky in a particular region during a certain season. This observation is comparable to modern epidemiology. The ancients developed the five *xing* (element) theory and *ziwu liuzhu* (comparable to chronobiology). They also attempted to quantify medicine and devised formulas for diagnosis and selection of acupoints for treatment with acupuncture.

The strategic loci, known as acupoints or acupuncture points, are located along 14 meridians (or channels) on the body. Qi (the essence or elixir of life) circulates along these meridians regularly and incessantly. If and when it is impeded, sickness results. Acupuncture needles inserted at the strategic loci or acupoints remove this impediment and thus cure the illness. Theoretically, we may regard the neurochemicals in conjunction with the biophysical effects of needling as components of qi.

HERBAL MEDICINE OR ETHNOBOTANY

Traditional Chinese medicine has used a vast variety of herbs for therapeutic purposes for several thousand years. The medicinal plants have many phytochemicals that may act additively and synergistically to exert multiple therapeutic effects. Only a small dose, therefore, is required. Their side effects, if any, are minimal and tend to be mild. Some herbs may contain antifree radical oxygen as well as antifree radical hydroxide. Thus, they may have divergent therapeutic effects. Such therapeutic herbs (e.g., ginseng) may cost much less than conventional drugs. With recognition of the great potential of medicinal herbs, increasing attention has been paid to their pharmacology.

HOMEOPATHY

Christian Frederich Samuel Hahnemann (1755–1843), a German physician and chemist, observed that quinine produced symptoms in healthy persons quite similar to those of the disease that it cured. This observation led him to formulation of the "law of similars" (similia similibus curantur), according to which drugs that produce similar symptoms of a disease in healthy people are used to treat that disease. He regarded symptoms as natural protective responses to a disease instead of malfunctions caused by the disease. In 1796, he published his findings, which included ideas from Hippocrates and Paracelsus.

At that time, medical practice emphasized utilization of huge doses of drugs that frequently made the sickness worse. Hahnemann advocated that much smaller doses of drugs would greatly enhance their therapeutic effects. The dilute solution is called "mother tincture." He termed his therapeutic system homeopathy. The use of small doses may be comparable to the current practice of immunization for allergies. Because of objections from the medical establishment and apothecary interests, he was forced to leave Leipzig, where he practiced.

At one time homeopathy flourished in Europe and the United States. About 22 homeopathic medical schools and more than 100 hospitals (some identified with the name of Hahnemann) were established in the United States. The

APPENDIX II

BROCHURE FOR PATIENT EDUCATION

In response to many questions from our patients about acupuncture, we have prepared this pamphlet to answer concisely some of the most commonly asked questions.

Q: What is acupuncture?

A: Acupuncture is a relatively new procedure in the United States, although it has been practiced for centuries in China and the Orient. It utilizes special, very thin stainless steel needles that are inserted at the acupuncture points on the body. These needles are solid and no fluid is injected into your body. They are usually only about half the diameter of the smallest-sized needles used by physicians for the injection of medicine. They are one-use, disposable, and presterilized by the manufacturer.

Acupuncture needles are no longer classified by the Food and Drug Administration as experimental devices as of March 1996.

Q: What conditions can acupuncture be used for?

A: First of all, acupuncture is *not* a cure-all. It is a good pain reliever. It brings about high degrees of success in treating low-back pain (even after surgery), neck pain (e.g., whiplash), myofascial pain, arthritic pain, migraine, tension and vascular headaches, trigeminal neuralgia (tic douloureux), temporomandibular joint (TMJ) syndrome, pain from shingles, menstrual cramps and pain, abdominal pain (e.g., spastic colon, colitis, ileitis), angina pain, and certain types of psychosomatic diseases. It has also been used very effectively to stop smoking, for drug addiction, alcoholism, and food "addiction" (overweight). It is quite helpful in psoriasis, cystic acne, poison ivy, genital herpes, cold sores, allergic dermatitis, eczema, and some other skin conditions. Tonsillectomy, tooth extraction, and other dental and surgical procedures have been performed in this country under acupuncture analgesia. Painless childbirth is feasible with acupuncture. It has been used in veterinary medicine. However, you should always try conventional Western medicine first. If it fails, acupuncture may be tried.

Q: Can acupuncture help everybody?

A: Like any other medical treatment, the results of acupuncture will not be known until after it is done. It is effective in as many as 85% of the patients who have failed to respond to conventional medicine or surgical management. There is a tremendous individual difference of response to acupuncture from patient to patient. There is no guarantee or warranty of how you are going to respond to acupuncture. But it is indeed a very valuable addition to our Western medicine.

Q: How should I feel after my first treatment?

A: That depends entirely upon the person. A few patients may have extremely satisfactory relief of pain after the very first treatment. For most people, several sessions of treatment are necessary before any kind of relief is felt. Just like any other kind of medical or surgical treatment, there is no way to predict the results.

Q: How often should I be treated?

A: The frequency and the number of treatments depend on your clinical status as well as your need and your response to acupuncture.

Q: Does acupuncture hurt?

A: Usually you will feel a slight prick. Whether it hurts or not depends entirely on you. If you are very afraid of needles, you may feel it more than other people. Actually the feeling is much less than having an injection or being pricked by a sewing needle.

After the acupuncture needle is inserted some kind of sensation is generated. It may be slight tingling, warmth, soreness, or numbness. It may appear locally or in a somewhat distant part of the body.

Q: Should I rest after the treatment?

A: After the treatment when some patients feel better, they tend to do things that they have not been able to do for quite some time. Thus, they overextend themselves, causing aggravation or recurrence of the pain-producing problem. No matter how good you feel after a treatment, you should take it a little easy for at least a couple of days.

Q: Will my pain get worse after acupuncture?

A: An apparent increase of pain may be coincidental because your attention is drawn to that specific area. It is also possible that your body may overrespond to the treatment. It is an exception rather than the rule. A clinical trial is the only way by which you can tell whether there may be additional pain after a treatment.

Q: Is there any bleeding?

A: Usually not. You may not even see a needle mark. Sometimes, however, a minute invisible blood vessel underneath the skin may be pricked during the insertion of the thin needle. Very rarely, there may be a black and blue spot.

Q: Are there any complications?

A: *Newsweek* magazine in July 1974 quoted the *Journal of the American Medical Association*, which reported cases of pneumothorax (air in the chest) and hemothorax (bleeding in the chest). A large epidemic of infectious hepatitis was reported in the *American Journal of Epidemiology* in March 1988. Forty patients contracted hepatitis in one acupuncturist's office. Cases of septic infections were also reported. There is also a possibility of AIDS infection. All of these infectious complications are traceable to the use of nonsterile, contaminated needles. However, when acupuncture is carried out with sterile needles and proper sterile precautions, these complications do not occur.

Q: May I drive my car immediately after the treatment?

A: We recommend that you have someone drive you to and from our office for the first visit. After that, it would be up to your best judgment. It is not unusual for some patients to feel very relaxed and maybe even sleepy after acupuncture treatment.

Q: Should I give up all my medications?

A: No. You should continue to follow your own physician's instructions. A sudden change of your medication regimen could possibly cause severe adverse effects. Acupuncture is used to complement and supplement your own physician's treatments. We work with physicians but do not replace them.

Q: What about a special diet after acupuncture?

A: At this point in time we do not know what effect any particular food has on acupuncture or vice versa. We therefore recommend that you keep your regular diet, especially if it is a special one, such as for diabetes.

Q: How does acupuncture work?

A: In the early 1970s, the National Institutes of Health sponsored research projects on acupuncture. Research has been done mainly in China, Sweden, and Canada, and only some in this country. Since 1975, we understand more about acupuncture scientifically. Basically, acupuncture releases morphine-like chemicals produced by our own body (endorphins) to suppress pain via certain neural mechanisms. Little research on its mechanism to counteract addictions to drugs, alcohol and nicotine, and skin diseases has been done. It is quite conceivable that acupuncture may be involved in the healing processes. A lot more research needs to be pursued. In 1993, the National Institutes of Health has again started to sponsor research programs on acupuncture through its Office of Alternative Medicine.

Q: Does my health care insurance cover acupuncture treatments?

A: It depends on your insurance policy. Although some insurance policies, such as Medicare and Blue Cross/Blue Shield, do not cover acupuncture treatment per se, they may cover a part of the office visits. Recently, a few major insurance companies and HMOs started to cover the expenses for acupuncture treatment in certain areas of the country. You should check with your insurance agent. If you are a Medicare patient, please check with our staff as to whether or not we participate in the Medicare program. The financial responsibility for our professional services is entirely yours.

If you have other questions concerning acupuncture, please do not hesitate to discuss them with us. We will do our best to answer them.

EDWARD M. PHILLIPS, MD

14

Physician Involvement in Subacute and Long-term Care

Perhaps the most critical change in health care today is the increasingly rapid discharge of patients from acute hospitals directly to home, rehabilitation, long-term care, and, more recently, subacute care. Continued decline in hospital lengths of stay and number of acute hospital beds should prompt astute physicians to observe a corollary of Sutton's law: Diversify your practice to alternate levels of care, "because that's where the patients are." Moreover, treating subacute patients and long-term residents at an extended care facility is an underappreciated, yet rewarding and remunerative activity.

Do not be fooled by the setting. Intensive medical and rehabilitative care is now pursued in subacute units, which are based in skilled nursing facilities (SNFs). The continued rapid expansion of subacute care programs has created a multitude of opportunities for physicians in both primary care and specialty-based practices. The focus of the unit, whether it is rehabilitation, postoperative recovery, ventilator support, complex medical, oncology, or wound care, dictates the need for specific physician specialties for both administrative and clinical work.

BACKGROUND

The advent of Medicare's prospective payment system, with the institution of diagnosis-related groups (DRGs) in 1983, provided a strong incentive for more rapid discharge of Medicare beneficiaries[23] with higher medical acuity[21] from acute care to rehabilitation units, long-term care, or home. As patients move "sicker and quicker" from acute hospitalization toward home or long-term placement, the necessary bridge is often subacute care. Managed care heavily affects the recent expansion of subacute care. As an example, SNFs were chosen more often than acute rehabilitation hospitals or units for beneficiaries of health maintenance organizations (HMOs) hospitalized for acute stroke compared with fee-for-service patients.[20] In some capitated settings, appropriate patients may be admitted directly to the subacute unit from the emergency department or outpatient clinic in lieu of acute hospitalization.[25] In addition, a large group of patients currently in acute care (10–20%) could be cared for effectively at the subacute level rather than in the acute care hospital.[6]

Lastly, the number of Americans 80 years of age and older is expected to double to six million by 2010.[26] This group accounts for the heaviest users of long-term care. Approximately one in four people 85 and older lived in a nursing home in 1990.[9] Thus, the reimbursement mechanisms, expansion of managed care, aging of the population, and boom in nursing home-based subacute units make the long-term facility a financially attractive venue for practice expansion.

DEFINITION

Subacute care is a relatively new phenomenon. Indeed, accreditation of subacute facilities by the Joint Commission on Accreditation of Healthcare Organizations (JCAHO) and the Commission on Accreditation of Rehabilitation Facilities (CARF) began as recently as 1995.[10] The federal government has not yet adopted a standard definition for subacute care, nor has it adopted a distinct reimbursement mechanism for subacute care.[24]

Several organizations involved in subacute care have adopted a definition. The American Health Care Association (AHCA), the Joint Commission on Accreditation of Healthcare Organizations (JCAHO), and the Association of Hospital-Based Skilled Nursing Facilities describe subacute care as follows:

> Subacute care is comprehensive inpatient care designed for someone who has an acute illness, injury, or exacerbation of a disease process. It is goal oriented treatment rendered immediately after, or instead of, acute hospitalization to treat one or more specific active complex medical conditions or to administer one or more technically complex treatments, in the context of a person's underlying long-term conditions and overall situation.
>
> Generally, the individual's condition is such that the care does not depend on high-technology monitoring or complex diagnostic procedures. Subacute care requires the coordinated services of an interdisciplinary team including physicians, nurses, and other relevant professional disciplines, who are trained and knowledgeable to assess and manage these specific conditions and perform the necessary procedures. Subacute care is given as part of a specifically defined program, regardless of the site.
>
> Subacute care is generally more intensive than traditional nursing facility care and less than acute care. It requires frequent (daily to weekly) recurrent patient assessment and review of the clinical course and treatment plan for a limited (several days to several months) time period, until the condition is stabilized or a predetermined treatment course is completed.[1]

FINANCIAL ISSUES

In dramatic contrast to the contraction of acute care hospital beds, subacute care is growing at an estimated rate of 20% annually and may generate 10 billion dollars annually in gross revenues in the next decade.[6] It is estimated that there are currently over 200,000 subacute beds in over 5,000 facilities in the United States.[19]

Most of the initial growth in subacute beds was in hospital-based units, where empty beds were converted to "transitional care units."[19] To physicians already working at the acute care hospital, the difference in treating patients in the transitional care unit versus the acute hospital may be transparent. Transitional care units are often distinguished from the acute hospital beds only by different regulations regarding reimbursement and decreased nursing intensity.

Within SNFs, subacute units are often separated from the residential portion of the facility and have a more clinical atmosphere. Whereas the residential area is often carpeted and nicely decorated as a home for residents, the subacute unit may have hospital beds, in-wall oxygen and suction, linoleum floors, and the general look and feel of a hospital unit.

The mounting financial pressures created by managed care necessitate provision of care at the least expensive venue. These pressures have proved a boon to subacute care in general and specifically to programs housed in extended care facilities. Moreover, the expansion of the elderly American population provides a burgeoning group of potential subacute care patients. The attraction of subacute units in nursing homes is that they can deliver intensive medical and nursing care at 30–50% below the costs of an acute care facility.[19] The savings accrue from decreased overhead related to factors such as administration, operating rooms, and emergency departments. In some states, because of regulations governing the number of long-term care beds, all subacute beds are housed within skilled nursing facilities.[4] Compared with competitive, physician-intense hospital settings, subacute units provide physicians with many untapped opportunities in extended care facilities.

EFFICACY

Beyond the cost savings, physicians should question the efficacy of subacute care in SNFs. One retrospective study comparing outcomes for stroke patients receiving acute medical rehabilitation and patients in a SNF subacute program demonstrated that the subacute program was substantially more cost-effective in terms of successful discharge and improved scores on the Functional Independence Measure.[12] However, a more recent study highlights marked differences in functional outcomes based on diagnosis as well as site of care.[13]

Specifically, functional outcomes of patients with stroke were higher at the acute rehabilitation setting, whereas results for patients with fracture were similar.

CONFLICTING CULTURES

The skills, experience, and outlook of providers working in SNFs are often in conflict when subacute care is introduced to the facility. Nursing home administrators, nurses, and aides trained in extended care are strong advocates for residents' rights and closely involve families and residents in decisions. The care is largely directed by nursing, and physician visits are required only monthly.

In marked contrast, rehabilitation professionals, such as occupational and physical therapists and speech-language pathologists, anticipate a functioning, goal-directed, interdisciplinary program of generally short duration. They provide rehabilitative services to both long-term residents and short-term subacute patients. The rehabilitation ethic of expecting patients to take care of themselves is often in conflict with nursing assistants trained to take long-term care of residents. Furthermore, the provisions of The Omnibus Budget and Reconciliation Act (OBRA) of 1987* designed to protect the rights of skilled nursing residents[16] often hinder true rehabilitation efforts for subacute patients.[18]

To complicate further the conflict of treatment styles, acute care nurses hired to treat medically complex, subacute patients often have a poor understanding and tolerance for regulations regarding residents' rights. Acute care nurses are geared toward quick-paced, medically intense interventions that usually are not dictated by an interdisciplinary team.[22]

The physician generally is welcomed by extended care nurses, taken for granted by acute care nurses, and critical to coordination of an effective team of rehabilitation professionals and to the interdisciplinary team for medically complex patients. The savvy physician understands the ethics and regulations of long-term care, provides guidance to the interdisciplinary team, and makes quick decisions in medically intense situations. Such physicians are uniquely suited to mend the conflict of cultures on a subacute unit.

ADMINISTRATIVE ISSUES

Opportunities to fulfill the OBRA '87 requirement for a medical director exist at all SNFs. According to the Health Care Financing Administration (HCFA), over

---

* OBRA '87 was an instrumental move to protect residents' rights at subacute facilities. This greater protection is due, in part, to restraint reduction and confidentiality protection. OBRA regulations also require on-site physical and occupational therapy and speech/language pathology services.

17,000 Medicare- and Medicaid-certified nursing homes in the United States house over 1.5 million residents.[15] Facility medical directors generally provide leadership in delivery of quality care. The American Medical Directors Association (AMDA) is the professional organization of long-term care physicians. The AMDA offers training toward designation as a certified medical director. The medical director may attend clinically to nursing home residents and expect Medicare reimbursement comparable to that in acute care hospitals.[24]

Doctors may work in subacute units as primary care physicians, consulting specialists, and medical directors of the subacute program. Although no regulations require a medical director for subacute units, many facilities hire program directors. Indeed, according to the AHCA, "the critical components necessary to ensure program quality and acceptable outcomes for the [subacute] patients include . . . a physician-directed program."[1]

The administrative roles in skilled nursing care and subacute units are distinct but may overlap: "The facility medical director may be a subacute physician program director, if qualified by virtue of education, experience, or training related to the program being offered."[1] The program director is expected to "assure the clinical integrity of the program through consultation and approval of the specific medical and rehabilitation protocols and provide guidance and implementation of the protocols. The physician program director participates in the steps to monitor and improve the quality of care and the appropriate utilization of services provided in the program."[1]

CLINICAL ISSUES

In general, subacute care demands more services than traditional long-term care. Therefore, in addition to higher-intensity nursing, more pharmacologic, and more frequent rehabilitative interventions, the need for physician services in general is increased. Although monthly physician visits may suffice for nursing home residents, subacute patients may require daily visits, with round-the-clock physician availability.[3] Subacute units care for both high- and low-acuity patients, but as cost pressures continue, low-acuity patients have been shifted to home care or noninstitutional residential settings.[26]

From a clinical perspective, specialists and primary care physicians attending a subacute unit can expand clinical work by seeing patients in the subacute unit as well as long-term residents in the extended care portion of the facility. For example, a physiatrist on site who oversees a subacute rehabilitation program probably will visit and treat long-term residents with functional decline and musculoskeletal pain. Psychiatrists have an added opportunity because of OBRA regulations requiring mental health services and oversight and review of all psychotropic medication use.

ACADEMIC ISSUES

Beyond administrative and clinical work, subacute facilities provide excellent sites for teaching postgraduate residents, medical students, nurses, and therapists. Nursing homes offer advantages as teaching sites in terms of time and space. Because the pace is less frenetic, "the opportunities for thoroughness and reflection abound."[11] Competition at the bedside for patient access as well as facility attention is significantly lessened.

Indeed, the residency review committees of both internal medicine and family practice have mandated geriatric experiences along the full continuum of care.[11] Increasingly, nursing homes and subacute units are popular sites for research.

REIMBURSEMENT FOR SERVICES

Reformation by the HCFA of Medicare payment policies to a resource-based relative value scale (RBRVS) in 1995 eliminated the prepayment screening system. Thus, "a physician providing frequent care to a subacute patient is required to file no more documentation than for comparable services in other health care settings."[3] Therefore, with appropriate documentation, patients in a subacute setting may be seen as often as is medically necessary.[7] Moreover, the reimbursement from primary care is essentially equivalent to hospital-based reimbursement.[7] Additional billing is allowed in recognition of the complexity of subacute patients and the additional regulatory burden associated with providing nursing home care.[24]

Subacute care is reimbursed at an inpatient care level whether it be in the hospital or in an SNF.[24] Specialty consultation in nursing facilities is actually reimbursed at a higher rate than a similar hospital service.[24] Some studies suggest that the presence of specialists (e.g., geriatricians treating frail elderly patients in subacute facilities) is cost-effective.[25] In general, liberalizing reimbursement for services provided in SNFs has helped the expansion of subacute care.

MARKETING YOUR SERVICES

In a competitive marketplace, third-party payors are more likely to award favorable contracts to subacute facilities that feature high-quality physician services.[3] Physicians on staff boost "clinical credibility."[5] Moreover, if your physician group covers capitated patients, the subacute programs may seek out your services for both clinical work and access to patients. Furthermore, your group may appropriately seek out the subacute facility as a less expensive venue than the local hospital in which to care for capitated patients.

OPPORTUNITIES

Major chains of subacute care providers have moved aggressively into acquisition or joint ventures with physician practices to care for a more medically acute group of patients.[5] Moreover, many of the major chains see physicians as the key to an effective continuum of care as patients progress from the acute care hospital, rehabilitation hospital, SNF, outpatient clinic, subacute facility, and home care. This is particularly true for elderly patients. An effective seamless continuum of care is again highly attractive to managed care companies. From the physicians' perspective, purchase of their practice by the subacute provider may allow sufficient capital to acquire sophisticated information systems or other infrastructure.

CREDENTIALING

Traditionally, medical care has been provided in either acute care hospitals or outpatient offices and clinics. Formal monitoring processes have lagged behind as care has shifted to new venues, including subacute units. Recently, JCAHO guidelines have been instituted to ensure higher quality in the subacute field.[14] Credentialing verifies an individual's capabilities and provides the basis for assessing actual performance, whereas privileging defines the scope of a practitioner's practice so that it is compatible with his or her areas of competence. As a physician, your license may allow you to perform surgery, but no hospital will grant privileges to perform the procedure unless you have adequate training and experience from residency, fellowship, or continuing medical education.

From a practical perspective, if you are already credentialed at a hospital or long-term care program, the subacute program may obtain copies of the primary source verification. Some argue for more stringent credentialing and privileging to ensure that physicians are prepared to meet the demands of multidimensional care required by the complex patients generally treated in subacute care settings. As Levenson points out, "Hospital privileges are typically specialty and procedure specific . . . subacute physicians may occasionally perform procedures, but most often they must manage the care of individuals with diverse problems in addition to the principal reason for admission."[14]

GETTING STARTED

Many SNFs welcome competent, well-trained primary care physicians available to treat long-term residents. Specialists willing to visit nursing homes are welcomed because they obviate patients' expensive and disruptive trips to the hospital. Opportunities for medical directorship may be advertised in local health care publications, or nursing facility administrators may be contacted directly.

Similarly, local subacute units are marketed in local health care publications. The American Subacute Care Association is dedicated to providing information and promoting subacute care. General insight into long-term and subacute care from the facility's perspective can be gained from the American Health Care Association (address below), which represents over 11,000 SNFs in the United States.

Resources
American Health Care Association
1201 L Street, NW
Washington, D.C. 20005-4014
(202) 842-4444

American Medical Directors Association
10480 Little Patuxent Parkway
Suite 760
Columbia, MD 21044
(410) 740-9743
(800) 876-AMDA
(410) 740-4572 fax

American Subacute Care Association
1720 Kennedy Cswy
Suite 109
North Bay Village, FL 33141
(305) 864-0396
(305) 868-0905 fax
http://members.aol.com/ascamail

REFERENCES

1. American Health Care Association: Nursing Facility Subacute Care: The Quality and Cost-effective Alternative to Hospital Care. Washington, DC, AHCA, 1996.
2. American Health Care Association: Subacute Care: Medical and Rehabilitation Definition and Guide to Business Development. Washington, DC, AHCA, 1994.
3. Bailis SS: The right stuff for subacute. Provider 21:27–29, 1995.
4. Fisher C: Facilities, hospitals, working together. Provider 21:45–46, 1995.
5. Fisher C: Long-term care companies add physician services. Provider 22:52–53, 1996.
6. Gonzalez C: Preparing for a new market. Provider 20:55–56, 1994.
7. Grossman SM: Physician reimbursement in the subacute environment. Presented at the American Subacute Care Association, California, 1996.
8. Haffey WJ, Welsh JH: Subacute care: Evolution is search of value. Arch Phys Med Rehabil 76:SC2–4, 1995.
9. Hobbs FB, Damon BL: 65+ in the United States. Washington, DC, U.S. Census Bureau, Current Population Reports, Special Studies, P23–190, April 1996.

10. Joint Commission on Accreditation of Healthcare Organizations: 1996 Accreditation Manual for Long-term Care. Oakbrook Terrace, IL, JCAHO, 1996.

11. Katz PR, Karvza J, Counsell SR: Academics and the nursing home. Clin Geriatr Med 11:503–516, 1995.

12. Keith RA, Wilson DB, Gutierrez P: Acute and subacute rehabilitation for stroke: A comparison. Arch Phys Med Rehabil 76:495–500, 1995.

13. Kramer AM, Steiner JF, Schlenker RE, et al: Outcomes and costs after hip fracture and stroke: A comparison of rehabilitation settings. JAMA 277:396–404, 1997.

14. Levenson S: Physician standards set for subacute care. Provider Mar:41–42, 1996.

15. Levenson S: Subacute and Transitional Care Handbook St. Louis, Beverly Cracom Publications, 1996.

16. Omnibus Budget Reconciliation Act of 1987. Fed Reg 54(21):5359–5373, 1989.

17. Pear R: New law protects rights of patients in nursing homes. New York Times, Jan. 17, 1988, 137:1 and 18.

18. Phillips EM: Rethinking OBRA regulations. Adv Direct Rehabil 6(6):98, 1997.

19. Reinhart D: Integrating sub-acute and home care. American Subacute Care Association–Website.

20. Retchin SM, Brown RS, Yeh SCJ, et al: Outcomes of stroke patients in medicare fee-for-service and managed care. JAMA 278:119–124, 1997.

21. Shaughnessy PW, Kramer AM: The increased needs of patients in nursing homes and patients receiving home health care. N Engl J Med 322:21–27, 1990.

22. Singleton GW: Overcoming culture conflict. Provider 21:27–30, 1995.

23. Steiner A, Neu CR: Monitoring the Changes in the Use of Medicare Posthospitalization Services. RAND MR-153-HCFA, 1993.

24. Stone D, Reublinger V: Long-term care reimbursement issues. Clin Geriatr Med 11:517–529, 1995.

25. von Sternberg T, Hepburn K, Cibuzar P, et al: Post-hospital sub-acute care: An example of a managed care model. J Am Geriatr Soc 45:87–91, 1997.

26. Willging P: The future of long-term care and the role of the medical doctor. Clin Geriatr Med 11:531–545, 1995.

KENNETH M. FINE, MD

15

Opportunities in Sports Medicine: The Team Physician

WHAT IS A TEAM PHYSICIAN?

Why don't you quit your job and become the team physician for the Metropolitan Cougars? Most often this question, when posed to a sports medicine specialist, shows a misunderstanding of the role of the team physician. Even for physicians who participate in the medical care of organized athletic teams, including professional or collegiate teams, the role of team physician is usually only part-time and contributes a small amount to a physician's patient volume. The exceptions are generally in large Division I universities, which may hire a full-time team physician whose sole role is to care for varsity athletes.[12,79] A more appropriate question might be: Can you supplement your routine office practice by serving as a team physician or consultant for any organized athletic teams?

What exactly does it mean to be a team physician? First, team physician must be distinguished from related positions such as competition physician, team consultant, and sports medicine specialist. The *competition physician* organizes medical coverage for a specific athletic event such as a soccer tournament or road race.[45,62] Many physicians who are interested in sports medicine become team physicians as well as competition physicians. A *team consultant* is a specialist who provides opinions or treatments when requested but does not follow the day-to-day medical matters of the team. A *sports medicine specialist* may or may not be a team physician. Some sports medicine specialists are interested and trained in the diagnosis and treatment of sports-related injuries but are not actually team physicians.

In contrast, the team physician is distinguished from other physicians by being available on and off the field, during practices as well as games, and by working outside the usual office hours.[27,34] According to the Committee on the

Medical Aspects of Sports of the American Medical Association, a *team physician* is a physician who is given authority by a team or school to make medical judgments relating to the participation and supervision of athletes on the team or in the school.[80,81] In some instances, the title "team physician" may be misleading. Physicians have been known to claim and subsequently advertise themselves as a team physician after consulting for only one patient. For some teams, the relationship is quite formal, with a written contract, scrutinized by lawyers, that dictates the responsibilities and benefits for the team and physician.[83] Other physicians who "hang out" at their child's games begin to help the coach or athletic trainer with injured players and grow into their role informally.[79,87]

Regardless of the manner in which one becomes a team physician, certain factors distinguish a team physician from a physician who simply treats athletic injuries. Most obvious is that team physicians have an interest in and develop experience with the care of injuries related to athletics. As already mentioned, a team physician spends at least some time treating athletes outside the formal office setting, often in a training room or game or practice facility. Usually, much of this treatment is conducted without direct financial compensation or billing. Team physicians are often responsible for covering games and/or practice sessions.[93] Sometimes schools or other teams arrange clinic schedules, during which the physician evaluates injured athletes in the training room at specified times.[9,67,79] Team physicians may spend a large amount of time corresponding by telephone and mail with athletes, athletic trainers, coaches, athletic directors, and management about the status of injured players.[34,91] The athletic trainer is usually the primary liaison between the team's medical staff and the coaching staff, and most team physicians know the athletic trainers much better than they know the coaches.[19,29,49,79] Physicians also may organize and conduct preparticipation physical examinations and sometimes provide recommendations about nutrition, training regimens, and medical red-shirt decisions and documentation.[9,45,69,79] With increasing frequency, doctors are also becoming involved with medical insurance issues regarding student-athletes. In addition, team physicians may become involved with administrative decisions, such as equipment purchases.[91]

The time required to fulfill the obligations of team physician varies, depending on the number of athletes and teams for which the physician is responsible. For example, the physician for a large university may be responsible for the care of hundreds of athletes. Some doctors in student health centers on college campuses also care for varsity athletes and spend a large percentage of their time doing so.[79] Football coverage is notoriously time-consuming because of the large number of players per team and higher injury rates. Football team doctors are usually responsible for being present at all home and away games. Some teams require the presence of a physician at all contact practices.[79,82] For basketball, the team physician usually does not go to away games; the home physician is also responsible for covering the visiting team.[30] Sports with a higher risk of injury such as wrestling and gymnastics are more likely to require a physician's presence.[79] The time commitment also varies with the traditions of the particular team and the personalities and abilities of the athletic trainers. Some athletic trainers take pride in calling the physician only for serious problems, whereas others consult more frequently with their doctors.[79] As a result of this and other factors (such as the number and types of teams covered), the time commitment of a team physician can be significant. Physicians who become affiliated with one or more athletic teams often find it helpful to work with a group of physicians to share the responsibilities.[56,93] Although the time commitment may vary, most team physicians devote many weekends and evenings to their team.[79]

SPECIAL EDUCATION FOR THE TEAM PHYSICIAN

What type of specialty training does one need to become a team physician? Most team physicians are orthopedic surgeons; many have formal postresidency fellowship training in sports medicine.[36,93] However, many other specialists are team physicians, including internists, family practitioners, physiatrists, pediatricians, emergency physicians, general surgeons, obstetrician/gynecologists, rheumatologists, and osteopaths.[9,10,12,14,15,18,20,27,28,30,55,58,60,71,73,79,86] Some specialties, including physiatry, family practice, internal medicine, and emergency medicine, have developed postresidency fellowship programs in sports medicine.[8,85] In a recent survey conducted in a Division 1 university, 88% of the medical problems reported to athletic trainers were related to the musculoskeletal system.[40] A study of high school athletes reported that more than 90% of injuries involved the musculoskeletal system.[75] Clearly, team physicians must have expertise with disorders of the musculoskeletal system, whether or not their practice is limited to nonoperative management.[30,34,67,86]

The team physician is often the primary care physician for all medical needs of the athletes and must have basic knowledge in areas such as nutrition, psychology, dentistry, infectious disease, dermatology, cardiology, pulmonology, and physiology in addition to knowledge of the musculoskeletal system.[17,21,34,51,52,67,68,79] He or she must also coordinate the medical care for the athletes and oversee appropriate follow-up, even if another specialist is treating the patient.[91] Communication with other health care professionals, including consultants, physical therapists, athletic trainers, and family physicians of the athletes is extremely important.[79] If the team physician disagrees with a decision made by an athlete's family physician, the team physician should be careful not to criticize the family physician in front of the patient. The team doctor should contact the other physician directly and try to reach a consensus.[4,33,34,56] Pharmacologic knowledge is also important, and specific knowledge of what drugs are banned by organizations such as the National Collegiate Athletic

Association (NCAA) and United States Olympic Committee (USOC) can be critical if drug testing is performed.[67,79] In a large city or university, the physician may have access to many subspecialists, but such consultants may not be readily available in some locations, especially if the team is traveling out of state or abroad. When the team physician of a professional baseball team was asked why he, an internist, was the official team physician instead of the orthopedic surgeon who was considered a consultant, he replied, "For the type of problems our guys get while on the road, you don't need an orthopedic surgeon." Team physicians are often required to treat communicable diseases and in the case of foreign travel should be responsible for ensuring that the proper vaccinations are performed.[45]

Regardless of his or her specialty, the primary team physician has the responsibility to organize an efficient system for consultation with other specialists.[18,34,79] If the primary team physician is not an orthopedic surgeon, an orthopedic surgeon must be closely involved with the team. There are roles for other consultants interested in athletic injuries, including cardiologists, neurologists, neurosurgeons, general surgeons, dermatologists, radiologists, dentists, oral surgeons, gynecologists, urologists, psychologists, psychiatrists, and ophthalmologists.[38,51,79] In some situations, the team physician functions as a typical primary care physician, to whom all medical problems are reported initially. Other teams or colleges develop systems by which certain problems are referred directly to the appropriate specialist. The referral pattern depends on the preferences and experience of the team physician and the athletic trainers as well as the availability of certain specialists. There is always a need for physicians in any specialty who are interested in treating athletes and willing to provide excellent service for athletic organizations. Because many physicians do not understand the medical and logistic needs of athletes, there will always be a role for doctors who are willing and able to accommodate the athletes' needs. However, regardless of the specialty of the team physician, certain problems inevitably fall outside his or her expertise; the team physician must know when to refer.[33] Conversely, if the team physician refers too many patients, he or she may be viewed merely as a triage mechanism and thereby lose the trust of the team.

RESPONSIBILITIES OF THE TEAM PHYSICIAN

Many responsibilities accompany the position of team physician. First, the team physician must gain knowledge and experience for optimal performance in his or her role.[79,93] Of course, the team physician must be enthusiastic about sports and sports medicine.[79] Formal fellowships have been developed in sports medicine, and ideally all new team physicians should be graduates of such programs.[8,79,85] Many specialties have Certificates of Added Qualification in Sports Medicine, including the American Board of Internal Medicine, Family

Practice, Emergency Medicine, and Pediatrics.[27] Another good way to develop experience as a team physician is to work for a period with an experienced team physician.[79] There are textbooks and team physician courses such as the course sponsored by the American College of Sports Medicine.[2,13,18,61,79,88] The team physician should make a commitment to staying current with the field by reading journals, going to meetings, and belonging to sports medicine organizations.[91] He or she also should commit to learning about exercise physiology, biomechanics, rehabilitation, and nutrition.[27,34,67,69,79,86] Although it helps if the physician has been an athlete, this is not absolutely necessary. Team physicians should learn about the sport with which they work and consider getting involved as participants in some type of athletic activity.[4,27,34,86,91] Team physicians must establish relationships with coaches, trainers, and management.[4,79,82,91] They also should develop an efficient network of consultants.[14,18,34] It is important to oversee on-site facilities for evaluation and treatment of injuries as well as confirming an efficient communication and transportation system for serious injuries.[18,30,34,67,75] Finally, team physicians should be involved with the education of athletes, coaches, and others in the community about the prevention and treatment of injuries and should contribute educationally by conducting or facilitating research related to sports injuries.[1,9,24,34,79]

FINANCIAL CONSIDERATIONS FOR THE TEAM PHYSICIAN

Being a team physician can be an enjoyable experience. The opportunity to work with young, motivated patients and to participate in the successes and failures of a team can be tremendously rewarding. The variety of supplementing office and in some cases operative practice with activities on the court or field is often enough reason to become a team physician. Sometimes other "perks" include game tickets and travel. The financial rewards are variable. Fewer and fewer physicians receive a salary, and most team physicians have a fee-for-service relationship with or without a formal contract.[79,83] Some physicians also believe that their practice is enhanced by community recognition of their role as physician for a certain team. When choosing a doctor for a sports injury, a patient may say, "I want to go to the doctor who treats the Metropolitan Cougars."

Ironically, some teams actually charge doctors for the "privilege" of being their physician. In some cases, the job of team physician is put up for bid.[64,70] For instance, Major League Soccer (MLS) set up a bidding process in which the highest bidder became the team physician in cities with soccer teams. In the Washington, D.C. area, MLS officials requested a sum of $150,000 from local doctors interested in becoming D.C. United's physician. Both the Charlotte and Jacksonville teams in the National Football League reportedly put the job of team physician out for bid.[37,48] The Orlando Magic of the National Basketball Association received money from their medical providers, and the Jacksonville

Jaguars of the National Football League reportedly received one million dollars from the group that became their team physicians.[37,42,63,64,72] The Carolinas Medical Center committed $150,000 per year to the Carolina Panthers and described their contract as a managed care contract, with the players steered toward their hospital.[90]

Some physicians believe that an association with a professional team is a useful form of professional advertising, especially in sports such as football, in which injury rates are high and the injuries often receive significant attention in local newspapers.[48] As part of these financial agreements, the physician or medical group becomes a "sponsor" and is given certain advertising rights, such as having their name on billboards. In addition, their name may be mentioned by the announcer at the game or on radio or television advertisements. Such advertisements are easily recognized at most professional and some collegiate athletic events. In some instances, large health care organizations negotiate contracts to take care of professional or college teams. The organization becomes responsible for choosing the team's athletic trainers, physical therapists, and physicians. Strategies in which teams choose their medical care by the ability of the doctor or health care organization to pay the team or by negotiating all-inclusive contracts with large health care organizations are becoming more common. Unfortunately, this method of choosing team physicians often relegates skill and experience to a less important position in the decision-making process. In addition, many physicians strongly believe that advertising, in general, is questionable from an ethical standpoint.[33,48,95]

The method whereby physicians pay money to the team may create additional ethical problems. In the past, the team physician was sometimes a friend of the owner or of someone in management. Gradually such physicians were replaced by people with expertise and experience in sports medicine. The new trend whereby physician selection is influenced by financial factors creates questions about the loyalty of the physicians: Are they loyal to the players or to the organization? Players may not like the concept that their team doctor was not chosen because of skill alone. Although this phenomenon has been seen mostly in professional sports, it may become more prevalent even in college sports. Some experienced physicians believe that this trend is not good for the specialty of sports medicine.[33,48,95]

MANAGED CARE AND THE TEAM PHYSICIAN

Managed care is an increasingly important factor for the team physician and may contribute to the unfortunate trend by which physician ability becomes less important in choosing a team physician. In the past, if a team physician provided good service and was well liked by the players, coaches, and trainers, most referrals obviously were referred to his or her office. However, many team physicians are now encountering the following scenario: A player who has been followed by the team physician for many years for minor injuries (no bills generated) is examined in the training room. The athlete has now twisted her knee and has an effusion and positive Lachman's test. The physician recommends a radiograph and possible anterior cruciate ligament reconstructive surgery. However, the athlete belongs to a health maintenance organization (HMO) that requires evaluation by a primary care doctor and referral to a different orthopedist. This and similar scenarios are becoming more and more frequent. As a result, many physicians are deciding that the decrease in financial compensation due to managed care precludes them from continuing their role as team physician. Managed care also may affect the treatment of college athletes who are unable to receive more than superficial treatment from their team physician. In a survey of two Maryland universities, 65 of 202 athletes were from out of state. Many had out-of-state primary care physicians. If the primary care physician does not allow out-of-network care, treatment may be delayed, often resulting in lost playing and practice time.[9] College athletes are allowed only four years of participation, and any loss of playing time is important. The team physician, who usually knows the athlete well and is most experienced with the treatment of sports-related injuries, may not be allowed by the insurance company to treat the patient. In such cases, the team physician must stand by as the athlete is treated by someone who may not know the athlete or not understand the subtleties of the injury or the time factors involved with college athletics.[78]

Another modern phenomenon is that athletic trainers, who have no formal training in medical insurance issues, are usually responsible for negotiating with insurance companies, obtaining permission for care, and filing claims. Many athletic trainers believe that they are spending more and more time dealing with insurance companies, which interferes with their ability to care for athletes.[9]

LEGAL CONSIDERATIONS FOR THE TEAM PHYSICIAN

Similar legal issues affect all physicians. In general, the principle that good medicine equals good law holds true.[67] The definitions of standard of care and medical liability are no different for the team physician.[7] However, there are some special legal considerations for the team physician, who is expected to have expertise in certain areas of sports medicine, such as the treatment of potential spine injuries in football. A physician must have the skill expected of a *reasonably competent practitioner in the same class to which he or she belongs.*[6] Some team physicians have had difficulty in getting malpractice coverage because of the risk of career-ending injuries in multimillion-dollar athletes.[83] Medical staff are often pressured to return the athlete to playing status as soon as possible.[42] Such pressure comes from coaches, management, and sometimes athletes themselves. The physician may allow the athlete to return to play sooner than other patients. If a decision is made to allow an athlete to play "hurt," informed consent must be thorough and well documented.[7]

The physician must discuss both the risks and benefits of medical intervention (including surgery) or sports participation with the athlete. Both doctor and athlete should be comfortable with the decision. The importance of communication and disclosure applies to all patients and should not depend on the patient's athletic status, despite the sometimes competing interests of coaches, fans, management, and athletes.[7,91] Athletes have sued their doctors, complaining that they were not completely informed of their condition or the risks of continued participation.[32,70] Athletes, because of their extreme competitiveness, may be particularly susceptible to "selective listening" when their situation is explained by the team physician and therefore may not fully grasp the risks of continued playing. Sports may be so important to the athlete's self-esteem that he or she is willing to risk injury or even death. Athletes' goals are usually short-term, and often a milieu of machismo and indestructibility influences their decisions.[3,23,35,36,92] Team physicians also have been sued by athletes who claimed that the doctor put the needs of the team above what was best for the athlete.[63,70] For most conditions that affect the extremities, the risk of continued participation is persistent pain or reinjury. However, for injuries to the head and neck or for cardiac problems, reinjury may result in permanent neurologic damage or even death. Therefore, treatment of such conditions should not be compromised, regardless of the skill of the athlete or the importance of the particular contest.

In making decisions about an athlete's participation, physicians have competing goals. It is most important that the athlete's future in athletics and in life not be unreasonably jeopardized by allowing him or her to compete. A physician must never guarantee to a patient that it is entirely safe to compete; some risk is always inherent in sports. It is better to say that a player does not have a significantly increased risk compared with peers or that no medical reason precludes participation. Conversely, an athlete should not be held back from participation unnecessarily.[81,91] Physicians have been sued for not allowing a player to participate. Recent legal cases have used the Americans With Disabilities Act to support the athlete's assertion that he or she should be allowed to play despite potential risk.[7,54,66] Team physicians have sometimes been sued by athletes who claim that the doctor wrongfully allowed participation and the team did not allow second opinions.[31,44]

In some cases, an athlete or parent tries to override a physician's restriction on athletic participation by signing a release or waiver. Such releases are problematic, however, and the physician still should not allow the athlete to participate. A parent generally has no authority to release future claims on behalf of a child, and the statute of limitations does not begin until the child reaches legal age. Moreover, selective listening problems, referred to above, also may affect the validity of a release. When an athlete continues to participate despite the physician's recommendation, the physician should write a letter reaffirming his or her belief that the athlete should not participate. Physicians are liable for inaction as well as action, and failure to try to prevent unsafe activity may be considered negligent.[43,54,81,89]

Are physicians legally liable, even when they are working in a voluntary capacity? The answer to this question has been affected by the fact that some areas of the country have had problems attracting doctors to become team physicians. To reduce physicians' legal concerns and thereby encourage them to work with teams, some states, such as Maryland, Arizona, Arkansas, Georgia, Florida, Kansas, Missouri, Ohio, Oregon, and Tennessee, have passed laws that provide immunity to team physicians who provide care in an emergency, in good faith, and without compensation.[27,30] However, even a volunteer physician may be liable under some circumstances, especially when it is determined that gross negligence has occurred.[7,43,53]

Another difference between routine office practice and team physician practice may have legal ramifications: some of the treatment rendered by team physicians is done in informal settings. Therefore, documentation is not as rigorous. Team physicians may not dictate or write a note every time they evaluate a blister or rash in the training room or a concussion or "burner" on the sideline. Sometimes medications such as antiinflammatory drugs are dispensed without a formal prescription. Such medications are sometimes dispensed by athletic trainers, utilizing "standing orders" from the physician. Team physicians must understand that they assume legal risk even when they treat players informally or when medicine is dispensed via standing orders by the athletic trainer.[32] Physicians may get a sense of security, thinking that players appreciate their helping the team and therefore will not take legal action against them. Although most team physicians agree that athletes are generally not litigious, unfortunately this is not always true. The team physician must be careful with every medical decision. In a survey of high school football teams in California, 6.6% of the schools had been involved in football injury litigation within the past five years.[93] Legally, a physician–patient relationship or contract is assumed whenever a physician renders care to a patient, even without verbal or written expression.[27] Many sports medicine groups such as the American College of Sports Medicine are developing written standards of care that may become an important risk-management response to the increase in litigation throughout all of medicine.[32]

Guidelines that help the team physician to function efficiently from a legal standpoint include the importance of good documentation of opinions, especially those relating to the ability of an athlete to continue sports participation. Physicians should learn the intricacies and common injuries of the sports for which they are responsible. Team physicians should try to be objective about their decisions and avoid being influenced by the coach, media, fans, or management.[56,84] As difficult as it may be to keep a star athlete out of play, the team physician must stand firm.[79] It is helpful to have objective tests and the opinions of consultants to back up difficult decisions. If an athlete's ability to reenter a game is in doubt, the decision usually should fall on the side of safety. In addition, appropriate malpractice coverage specifically for activities as a team physician is essential. Some experts recommend that team physicians have a high limit on their plans.[27,34,67,81,96] Although team physicians have a tendency to render treatment in more informal settings, it is wise to get written consent for any procedure or medication that is dispensed. Failure to prove that proper consent was obtained prior to a procedure, even a minor one such as an injection, may result in a charge of assault and battery in addition to malpractice. Some experts recommend obtaining a formal written contract with the advice of lawyers before agreeing to become a team physician. However, the best way to avoid legal difficulties is to practice good medicine, which includes developing rapport with one's patients, being careful and thorough, following through, keeping good records, and consulting or getting second opinions when necessary.[81,96]

SPECIAL CONSIDERATIONS FOR THE TEAM PHYSICIAN

Certain stresses and pressures are unique to team physicians. As discussed earlier, they face pressure to get the player back in the game as soon as possible.[42] Many team physicians feel that they may lose their job if they keep players out too long. The decision whether to allow an athlete to play can be difficult but must be made often by a team physician.[79] Unnecessary restrictions may be harmful and frustrating for the athlete.[33] Decisions to restrict an athlete are more likely to be made by physicians not experienced in sports medicine, who tend to be more conservative.[79] Another unique pressure on team physicians is the degree of attention that their decisions or treatment may receive. When a player is treated surgically or nonsurgically, the player's progress is scrutinized by teammates, trainers, coaches, management, fans, and media. The physician's responsibility is primarily to the patient, despite pressures from the coach, management, or fans.[33,56,95] Because of the publicity that some athletes' injuries receive, the team physician may be inundated with suggestions or advice from general managers, coaches, trainers, and even fans. The team physician may have to deal with second guessing and criticism.[18,22,23,26,41,50,57,76,83] In extreme circumstances, physicians have received death threats because of decisions about high-profile athletes.[77] Depending on the relationship between the physician and team management, the physician's position may be vulnerable. Sports injuries are rarely life-threatening, but there are high standards of precision for both diagnosis and treatment.[75] A poor outcome or prolonged recovery can damage the physician's ego and reputation. The team physician may be forced to make instantaneous decisions about how long an athlete will be disabled because of the need for teams to fill their rosters while an injured player is relegated to a disabled list.[83] Potential conflicts between coaches and team physicians can be avoided by a clear understanding that the physician has absolute authority concerning medical decisions.[86] Usually, good coaches and physicians come to realize that what is best for the individual player is best for the team.

The high stakes and time constraints of some sports may result in a higher likelihood of surgery for certain conditions and more frequent use of certain tests, such as magnetic resonance imaging.[83] The physician also may be more likely to choose operative interventions when certain conditions occur in team members. Examples include anterior cruciate ligament injuries and stress fractures of the fifth metatarsal.

Another source of stress relates to difficult confidentiality issues, which may arise when the team physician of a high-profile professional or collegiate team has to deal with the media. It is important to remember that the same standards of confidentiality apply to all patients, even a celebrity athlete.[33] Although team physicians have benefited from publicity that they receive, many experienced team physicians believe that it is most ethical for physicians to discourage references to themselves in the media and not to use the media for personal gain.[83]

Another consideration for the team physician is that a player's response to injury is sometimes influenced by contractual matters; team physicians may not be informed of the specific details. For example, a collegiate athlete on scholarship may exaggerate an injury to be declared medically unfit, thereby continuing to receive a scholarship without continuing to play. Conversely, a physician may be influenced by the athletic department or management to declare a poorly performing athlete medically unfit to clear a space for another scholarship athlete or another player on the team.[35] In professional sports, contract incentives may influence a player to hide or exaggerate an injury. A team physician may decide to operate on an athlete without having received an honest history.[83] As athletes progress to the collegiate and professional level, they often develop medical habits that are difficult for a physician to change, and they may distrust medical advice that does not correlate with what they already believe.[36]

Despite the time involved and the possible financial, legal, and political drawbacks, many physicians still find the experience of being a team physician rewarding. The average length of time that team physicians remain on the job is 11 years, according to a survey conducted by the American College Health Association. This record indicates the physicians' satisfaction with their role. Many physicians report that their personal relationships with the players and the ability to see their patients perform are especially enjoyable.[79] However, some physicians may find the stress unpleasant when they cover a game while worrying or hoping that no player gets hurt.[11] There may be little or no direct financial benefit, but becoming a team physician may help to build one's practice and is a good community service.[34,60,79,86]

WHERE TO START

For a physician entering a new community, many paths may lead to becoming a team doctor; the most important factors are willingness and availability.[34] Some physicians may join a group that already cares for one or more teams. For someone with no previous connections, a good way to start is to contact local coaches, athletic trainers, and athletic directors.[30,67] It also may be useful to contact physicians already involved with local teams and let them know of one's interest and availability, especially if one is interested mainly in working as a consultant rather than as a primary team physician. It may be prudent for a prospective team physician to obtain the approval of other physicians in the area, especially because cooperation between the team physician and family physicians is important.[18] One may contact schools as well as nonschool leagues, such as children's soccer, football, baseball, and basketball. There are niches for physicians willing to develop a specific area of interest, particularly in specialized sports such as gymnastics, diving, and swimming. A physician may become involved by volunteering to give lectures to coaches, cover games, or give preparticipation examinations. A true sports medicine physician should not be concerned with the level of competition of the teams for which he or she cares; Michael Jordan gets the same injuries as a mediocre high school basketball player. The skill of the athlete is no reflection on the skill of the physician. The athlete, not the physician, is the one who wins the medals.[46] And never forget that sport is "only a game."[47]

REFERENCES

1. Albright JP, Noyes FR: Role of the team physician in sports injury studies. Am J Sports Med 16(Suppl 1):S1–4, 1988.
2. American Academy of Orthopaedic Surgeons: Athletic Training and Sports Medicine, 2nd ed. Rosemont, IL, American Academy of Orthopaedic Surgeons, 1991.
3. Bass A: Success can spur denial. Boston Globe, July 29, 1993, 1:63.
4. Bedo AV: Thoughts of a team physician. Mich Med 75(12):690–692, 1976.
5. Benda C: Sideline samaritans. Physician Sportsmed 19(11):132–142, 1991.
6. Bianco E, Walker E: Legal aspects of sports medicine. In Birrer R (ed): Sports Medicine for the Primary Care Physician, 2nd ed. Ann Arbor, MI, CRC Press, 1994 [referencing *Shilkret v. Annapolis Emergency Hospital Association*, 349 A.2d 245 (MD 1975)].
7. Bianco E, Walker E: Legal aspects of sports medicine. In Birrer R (ed): Sports Medicine for the Primary Care Physician, 2nd ed. Ann Arbor, MI, CRC Press, 1994, pp 27–35.

8. Birrer R (ed): Sports Medicine for the Primary Care Physician, 2nd ed. Ann Arbor, MI, CRC Press, 1994, pp 589–590.

9. Brandon T, Lamboni P: Care of collegiate athletes. Md Med J 45(8):669–675, 1996.

10. Brown DG: Perspectives of a rheumatologist team physician. Baillieres Clin Rheumatol 8(1):225–230, 1994.

11. Brown S: I'll pass: Why being team physician is not for me [letter]. Postgrad Med 89(3).24, 1991.

12. Butcher JD, Zukowski CW, Brannen SJ, et al: Patient profile, referral sources, and consultant utilization in a primary care sports medicine clinic. J Fam Pract 43:556–560, 1996.

13. Cantu R, Micheli L (eds): ACSM's Guidelines for the Team Physician, 2nd ed. Malvern, PA, Lea & Febiger, 1991.

14. Cantwell JD: The internist as sports medicine physician [editorial]. Am Intern Med 116:165–166, 1992.

15. Clinger RD: The 1981 Outstanding Team Physician Awards. Ohio State Med J 77(11): 649–651, 1981.

16. Cole L: Death, lies, and basketball. Washingtonian 25(1):123–136, 1989.

17. Cooper T: Contact sports and cardiac injury: What a team physician might be called upon to do. College Health 17:64–67, 1968.

18. Culpepper MI, Niemann KM: Professional personnel in health care among secondary school athletics in Alabama. South Med J 80:336–338, 1987.

19. DeLee JC, Farney WC: Incidence of injury in Texas high school football. Am J Sports Med 20:575–580, 1992.

20. Dick AD: Chalktalk for the team physician. Am Fam Physician 28(3):231–236, 1983.

21. Eathorne SW: Medical problems in a sports medicine setting. Med Clin North Am 78:479–502, 1994.

22. Eller D: The death of Reggie Lewis. Am Health 12(9):88–89, 1993.

23. Fainaru S: Hard questions remain on death. Boston Globe, July 29, 1993, 1:1.

24. Fields KB: Sports medicine: A research agenda for primary care [editorial]. Fam Pract Res J 12(2):101–104, 1992.

25. Foreman J: Autopsy shows Lewis had scar tissue in heart. Boston Globe, August 5, 1993, 1:2.

26. Foreman J: Two cardiologists come to Mudge's defense. Boston Globe, August 5, 1993, 1:16.

27. Garfinkel D, Birrer R: The team physician. In Birrer R (ed): Sports Medicine for the Primary Care Physician, 2nd ed. Ann Arbor, MI, CRC Press, 1994, pp 9–14.

28. Geiringer SR, Bowyer BL, Press JM: Sports medicine. I: The physiatric approach. Arch Phys Med Rehabil 74(5S):S428–S432, 1993.

29. Gertsen K, Lopez J: The relationship of the certified athletic trainer and the team physician in sports medicine. Md Med J 45(8):675–677, 1996.

30. Harries T: Medical coverage of high school sports. Md Med J 45(8):686–689, 1989.

31. Herbert D: Legal Aspects of Sports Medicine. Canton, OH, Professional Reports, 1990.

32. Herbert D, Herbert W: Medical-legal issues. In Kibler WB (ed): ACSM's Handbook for the Team Physician. Baltimore, Williams & Wilkins, 1996, pp 452–461.

33. Howe W: Ethical considerations in sports medicine. In Birrer R (ed): Sports Medicine for the Primary Care Physician, 2nd ed. Ann Arbor, MI, CRC Press, 1994, pp 37–39.

34. Howe W: The team physician. Primary Care 18:763–765, 1991.

35. Huizenga R: Winning at all costs—NFL football and doctors' dilemma [transcript]. ABC News Nightline, November 1, 1994.

36. Jaffe L: Perspectives of an orthopaedist team physician. Baillieres Clin Rheumatol 8:221–223, 1994.
37. Keteyian A: Winning at all costs—NFL football and doctors' dilemma [transcript]. ABC News Nightline, November 1, 1994.
38. Kilhenny C: Improving communications between team physician and radiologist. J Sports Med 1(1):2, 1972.
39. Kirk K: How to be a sports medicine physician: The old tape and go. Ohio Med 86(2):128–131, 1990.
40. Klug R, Hunt M, Westerman B, Fine K: Evaluation of injuries and illnesses at an NCAA division I athletic program. Presented to the Society for Academic Emergency Medicine, San Antonio, TX, May, 1995.
41. Knox R: A look at a doctor on the spot. Boston Globe, July 29, 1993, 1:1.
42. Koppel T: Winning at all costs—NFL football and doctors' dilemma [transcript]. ABC News Nightline, November 1, 1994.
43. Kronisch R, Flowers F, Ball R: Medicolegal challenges of advising at-risk patients: The example of Marfan's syndrome. Physician Sportsmed 22(9):37–44, 1994.
44. Krupa G: Issues of liability are not clear-cut. Boston Globe, July 29, 1993, 1:63.
45. Kujala UM, Heinonen OJ, Lehto M, et al: Equipment, drugs, and problems of the competition and team physician. Sports Med 6(4):197–209, 1988.
46. Leach R: How many medals? [editorial]. Am J Sports Med 20:495, 1992.
47. Leach R: It's only a game [editorial]. Am J Sports Med 25:1, 1997.
48. Leach R: Job auction [editorial]. Am J Sports Med 23:379, 1995.
49. Leach RE: Athletic trainers [editorial]. Am J Sports Med 19:565, 1991.
50. Lehman B, Foreman J: Lewis got 3rd opinion. Boston Globe, July 29, 1993, 1:1.
51. Lephart S: Emergency treatment of athletic injuries. Dent Clin North Am 35:707–717, 1991.
52. Levine N: Dermatologic aspects of sports medicine. Dermatol Nurs 6(3):179–186, 1994.
53. Lubell A: Questioning the athlete's right to sue. Physician Sportsmed 17:240–244, 1989.
54. McCallum J, Kennedy K: The heart of the matter. Sports Illustr 83(23):26, 1995.
55. McClain LG, Reynolds S: Sports injuries in a high school. Pediatrics 84:446–450, 1989.
56. Macleod DA: Team doctor. Br J Sports Med 23(4):211–212, 1989.
57. MacMullan J: Scheller's worst fears came true. Boston Globe, July 29, 1993, 1:64.
58. Malacrea RF: Injuries on the field: The pediatrician as team physician. Pediatr Ann 7:716–729, 1978.
59. Mason B: Winning at all costs—NFL football and doctors' dilemma [transcript]. ABC News Nightline, November 1, 1994.
60. Menna VJ: The pediatrician as team physician. Pediatr Rev 9(2):35, 1987.
61. Miller M: The Team Physician's Handbook. St. Louis, Mosby, 1990.
62. Monto RR, Bassett FH III: Team physician 9. The role and responsibilities of the competition physician. Orthop Rev 19:1015–1020, 1990.
63. Munson L: Crippling indifference. Sports Illustr 83(20):81, 1995.
64. Munson L: Fast operators. Sports Illustr 83(20):84, 1995.
65. Nadis S: Cardiac alert. Omni 17(3):38, 1994.
66. Naughton J: Judge backs student in medical dispute. Chron Higher Educ 43(6):A46, 1996.
67. Niedfeldt MW, Young CC, Leshan L: Establishing a high-school-based training room clinic. Wis Med J 95(96):356–360, 1996.

68. Nixon JE: The many hats of the team physician. J Sports Med 1(2):53, 1973.
69. Noble HB, Porter M: The role of the team physician in school athletics. Il Med J 161(2): 112–113, 1982.
70. Nocera J: Bitter medicine. Sports Illustr 83(20):74–88, 1995.
71. Patterson PH: Being a team physician. Pediatr Ann 26:13–16, 1997.
72. Pearce F: Winning at all costs—NFL football and doctors' dilemma [transcript]. ABC News Nightline, November 1, 1994.
73. Press JM, Akau CK, Boyer BL: Sports medicine 5. The physiatrist as team physician. Arch Phys Med Rehabil 74(5S):S117 449, 1993.
74. Pro team physician describes athletes' peculiarities. J Med Assoc State Ala 36:1419–1429, 1967.
75. Quigley TB: Becoming a team physician [editorial]. Postgrad Med 48:284–285, 1970.
76. Rovner S: A clash of diagnoses: Celtics' Lewis benefits from 2nd opinion. Washington Post May 12, 1993, C, 1:1.
77. Ryan E, Tye L: Mudge threats reported. Boston Globe, July 29, 1993, 1:64.
78. Sallis RE, Massimino F: Sports medicine and managed care. A positive partnership. Physician Sportsmed 23(4):33–35, 1995.
79. Samples P: The team physician: No official job description. Physician Sportsmed 16:169–175, 1986.
80. Savastano AA: The team physician and the law. R I Med J 51(9):558–560, 1968.
81. Savastano AA: The team physician, trainer, instructor, coach, and the law. Good medical judgment and adequate malpractice insurance are important components of protection. R I Med J 62(9):367–372, 1979.
82. Shaughnessy C: The football coach and the team physician. J Am College Health Assoc 15(2):113–120, 1966.
83. Silberstein CE: The professional sports team physician. Md Med J 45(8):683–685, 1996.
84. Sperryn PN: Ethics in sports medicine—the sports physician. Br J Sports Med 14(2–3). 84–89, 1980.
85. Sports medicine fellowships for primary care physicians. Physician Sportsmed 22(3): 117–118, 120, 123–124, 1994.
86. Stackpole JW: The team physician. Pediatr Ann 13(8):592–594, 1984.
87. Steele M: Caring for athletes in youth sports. Md Med J 45(8):689–691, 1989.
88. Strauss R (ed): Sports Medicine, 2nd ed. Philadelphia, W.B. Saunders, 1991.
89. Strosnider K: Court says university may keep player with heart ailment off its basketball team. Chron Higher Educ 43(15):A62, 1996.
90. Taylor A: Winning at all costs—NFL football and doctors' dilemma [transcript]. ABC News Nightline, November 1, 1994.
91. The team physician. A statement of the Committee on the Medical Aspects of Sports of the American Medical Association, September 1967. J Sch Health 37(10):497–501, 1967.
92. Trainer J: Shroud of mourning surrounds loved ones. Boston Globe, July 29, 1993, 1:63.
93. Vangsness CT Jr, Hunt T, Uram M, Kerlan RK: Survey of health care coverage of high school football in southern California. Am J Sports Med 22(5):719–722, 1994.
94. VanHelder WP: Sports medicine in the emergency room [editorial]. Can J Sport Sci 16(2).86–87, 1991.
95. Warren R: Winning at all costs—NFL football and doctors' dilemma [transcript]. ABC News Nightline, November 1, 1994.
96. Willis GC: The legal responsibilities of the team physician. J Sports Med 1:28–29, 1972.

DAVID T. BURKE, MD, MA
MICHAEL BURKE, MA

16

Using a Medical Newsletter to Promote Your Practice and Reputation

With the advent of the information age, many of us in the medical field feel the stress of information overload. The National Library of Medicine reported a 30% increase in the number of available periodicals over the past 20 years. In addition, there has been a 56% increase in the average number of articles in each journal. Internet accessibility has many benefits, including the ability to retrieve updated information literally at the tip of your fingers. However, accessing the precise information that we need at any given time can be challenging as we try to access the meaningful and eliminate the superfluous. More and more, we rely on others to triage this information and to present only the most relevant portions. Topic-specific newsletters perform just such a function.

Newsletters are an efficient method for medical societies to transmit information about upcoming meetings, current topics of interest, opportunities for continuing medical education, research developments, and employment opportunities. Individual physicians or group practices may wish to advertise their practices in a newsletter form that can be distributed to referral or potential referral sources. Well-written newsletters can be a welcome mailing that keeps the provider's name and specialty interest in the forefront of the reader's mind. Newsletters that are professionally presented with up-to-date information lend credibility to an individual physician as well as a group practice. A newsletter provides a physician or group of physicians with a forum to disseminate information to the public and can be a useful means of advertising a medical practice.

Because the cost of medical journals has sky-rocketed over the past few years, pressure on medical libraries to cut the subscription list has increased. As a result of this reduction in available journals at medical libraries, physicians have less access to traditional medical journals. Because the medical system is constantly in flux, physicians are seeking to redefine and to master their new specialty interests. Faced with this daunting task, more and more physicians rely on information services to process some of the important information into meaningful and digestible bits. With fewer journals available and an increased need for state-of-the-art information, the introduction of electronic virtual libraries or surveillance journals has been proposed as a solution.[1] Finally, while most physicians have access to the Internet, this is not necessarily true of potential patients. Thus, newsletters are an easy and convenient way to convey important information in both medical and lay communities.

DEFINING YOUR TARGET AUDIENCE

The first task in creating a newsletter is to define your target audience. You want to decide whether your audience will be a lay audience or a medical audience. Next, decide whether you are targeting a specific demographic region. You also want to define whether you are interested primarily in reaching a particular age group, medical specialty, or other demographic subgroup. Defining your target audience is key to the success of your newsletter and will enable you to reach the audience for whom your newsletter is designed. This will limit the amount of unnecessary money spent on production and mailing to people who may not be interested in your product.

DEFINING YOUR SUBJECT

The second step in creating a newsletter is to define your subject matter as clearly as possible. The reader should have no doubt about what to expect from a publication once it is picked up. Providing too broad a subject matter often results in failure to convey appropriate information successfully. Moreover, when the subject is excessively broad, the utility of the newsletter as a concise source of information becomes diluted. Once this occurs, the value of the publication is undermined, and it probably will lose its audience. Therefore, defining your subject matter as clearly as possible is critical in the early stages.

PRODUCING AND REPRODUCING YOUR NEWSLETTER

The third step is to determine the parameters of producing and reproducing your newsletter. Take the time to plan how often the newsletter should be circulated. You need to consider the amount of potential information that you intend to transmit as well as the amount of information that your audience can digest. For a medical society newsletter, a quarterly basis may be sufficient to keep the membership apprised of upcoming events and important specialty-related issues. If you are producing a newsletter to promote your practice, you may want to circulate the newsletter monthly, bimonthly, quarterly, biannually, or even annually. Although there may be many things to say, remember that the purpose of your newsletter is to triage and present only the most important information to your readers. One of the advantages of the newsletter format is that it allows presentation of a reasonable amount of information so that your reader is not overwhelmed. If editorial restraint is insufficient, the size of the newsletter may be excessive, and you risk having it get lost among the volumes of other information that your reader may be receiving. Cost per page also may be a limiting variable and needs to be carefully considered.

PRESENTATION OF YOUR NEWSLETTER

The fourth step is to consider the general look of your newsletter or its presentation. The layout transmits a message about the content. Drama and artistic flair may project a message contrary to the seriousness of a medical newsletter. Society newsletters may lend themselves to a more light-hearted and artistic format, but if the message is solemn or scientific, a more staid format may be appropriate.

Presentation is also important in considering cost. The use of color will probably escalate the cost of reproduction up to threefold. In addition, the importing of pictures or graphics will complicate the production of the newsletter and require a bit more sophistication and time in the initial creation. Sophisticated and colorful presentations may introduce a problem with reliable reproduction. If a portion of the newsletter needs to be identical with every issue (such as the banner or a logo), it becomes a real concern in terms of quality. When quality of presentation is compromised, the quality of the content becomes suspect. Therefore, carefully consider the content of the newsletter as well as the cost for production and reproduction.

FINDING THE RIGHT PEOPLE TO HELP YOU PRODUCE YOUR NEWSLETTER

The fifth step in starting a medical newsletter is to find appropriate production people who will be able to work reliably and skillfully within your requirements and deadlines. The proliferation of desktop publishing programs has expanded the list of people to work on your production; however, as with any business venture, the skill level of publishers may vary greatly. Because many publications are under a tight deadline, flexibility and response time are critical.

Printing companies who provide services to a number of other publications may not provide a quick response for last-minute changes, thereby jeopardizing your distribution deadline. Alternatively, a company that is too small may not be able to provide as many services as a larger company. Publishing companies that specialize in medical journals have the advantage of an available staff already familiar with medical language. They also may be useful in providing editorial as well as logistic support in the production process. Such companies should have the ability to assist with all aspects of production and reproduction, which can greatly simplify the process. The cost of this package service may be prohibitive, however, and budget considerations may necessitate that each phase is completed separately. Given the proliferation of desktop publishing, the production phase of the newsletter can easily be done in many office settings in a reasonably efficient manner. If you are able to produce a newsletter in your office, you may have to outsource only the reproduction of the newsletter.

Reproduction also can be done at a variety of businesses. Cost varies significantly and often fluctuates based on the size of your order and the flexibility of your production schedule. Introduction of color and standardized graphics that need to be reproduced identically from issue to issue leads to a predictable loss in reliability of quality. There is no substitute for explicit instructions and good quality control steps. Knowing up front the minimal quality requirements and being prepared to enforce them will help to ensure that your newsletter is reproduced accurately and professionally.

DISTRIBUTING YOUR MEDICAL NEWSLETTER

The sixth and final step in creating a medical newsletter is to distribute the newsletter efficiently to your target audience. In choosing the method of distribution, a number of decisions affect presentation, timing, speed, and cost. The most cost-efficient mailing method is to place the stamp or meter the stamp on the newsletter itself and to mail it third class. Although this method is common, it often results in damaged newsletters and reduced quality. To avoid damage, the newsletter may be placed in an envelope, which increases the cost in two ways—by increasing the weight and therefore the cost of the mailing and by requiring purchase of envelopes. In addition, adding an envelope means an extra step in preparing the newsletter for mailing. This process can be simplified by an automated process of printing the addresses on the envelopes and placing the envelopes in order of zip code. Organizing the mailing by zip code is essential for mailing by third class. In general, the post office is very strict with the regulations of how the mail must be ordered and bagged. The time and effort spent sending a newsletter third class must be weighed against the additional expense of mailing first class. Mailing services charge extra for the labor of this organization, thus reducing some of the cost savings realized by third-class postage. To obtain a better rate with other postage options, you must meet the strict requirements of the post office for a minimal number of pieces of mail per zip code. Checking with the post office to determine the best method of distribution will enable you to stay within your budget and at the same time allow you to send your newsletter in a timely and efficient manner.

Additional considerations must be addressed for mailing overseas. You need to be certain that you have obtained proper addresses and appropriate postage rates for each country. If your newsletter depends on timely arrival, there is a significant increase in expense for mailing either first class or by airmail. This increase can be tempered a bit by using bulk mailing with individual preparation at the target country. This service can be purchased at an overall cost less than mailing directly by first class from the United States. If you choose third class, expect a delay of over one month in arrival time.

CONCLUSION

Deciding to embark on the production and distribution of a medical newsletter can greatly enhance your medical practice. Although the task may seem daunting, following the six steps outlined above will enable you to produce a professional newsletter that targets a specific audience in a cost-efficient and timely manner.

REFERENCE

1. Humphrys BL, et al: Growth patterns in the National Library of Medicine Serials Collection and Index Medicus Journals, 1966–1985. Bull Med Library Assoc 82(1): 18–24, 1994.

JERRY C. PARKER, PhD
RICHARD T. KATZ, MD

17

Strategies for an Academic Career

By most criteria, science is a noble calling. The modern term *science* derives from the Latin root *sciens*, which means "knowing." Yet there are many ways of knowing, including intuition, rationalism, and empiricism. Of interest, the unique combination of rationalism and empiricism has evolved into the powerful tool called the "scientific method." The scientific method involves a cycling from direct observation (empiricism) to an attempt to understand cognitively (rationalism) and then back to further direct observation. Thus, the scientific process systematically spirals to increasingly higher degrees of comprehension of the natural world. Accordingly, a new member of the scientific community steps into a long history replete with the names of persons who have devoted their lives to the pursuit of knowledge—Galileo, Newton, Darwin, Curie, Einstein, and legions of others who, albeit less famous, have been equally dedicated. In short, one should not pick up the mantle of science lightly. Hard work, persistence, dedication, and, above all else, integrity are required to contribute meaningfully to the body of scientific knowledge. Ulterior motives of any kind—acclaim, recognition, financial rewards—will prove insufficient.

SCIENTIFIC ETHICS

Although brilliance, creativity, and mathematical giftedness are desirable, the simple intention to do careful, ethical work is probably a scientist's most valuable asset. Hence, keen attention to the principles of scientific ethics is the starting point for a research career. Any doubt about the veracity of this statement should be quickly dispelled by cursory reflection on the history of scientific projects gone awry. The Nuremberg Trials after World War II revealed the horrific potential for harm to humans in the context of scientific inquiry; Nazi doctors placed their desire for experimentation, most shockingly, above the human rights and welfare of subjects.

Florid examples of unethical research are not confined to totalitarian regimes. In the early 1940s, when penicillin was first discovered, African-American men enrolled in an ongoing naturalistic study of syphilis (the Tuskegee Syphilis Study) were not treated with the newly available antibiotic medication because of the desire to continue the longitudinal research program; the trial was not stopped until 1972. In the 1950s, at the Willowbrook School in New York, a state institution for persons with mental retardation, children were deliberately infected with the hepatitis virus to study the natural history of the disease; in some cases, children needing admission to the school were not accepted unless their parents consented to the studies. In the 1960s, at a San Antonio contraception clinic, disadvantaged Hispanic women seeking contraception were placed in a cross-over trial (involving a placebo) that resulted in unwanted pregnancies; the women were not informed of the placebo arm of the trial. More recently, studies involving radiation exposure to unsuspecting military personnel have been revealed. There are simply countless ways in which well-intending scientists can make appalling errors in ethics. Therefore, a penetrating exploration of ethical concepts is a required exercise for all scientists.

At the most fundamental level, ethical behavior is regulated. The regulations of the U.S. Department of Health and Human Services require that all institutions competing for federal research funds must utilize an institutional review board (IRB) to review and monitor experiments involving human subjects. The regulations cover many diverse topics, such as determination of risk, review mechanisms, informed consent, research with disadvantaged populations, and criteria for IRB approval. A new researcher must be cognizant of IRB regulations and capable of full compliance before a research program can begin. An excellent overview of IRB regulations has been provided by Levine.[3]

Beyond the specific domain of IRB regulations, however, lies the broad issue of professional and scientific ethics. Most researchers, if not all, are members of multiple organizations that restrict their activities through the mechanism of professional codes of ethics. For example, the American Psychological Association has published both a generic ethical code and a specific supplement that covers research ethics. Many medical, academic, and professional societies also embrace ethical codes that are binding on their members. Similarly, most institutions of higher education have policies addressing ethical codes that govern the academic and research behavior of faculty, staff, and students. Any prudent researcher, as a matter of professional responsibility, must maintain complete familiarity with the particular matrix of ethical codes that impinge on his or her scientific behavior.

Even beyond both IRB regulations and ethical codes, however, dwells the broad issue of human values in science. Researchers attempting to act in good faith regarding regulations and ethical codes can, nevertheless, make serious ethical errors because of failure to recognize the potential for intrusion of their own personal biases into their work. At the most basic level, there is always the risk of self-deception because of the tendency to see what we want to see. Yet researchers must be devoted to a relentless search for scientific truth—completely unadulterated by personal biases and beliefs. Because philosophical, religious, cultural, political, and economic values have the potential to affect the judgments of an unsuspecting researcher, extreme vigilance is necessary. Similarly, financial conflicts of interest can easily conspire to cloud objectivity, especially when funding from pharmaceutical companies is involved. Lastly, unchecked motivation for speed of publication or public dissemination may run counter to the thoughtful deliberation and caution required in the search for scientific truth. The pressure to accelerate publication, the compulsion to strengthen a promotion dossier, or a strong desire to attend a particular scientific conference may impinge on the judgment of an otherwise careful investigator.

For all of these reasons, the simple but unflagging "intention to do careful, ethical work" is a genuinely critical asset for any researcher.

RESEARCH TRAINING

For the mastery of most complex skills, in-depth education and training are required; this requirement also applies to aspiring researchers. During the course of traditional graduate training for advanced research degrees (e.g., doctorate of philosophy [Ph.D.]), students spend several years in focused study of the state of their particular scientific discipline. Specifically, students must learn what is already known about their individual disciplines so that they will be able to recognize the cutting edge of their literature; they must be able to formulate scientifically important research questions. Ph.D. students also receive in-depth instruction in the requisite skills of the successful scientist (e.g., research design, statistics, measurement theory). Lastly, students in research-oriented degree programs are required to conduct an independent research project, which permits them to acquire through direct experience the basic skills required of a scientist. Throughout their academic experiences Ph.D. students have the advantage of working with a major professor/advisor who spends several years serving as a research mentor.

For the typical physician entering the academic community, the graduate training experience has been much different. The medical school years are spent learning the fundamentals of clinical medicine; internship and residency are spent developing the skills and knowledge required for a particular medical specialty (and for the passage of specialty boards). Some physicians may have been exposed to a few peripheral research involvements along the way, but typically graduate medical education does not even remotely approximate the type of academic and research training necessary for success as an independent investigator. Therefore, most new physician/academicians have much catching-up to do. Accordingly, one of the first orders of business for a new physician embarking on an academic career is to pick carefully and establish a close relationship with a research mentor.

Of interest, the mentor does not necessarily have to be a person from the aspiring researcher's own professional speciality—or even a physician. More important than professional identity is a track record of successful research accomplishments. Ideally, the mentor should be widely published and have a strong history of extramural funding. For practical reasons, the mentor also should have a genuine interest in the physician's field of study so that the professional relationship will be reciprocally rewarding. Once a mentor has been selected, the young physician can begin to receive advisement about the best strategies for progressing toward his or her research objectives.

Beyond a mentor, a systematic training experience in the form of a research fellowship or some alternative research training program is also highly desirable. The research fellowship can function somewhat like the dissertation year for Ph.D. students. In effect, a structured, hands-on research fellowship can be extremely valuable because the experience is primarily "learning by doing" and, therefore, a helpful contrast to textbook learning and other structured didactics. Many potential funding sources for research fellowships exist; the mentor and the researcher's colleagues can offer specific advisement and recommendations. Nevertheless, in some combination, a new physician researcher must pursue mentoring, fellowship training, and other intensive research training experiences to acquire the core research skills that are typically lacking after a traditional program of graduate medical education.

RESEARCH DESIGN AND METHODOLOGY

One topic of particular educational importance for the aspiring researcher pertains to research design and experimental methodology. Few short-cuts are possible in the mastery of this topic. The central methodologic concept for the beginning researcher involves the ability to ask an appropriate research question. It is insufficient for scientific purposes to pose broad, vague, untestable hypotheses. The keen art of articulating straightforward, unambiguous, focused, testable research questions is an imperative skill. Without this basic ability, researchers do not succeed.

Prospective researchers also must understand the hierarchy of research design, beginning with the "true" experiment, which involves randomized groups and manipulation of a single, independent variable. Furthermore, the researcher must be able to distinguish between true experiments and quasi-experiments, for which complete experimental control is lacking. In the quasi-experimental situation, experimenters must make accommodations for preexisting groups and otherwise accept that the desired degree of experimental control cannot be achieved. In addition, prospective researchers must be able to recognize the strengths and limitations of correlational studies in which the relationships among two or more variables are examined. Finally, aspiring researchers must be able to appreciate the appropriate application of observational studies and single-case designs. Each of these experimental levels is a major topic in its own right, and each level demands in-depth understanding on the part of a prospective investigator.

For human experimentation, in particular, researchers must understand the key principles of random sampling and the techniques for maximizing the representativeness of an experimental cohort. Specifically, a researcher must appreciate how to facilitate the generalizability of research findings and the extrapolation of results to a broader population. Similarly, both internal and external validity of a study must be assured. Therefore, researchers must understand how to create the conditions for a valid, reproducible experiment.

Another important methodologic principle pertains to levels of measurement. Researchers must be able to differentiate categorical measures, which simply attach an identity or characteristic to a subject or a group, from ordinal, interval, and ratio levels of measurement. At the ordinal level, only distinctions of higher versus lower can be made. At the interval level, the units of measurement are presumed to be equal (e.g., temperature on the Fahrenheit scale), whereas at the ratio level the units of measurement are equal and the zero value represents a true absence of the variable (e.g., height in inches). Each level of measurements has unique characteristics that affect experimental methods and statistical possibilities.

Several excellent texts help researchers to master the fundamentals of research design and basic experimental methodology. A particularly excellent source is *Designing Clinical Research* by Hulley and Cummings.[2]

STATISTICAL STRATEGIES

The fundamental principles of statistics are fairly straightforward; most physicians will have already completed one or two statistical courses during their undergraduate years. Yet the statistical literature is evolving daily. New ways of approaching statistical problems, new tests, and new statistical outlooks are published regularly. In addition, as a result of the revolution in computer technology, there is essentially no end to the complex mathematical calculations that can be accomplished in support of applied biostatistics. For the typical nonstatistician, mastery of statistical principles is a daunting task indeed—not to mention the process of keeping abreast of the latest developments.

Fortunately, physicians do not have to become statisticians to succeed as researchers; they simply have to collaborate with a well-trained, professional statistician. Research institutions inevitably have statisticians on faculty, although their accessibility varies widely across settings. In some institutions, statistical consultants are readily available at little or no cost. At other institutions, statistical services must be purchased from grant funds or departmental resources. Given the challenging fiscal climate of medical schools, the most common scenario requires some form of monetary support from users of statistical services. Nevertheless, statisticians are almost always accessible in research settings, and they are invaluable colleagues.

As a cautionary note, there are numerous personal computer-based statistical packages on the market; most are excellent in terms of generating statistical solutions. The problem is that statistics is a cognitive specialty. Skill comes not from the operation of a software package but from the knowledge of what statistical approaches are required in a given situation. In the hands of an unsophisticated user, a statistical software package can be dangerous (i.e., can yield potentially false conclusions). Therefore, the aspiring researcher should not confuse statistical computation skills (which almost anyone can acquire) with the cognitive skills of a statistical consultant (which only a professional statistician can provide). The astute researcher will find a good statistician and cultivate a close, collaborative relationship.

Finding a good statistician is just the first step; researchers also must learn how to become effective statistical consumers. For effective collaboration, the researcher must understand what the statistician has to offer. Specifically, early in the collaborative process the statistician typically focuses on the research question and may be able to help the researcher define or clarify the exact hypothesis. The statistician also explores the proposed research design to make sure that the necessary data are collected to answer the specific research question. The statistician helps to calculate the needed sample size, designs the data collection format, and helps to devise strategies for ensuring data quality. When a project is completed, the statistician oversees the data analyses, helps with the interpretations of results, and typically cowrites the statistical sections of a research paper.

In turn, a researcher must facilitate the tasks of the statistician. Most importantly, the researcher should initiate the statistical consultation *before* data collection begins; the researcher should avoid presenting already collected data to the statistician because there are simply too many ways to make fatal mistakes in the data collection process. Statisticians do not like to work on salvage jobs, in which they are asked to try to save something from a flawed method. They want to be involved from the start. Statisticians also expect researchers to make an adequate time commitment to their own projects and to be knowledgeable about exactly what they are doing. Statisticians do not want to be in a position of knowing more about the details of a research project than the researcher.

Research assistants come and go; therefore, researchers must assume responsibility for knowing the details of their own projects.

The statistician also expects the researcher to have a basic mastery of the scientific literature pertaining to the research question; issues in the literature often affect statistical decisions. In addition, the researcher must have preliminary knowledge of fundamental statistics (or be willing to acquire it) so that the necessary professional communication can take place. Several excellent introductory biostatistical textbooks are available; Shott[5] and Colton[1] are excellent sources.

SCHOLARSHIP AND THE SCIENTIFIC LITERATURE

One of the fundamental keys to a successful research program is the ability to position one's work on the cutting edge of a field of scientific inquiry, but finding the cutting edge is more difficult than meets the eye. In most cases, a researcher's ideas are not completely novel; someone probably has pursued similar studies before. Therefore, mastery of the scientific literature is imperative for truly scholarly work; a researcher needs to learn from the mistakes and successes of others to conceptualize and design optimal experiments. Beginning researchers must remember that science is a shared endeavor and that progress is made through collaborative efforts and the synergy of the scientific community. Accordingly, aspiring researchers must resist the temptation to work (and think) in isolation. The scientific literature constitutes a rich source of ideas, an introduction to state-of-the-art methodology, and a way to discover relevant theories. Science is greatly enhanced by theories that (like straw men) are set up to be knocked down. Theories lead to predictions that, in turn, may evolve into compelling research projects. Specifically, the scientific method is more than just data collection; a scholarly process is required to motivate and direct empirical efforts.

The information explosion is a fact of modern life, particularly for scientists. New scientific articles are published daily, and keeping up with one's field can be quite difficult. Fortunately, electronic aids are available, but the place to begin is typically with an experienced medical librarian. As is the case with statistics, an effective literature search involves a cognitive process, not just software gymnastics. An inexperienced searcher can waste countless hours using ineffective strategies and end up with incomplete information. For example, MEDLINE is only one of numerous scientific databases; typically the medical librarian can markedly expand a researcher's source of information by examining additional databases. In short, a medical librarian often gains access to the pertinent scientific literature for a given research topic more quickly and accurately.

One particularly useful strategy is to establish a recurring literature search that identifies new articles as they appear in the literature. In this way, up-to-date information (typically monthly) can be transmitted to the researcher based on his or her preset search parameters. Such automated strategies are extremely valuable because they can save enormous amounts of time, which is one of a researcher's most precious commodities.

An inevitable problem arises when a researcher seriously delves into the scientific literature; namely, large numbers of reprints begin to accumulate. Fortunately, reference manager software dramatically eases the burden of sorting, organizing, and filing reprints. Each new reprint is given an identification number and entered into a database; reprints are simply filed in numerical order by identification number. Retrieval is accomplished by either author name or subject heading; the identification number always makes access easy. The best advice is to start with the reference manager system early in one's career before the random, disorganized stacks of reprints begin to accumulate. An additional advantage of reference manager software is that reference lists for publications can be easily and accurately constructed from the database, which saves much valuable time for the researcher. Most reference manage software can format references in a wide range of bibliographic styles, which makes changing from one style to another an easy matter.

The bottom line is that successful researchers must be good scholars. They must be keenly aware of what is occurring in their scientific fields, and they must be able to place their studies in a broader scientific context.

CRITICAL PEER REVIEW

In the research process, an openness to critical feedback from peers is a valuable asset. In many situations, researchers are required to commit their ideas to paper and to solicit feedback from their peers: namely, when they write proposals, when they apply to IRBs, when they submit to local research committees, when they forward manuscripts for publication, and when they prepare grant applications. In each instance, the researcher risks (and probably will receive) critical feedback. In some ways, human nature tends to induce defensiveness and frustration when one's hard work is reviewed critically, or even rejected, by peers. Yet the process of opening up scientific products to critical review has the potential to be extraordinarily constructive. If approached correctly, each critical review has the potential to improve the quality of scientific work. The most successful researchers do not try to avoid constructive criticism; in fact, good researchers actively solicit peer reviews as a way of sharpening their own scientific rigor. In general, the optimal way to get feedback is to produce one's best scientific product and then to ask directly for critical review. Researchers who send out rough drafts of their manuscripts or grants are less apt to get useful commentary in return. Colleagues do not usually want to devote their time to the review of an incomplete scientific product or, in essence, to rewrite a scientific document themselves. In contrast, colleagues are much more likely to respond constructively when they can see that a researcher has put forth his or her best effort on a scientific product; then they typically contribute their energies to help move a manuscript to a higher scientific level.

In its purest form, research is simply a search for scientific excellence; a genuine openness to critical peer review can be a valuable strategy in helping a researcher to achieve his or her best scientific potential.

DATA MANAGEMENT SYSTEMS

The beginning researcher should be meticulous about the establishment of data collection systems; good habits in this area will serve a researcher well over an entire career. Data collection errors occur in numerous ways. Forms can be filled out incorrectly by subjects; numbers can be incorrectly transcribed, or data entry errors can occur. Similarly, summary scores can be calculated incorrectly, or mistakes can be made in the electronic manipulation of data. In the worst case scenario, data (or even entire data sets) can be misplaced or even lost.

Good researchers simply do not let data collection errors of these types occur. Instead, they develop precise, meticulous systems for managing their data sets; in fact, all researchers have an ethical obligation to do so. Successful researchers typically involve a statistician in the development of data management systems because most errors can be avoided by careful design of forms, double entry of data, and statistical programming to identify out-of-range data points. In the field of research, careless management of data is completely unacceptable and unethical; one or two erroneous outliers can dramatically alter the results from studies that involve only small-to-moderate sample sizes. A researcher should never be in a position of doubting the validity of his or her data; thus, beginning researchers should possess a thorough understanding of the need for meticulous data management.

SCIENTIFIC COMMUNICATION

Success as a researcher involves extensive writing and other forms of scientific communication. Clearly, a researcher must be able to convey effectively his or her ideas, plans, proposals, and outcomes to others in the scientific community. Therefore, lucid scientific writing and effective public speaking assume extreme importance for the aspiring researcher. Yet, for many scientists endowed with extraordinary quantitative gifts, truly professional writing skills are not fully developed. Indeed, the precision and clarity required for optimal scientific communication demand more writing expertise than many researchers have previously been required to exhibit. Therefore, aspiring researchers typically can benefit from a commitment to the enhancement of their writing skills as a life-long learning process. Possibly the most notable example of an exceptional scientific writer is Edward O. Wilson, the Harvard biologist, who twice won the Pulitzer Prize in General Non-Fiction; the 1991 prize was for a scientific textbook entitled *The Ants*. Wilson appears to have little room for improvement in his scientific writing, but most researchers have ample opportunity for growth as scientific writers.

Of interest, in his memoir[6] Wilson compared his approach to scientific communication to that of a storyteller. Simply put, his life-long scientific quest was to find scientific stories and to tell them with exceptional clarity. Aspiring researchers would do well to emulate Wilson's straightforward, honest, unembellished approach to scientific writing.

RESEARCH FINANCING

Research costs money. At the least, the time that a researcher devotes to a project has a monetary value. More typically, research also involves additional personnel, space, equipment, clerical support, subject fees, computing time, and a host of other potential cost categories that, in some combination, are part of the expense structure for a given project. To a great extent, a researcher must be adept at both obtaining and conserving money.

With few exceptions, successful research programs are funded by extramural grants from sources such as the National Science Foundation, National Institutes of Health, Institute on Disability and Rehabilitation Research, private not-for-profit foundations, and/or private industry. In most cases, grant applications are highly competitive, and only the top-ranked submissions (5–25%) are typically funded. Accordingly, talented researchers who wish to see their research programs survive over time must be constantly planning for the financing of their scientific work.

Funding dilemmas are a never-ending reality for most researchers. The aspiring investigator should bear no illusions about the necessity for winning extramural funds; without such monetary support, a researcher's career will end quickly. Unfortunately, there are no short-cuts in the competition for extramural funds; well-conceived, cutting-edge research proposals generally will be funded, whereas mediocre proposals will not.

At the inception of a research career, start-up funds from a researcher's department or institution can sometimes be arranged, but such funds are almost always time-limited. Deans and departmental chairs expect a return on their investments; extramural awards eventually have to arrive for institutional support to continue. For physicians, in particular, the fiscal pressures are intense. Relatively speaking, the salaries of physicians are high, and their clinical skills have the potential to generate money. Thus, a physician who cannot successfully compete for extramural funds usually will be reassigned to clinical duties fairly quickly.

Although private industry is sometimes a less competitive source of research funds, there are many potential problems. First, the lower level of critical peer review does not serve a researcher well in the long run; successful researchers must receive the critical support of scientific peers to function effectively within the scientific community. Otherwise, the researcher's efforts will yield little in terms of publications and contributions to the scientific literature. Second, private industry typically has its own agenda; industry tends to expend funds on the basis of economic potential, not necessarily on the basis of scientific appeal. Therefore, with funding from private industry, a researcher often is gradually pulled from cutting-edge research endeavors into commercial ventures that typically have little or no scientific value. In short, the aspiring researcher should be somewhat skeptical about financial support from private industry. At most, industry funds should only augment funding from competitive, peer-reviewed sources, not replace it entirely. The reality is that aspiring investigators must commence planning for the funding of their scientific work at the inception of their research careers.

ADMINISTRATIVE SKILLS

Successful researchers are typically good administrators (or at least wise enough to hire someone who is). At the practical level, research is a major administrative task in which time and money are central elements. In some combination, the processing of paperwork, meeting of deadlines, management of time, conservation of resources, and cultivation of a harmonious work environment are inherent in the process of research administration; the cycle never ends. Following the awarding of a grant, a researcher must establish the infrastructure for a protocol, recruit subjects, collect data, manage information, arrange for statistical analyses, and present or publish the results of the study—all within a relatively short time. Otherwise, future awards are unlikely. Review boards are not inclined to give additional funds to a researcher who has not used a previous award wisely. Therefore, researchers must confront the reality that the operation of a research program is much like the operation of a small business, except that scientific excellence must be a key part of the equation.

There are many strategies for administrative success. In fact, self-proclaimed gurus on the subject are ubiquitous, but each researcher must find his or her own way. Clearly, time must be used wisely, funds must be managed carefully, and personnel must be supervised optimally to achieve success in a research program. There are no easy solutions, but the aspiring researcher must realize that long-term success is unlikely unless effective administrative strategies can be brought to bear on the complexities of the typical research program.

CONCLUSION

Experimental researchers acknowledge that research is hard work, especially in the context of Western society, where capitalism and productivity are dominant values. In some ways, the necessity for researchers to survive in a highly competitive environment runs counter to the optimal conditions for creativity. Playwright Arthur Miller points out that the plight of the aspiring scientist is much like that of the aspiring artist.[4] In both cases there is great pressure to produce products that are saleable in order to garner the necessary funds to continue. For the artist, the sales are to the commercial establishment, which is willing to pay for products that are marketable to the masses. For the researcher, the sales are to granting agencies and review boards that have the power to fund a research program, but the granting agencies and review boards often have their own preferred themes or special priorities that affect the selection process. Accordingly, researchers are often forced to focus on the special interests of the granting agency, not just on their own creative process.

Yet, despite all of these pressures, the life of a researcher can be genuinely rewarding. Much like an artist, a researcher has the prerogative to pursue an area of special interest, and this process can be highly self-actualizing. In fact, besides researchers and artists, few persons are afforded the opportunity to be paid to pursue their own intellectual interests, and the satisfaction to be derived from producing an intellectual product of enduring value is truly great. When a researcher publishes a paper, the work exists for the benefit of society, and it exists for all time. The personal rewards for the researcher can be great indeed.

Lastly, aspiring researchers should remember that there is more to life than research alone. The greatest research productivity probably comes from investigators who are able to maintain balance in their lives. Family, friends, exercise, sleep, and recreational pursuits factor into the research equation in some way. The best strategy is not to focus on research (demanding as it can be) to the exclusion of everything else. Beyond a point, the obsessive researcher typically loses effectiveness, creativity, and perspective. With a balanced life and a healthy pursuit of academic excellence, a research career can be extraordinarily rewarding and genuinely self-actualizing.

ACKNOWLEDGMENTS The authors gratefully acknowledge the intellectual contributions of their colleagues: Thomas Findley, Lynn Gerber, Gary Goldberg, John Hewett, Jane Johnson, David McDonald, Gregory Petroski, Michael Priebe, Elliot Roth, Gordon Sharp, Richard Harvey, Steve Gnatz, and Steven Stiens. The assistance of Barbara Cullen and Kathleen Koch in the preparation of this manuscript is also appreciated.

REFERENCES

1. Colton T: Statistics in Medicine. Boston, Little, Brown, 1974.
2. Hulley SB, Cummings SR: Designing Clinical Research: An Epidemiologic Approach. Baltimore, Williams & Wilkins, 1988.
3. Levine RJ: Ethics and Regulation of Clinical Research, 2nd ed. New Haven, CT, Yale University Press, 1988
4. Miller A: On creativity. Arthritis Rheum 35:985–989, 1992.
5. Shott S: Statistics for Health Professionals. Philadelphia, W.B. Saunders, 1990.
6. Wilson EO: Naturalist. New York, Warner Books, 1994.

W. MICHAEL ALBERTS, MD, MBA

18

Business and Management Training for Physicians

In a recent issue of *American Medical News*, Borzo noted, "No longer is it enough for a physician to be a well-trained professional, a good scientist, and a caring person. Increasingly, medicine depends on financial skills and business sense."[1] Some say that this reality is a sad commentary on the state of health care today. Nevertheless, it is a reality, and the prudent physician should attempt to acquire the skills and knowledge necessary to ensure his or her success.

Business and management issues may consume a significant component of a physician's day. The pulmonologist who is medical director of the intensive care unit, the cardiologist in charge of the cardiac catheterization laboratory, the family physician who is chair of the hospital quality assurance committee, the urologist who heads the medical group compensation committee, and the pediatrician who is a member of the group practice board of directors require expertise outside the field of medicine. On a wider scale, each and every physician is faced with staffing and organizing his or her office, meeting government regulations, and dealing with third-party payors (and do not forget personal finances). Business and management skills and knowledge will prove beneficial for physicians in the 1990s and beyond.

For some physicians, medical management is now a legitimate career choice. Until 10–15 years ago, if you asked the average physician why any doctor would choose to assume management duties or even a full-time managerial role, the traditional response was that the physician was seeking a more relaxed lifestyle or escape from the rigors of clinical medicine.[2] Management roles were primarily titular or liaison positions that lacked real authority or responsibility. Such positions were thought to be a stepping stone to retirement or a safe haven for doctors who failed to build a successful practice.[2] Things have changed.

The need for physician managers and leaders is great. As Rice noted:

> [F]ifty years ago, most positions of influence in the U.S. healthcare sector were held by physicians. Today, in sharp contrast, most positions of power are held by nonphysician managers and policymakers. Physician leaders were pushed— or chose to step—off to the side as business, finance, and insurance specialists assumed positions of influence during the period of health-sector expansions in the 60's, 70's, and 80's. Recent assessments seem to indicate the erosion of physician influence has turned a corner. A new era of physician power seems increasingly likely, particularly if individual physicians conscientiously prepare for their new opportunities, and if medical schools and journals increase their attention to the formal development of needed leadership knowledge, skills, and attitudes.[3]

Although the need is great, until recently medical school and postgraduate curricula did not sufficiently address everyday, practical business and management issues; indeed, such issues were often ignored completely. Solomon has even suggested that "the medical education establishment owes physicians an apology":

> By ignoring the business side of medicine, medical schools and training programs have produced a profession that is ill prepared to knowledgeably participate in the national debate on health care reform, to develop new forms of practice better suited to the new environment, and to assume management roles and responsibilities.[4]

Fortunately, business and management training is gradually assuming a place in the curriculum for medical students[5] and postgraduate trainees.[6] A few medical schools now offer joint M.D./M.B.A. (e.g., Wake Forest University, University of Pennsylvania) or M.D./M.P.H. (e.g., Tufts)[7] programs. Although this new emphasis on the business of medicine may benefit future graduates, most physicians currently in practice lack sufficient business and management training.

Given the need for business and management education and the fact that most practicing physicians did not receive such training, how can the prudent physician obtain these beneficial skills? The goal of this chapter is to answer that question. In doing so, three topics are discussed: (1) why physicians might be interested in management, (2) why management is a different science from clinical medicine, and (3) what options are available for obtaining business and management training.

WHY THE INTEREST IN BUSINESS AND MANAGEMENT?

Why might physicians be interested in the business and management side of medicine? Most survey studies addressing this question have found that the three most common reasons for assuming a managerial role or responsibilities are (1) desire to improve health care ("I had a need to plan and fix things."), (2) desire to influence others ("I had ideas that I wanted to see implemented."), and (3) desire to develop policy ("It is important for physicians to become involved in the larger policy issues in health care.").[2]

Another survey found that the most common reasons for physicians seeking or accepting management positions were a desire (1) to be challenged, (2) to lead others, (3) to achieve more professional growth, and (4) to maintain continued autonomy.[3] Physicians entering a master of business administration degree program were asked how they expected their degree to affect their financial status: 10 expected their income to decrease, 19 anticipated no change, and only 9 expected an increase (VA Syperda, personal communication, 1993). Most studies confirm the fact that physicians do not assume managerial positions or duties merely for monetary compensation. Of note, Kirschman recently reported the results of a survey indicating that the average annual salary base for a full-time physician executive in 1995 was $180,930 for hospitals, $206,704 for group practices, and $182,633 for managed care organizations.[8] Top-level positions may command a base well over $200,000 with a potential bonus package of 9–37% of the base.[9]

MANAGEMENT: A DIFFERENT SCIENCE

Business and management skills are different from clinical skills. The best clinician will not necessarily be the best manager and leader. The converse, however, is usually true: the best manager and leader is most often an outstanding clinician. Table 1 contrasts the skills and attributes needed by a skilled clinician with those needed by the effective physician manager.[10] Many are polar opposites. For example, Kissick noted that the medical practitioner is compelled to master a body of knowledge to ensure expertise, whereas the manager is trained to orchestrate the expertise of others.[11] According to Roth, "Management skills are not an inherent part of anyone's abilities. They have to be acquired."[12]

Several studies have looked at the common attributes demonstrated by successful medical leaders. In 1987, Brown and McCool interviewed a number of

TABLE 1. Major Differences between Clinicians and Managers

Clinicians	Managers
Doers	Planners, designers
1:1 interaction	1:N interactions
Reactive personality	Proactive personality
Require immediate gratification	Accept delayed gratification
Deciders	Delegators
Value autonomy	Value collaboration
Independent	Participative
Patient advocate	Organization advocate
Identify with profession	Identify with organization

From Kurtz ME: The dual role dilemma. In Curry W (ed): The Physician Executive. Tampa, American College of Physician Executives, 1994, pp 81–88.

health care leaders, not all of whom were physicians. The successful medical manager was characterized as energetic, hard-working, calm in the face of a crisis, visionary, and entrepreneurial.[13] In a similar survey study, Leider and Bard asked physician managers throughout the country the following questions: What are the key skills or core competencies for physicians looking to undertake management or leadership roles? Clinical credibility, communication skills, team-building ability, experience in negotiation and conflict resolution, and expertise in quality management were the items most commonly listed.[2] Table 2 gives a more comprehensive list.

In a recent study, physician executives were asked to identify desirable traits in an effective medical director.[14] Communication and interpersonal skills were found to be the most important. Clinical credibility, ego strength, concern about quality, and being a team player were listed frequently. In this particular study, formal training was not considered of great importance. Most surveys, however, have found that the physician manger should become knowledgeable in financial analysis, cost-accounting, economics, decision analysis, marketing, and strategic planning.[15] In most organizations, nonphysician managers are usually responsible for such functions, but the physician manager must "speak the language."

OPTIONS FOR OBTAINING BUSINESS AND MANAGEMENT TRAINING

When a physician recognizes the need for business and management education, either to serve current needs or to pursue future career goals, the applicable

---

TABLE 2. Key Competencies and Skills for Physician Managers

Communication skills	Negotiation and conflict resolution
Listening	Striving for "win-win" situations
Speaking	Focusing on interests rather than
Writing	positions
	Encouraging others to communicate
Leadership skills	and resolve conflict
Articulating a vision for the future	Serving as a facilitator
Creating an environment of shared responsibility	
Developing the skills of others	Quality management
Framing and facilitating critical conversations	Articulating a philosophy of continuing
	improvement
Team building	Embracing the "good apple" approach
Embracing a participatory leadership style	Focusing on processes as the cause of
Developing a common goal or purpose	problems
Creating a climate of communication and trust	Empowering the people who do the work
Effectively leading meetings	to solve problems
Recognizing and encouraging synergy	Using data to gain insight into problems

From Leider HL, Bard MA: Leadership in managed care organizations: The role of the physician manager. In Nash DB (ed): The Physician's Guide to Managed Care. Gaithersburg, MD, Aspen Publishers, 1994, pp 63–94.

question is not whether to obtain business and management training, but rather how to obtain it. That decision presents a new series of questions. What is the appropriate setting for training? What level of knowledge is sufficient? What level of knowledge is recommended? How valuable or necessary is a formal degree in management? How practical is it for a busy physician to obtain this education?[16] The answers to these questions depend on the individual but hinge on background, prior training, prior experience, current job responsibilities, and future aspirations.[16]

There are several options for acquiring business and management training. Self-study and on-the-job training are the traditional approaches and continue to be common. Numerous textbooks addressing general business and management issues and issues specific to health care are available. Computer-based learning opportunities are becoming increasingly available. For example, the Society for Medical Decision Making offers a CD-ROM program entitled "Health Economics." Look for an explosion in this type of computer-based training. The American College of Physician Executives has recently piloted a course for physicians delivered over the Internet. Look for an explosion in long-distance learning as well.

Many larger insurance companies, managed care organizations, and group practices offer in-house management training programs for employees and affiliated physicians. The Department of Internal Medicine at the University of South Florida in cooperation with the College of Business Administration recently developed a business administration skills certificate program for division directors and departmental leaders. The program is delivered in four modules: (1) economics and the environment of business; (2) finance and accounting skills; (3) managing and negotiating; and (4) marketing, service operations management, and management of quality. An optional fifth module (computer skills and management information systems) will be offered to those who lack computer skills and fundamental understanding of the role and scope of information systems in the medical management environment. Each module consists of four sessions, four hours each, meeting once a week.

A second popular option is attending short-course programs similar to those in continuing medical education (CME) that address business and management issues. A more formal option is participation in fellowship, sabbatical, or certificate programs. The most structured and intense option is pursuing the third degree (i.e., M.B.A., M.P.H., M.H.A., M.S.)

SHORT-TERM WORKSHOPS OR SEMINARS

The pursuit of a formal graduate degree is an expensive and time-consuming process and should not be undertaken lightly.[17] For physicians with little or no management experience, it is often a good idea to assume some part-time administrative duties to test the waters. Such opportunities permit the physician to acquire key management skills and competencies by involvement in progressively more challenging management roles.[17]

If the physician discovers that he or she enjoys such activity, a good place to begin to obtain advanced education is short-term workshops or seminars, which are commonly offered by professional associations, universities, and private sector accounting, management, or consulting firms. Such seminars are generally of short duration (1–5 days) and tend to stress problem-solving and skills-building rather than theoretical or in-depth analysis.[18] An example is the three-part "Physician in Management" series of seminars developed by the American College of Physician Executives. These seminars are basic, sampler-type courses, but they are outstanding for the curious and those whose background in management is minimal (Table 3). A number of other professional associations offer similar CME-type productions, including the Medical Group Management Association, Society for Physicians in Administration, American College of Medical Practice Executives, American College of Healthcare Executives, American Board of Quality Assurance and Utilization Review Physicians, and the American Group Practice Association.

Colleges and universities provide an excellent source of short-term educational opportunities. The University of Southern California Center of Excellence in Health Care Management has offered a five-day Executive Management Institute in Health Care. The Wharton School of Business of the University of Pennsylvania has offered a $4\frac{1}{2}$-day program entitled Management Development for Physician Executives. The cost of this program was approximately $3000. The Harvard Medical School's Department of Continuing Education offers a program entitled Leadership for Physician Executives—A Seminar for Health Care Administrators. The cost for this one-week session is approximately $4000. The Owen Graduate School of Management at Vanderbilt University offers a number of health care management executive programs, ranging from the Management Program for Health Care Professionals and Managers, which meets weekly for four months, to a two-day course entitled Activity-based Costing and Management for Health Care Organizations. The University of North Carolina Kenan-Flagler Business School, in association with several organizations, offers a "mini-MBA" program entitled Medical Management for Physician Executives. Four separate one-week sessions are conducted on the Chapel Hill campus. These are but a few examples of many such programs.

FELLOWSHIPS, SABBATICALS, AND CERTIFICATE PROGRAMS

An opportunity that may require less downtime than a formal degree but that provides more advanced course work is short-term sabbaticals or fellowships. Berman has described one such nondegree program offered by the Harvard Business School.[19] This program is a well-regarded, 12-week, intensive learning experience that provides contact with managers from all fields.[19] The benefits

---

TABLE 3. Physician in Management Seminars Sponsored by the American College of Physician Executives*

Seminar I	A Systems Perspective of Health and Medical Care
	The Economics of Health Care
	The Economics of Organizations
	The New Environment of Regulated Competition
	Strategic Planning and Marketing
	The Physician as Manager
	Management Skills for Physician Managers
Seminar II	Competition and Conflict
	The Shifting Sources of Power and Influence
	Influence Through Effective Communication
	The Fundamental Principles of Negotiation
	Successful Strategies and Tactics of Negotiation
	Building Strategies for Success in Health Services
	Planning That Works for Healthcare Organizations
	Ethical Challenges of Physician Executives
Seminar III	Implementing Change
	Managing Quality of Service
	Creative Problem Solving
	The Physician's Role in Managing Organizations
	Putting It All Together

---

* For more information, contact the American College of Physician Executives, 4890 West Kennedy Boulevard, Suite 200, Tampa, FL 33609-2575. Telephone: 813-287-2000, fax: 813-287-8993.

of such a program include (1) a limited but intense time commitment, (2) the opportunity to immerse oneself totally in the discipline, and (3) strong linkages to high-level managers from nonmedical fields.[16] Drawbacks include (1) the need to be away from family and work for a certain time, (2) the large immediate cash expense, and (3) the lack of a formal degree after completion.[16] Various colleges, universities, and private foundations offer similar programs.

The American College of Physician Executives has developed a program called the Graduate Program in Medical Management. The program is billed as an alternative to traditional graduate degree programs in management and attempts to recognize CME activities. The graduate program requires completion of the Physician in Management Seminars I and II plus focused seminars in management of professional performance, quality management, management of change, health care finance, medical informatics, ethics, health law, and additional electives. These requirements are followed by a 72-hour, on-campus Capstone Course at Tulane University in New Orleans.

THE THIRD DEGREE

After completing these introductory steps, many individuals are committed to a career in medical management or making management a larger part of their job description. A legitimate question at the this point is whether they should pursue a formal graduate business and management degree. In 1986, the

Physician Masterfile from the AMA listed 14,399 physicians whose "primary professional activity" was administration. A survey of this group found that only 12.7% reported a management master's degree.[20] Moreover, 9.8% had obtained M.P.H. degrees an average of 17 years previously. Such a degree program would have been unlikely to include management education as we currently understand it. The other 2.9% reported M.B.A. or M.S. degrees within the previous 10 years or so. These degrees probably correspond more closely to current management training.[17] Although a minority of those sampled in the study held a graduate degree, 22% of respondents indicated that formal graduate coursework or an advanced degree would be required for administrative positions in the future and 62% indicated that such management training would be advisable.[20]

In a 1994 survey conducted by Hay Management Consultants of 2468 members of the American College of Physician Executives, 22.0% of respondents held advanced degrees (41%, M.B.A.; 31%, M.P.H.; 9%, M.H.A.; 3%, M.P.A., and 15%, others).[9] When asked if a management degree was beneficial, 22.6% said very beneficial, 34.1% said beneficial, 37.6% said somewhat beneficial, and only 5.7% said not beneficial. In a broader study by Witt/Kieffer, Ford, Hadelman, and Lloyd, 9.4% of physicians in management positions reported having an M.B.A. This figure is up from 6% in 1990 and none at all in 1979. Moreover, 38% of physicians in the survey were working on or intended to pursue an M.B.A.[21]

Therefore, physicians serious about spending a good portion of their professional day in management should consider an advanced degree or advanced business and management course work. Most executive search firms believe that an advanced degree is not critical in the selection process for physician executives.[22] Experience is every bit as important. Lyons has stated that "it is evident that management know-how and proven experience always count for more than the 'initials' alone when clients offer a management job. Nonetheless, roughly half of the physician executives hired today are physicians with two degrees."[23] Kindig and Sanborn stated that by 1998 some kind of formal management degree will be expected by most organizations when they hire physician executives.[17] The physician who completes an advanced business or management degree program demonstrates seriousness, motivation to excel that is outside the norm, and true commitment to mastering business and management principles and theory.[23]

A recent review of the demographics of the M.B.A. for Physicians Program at the University of South Florida revealed that the average age of participants was 44 years with a range of 30–63 years. The average clinical experience was 12 years, and the average administrative experience was 9 years. Most were affiliated with a hospital or clinic (31%), 25% were solo practitioners or in small groups, and 22% were in a group practice. Only 9% were from academic medicine. The most common specialty of enrollees was internal medicine (21%), followed by surgery (10%) and emergency medicine (9%). Most other specialties were represented in the remaining 60%.

BASIC QUESTIONS IN LOOKING FOR
A SPECIFIC ACADEMIC PROGRAM

If the decision is made to pursue a formal degree program, several basic questions must be answered: (1) which degree?, (2) which educational format?, (3) which university?, and (4) what is the cost?

The most common third degrees are Master of Hospital or Health Service Administration (M.H.A), Master of Business Administration (M.B.A.), Master of Public Health (M.P.H.) and Master of Science (M.S.) in administrative medicine, management, or related titles. The course work leading to a law degree (J.D.) rarely includes sufficient training in business and management. Although this degree may provide a physician with unique skills (such as negotiations and contracting), a masters degree will likely prove more useful for physician executives. The choice of a specific master's degree revolves around a number of factors.

There are several types of educational format. The traditional full-time, on-campus format is difficult for most mid-career clinicians. Although it may be the most stimulating and satisfying way of getting a degree, time and financial constraints make it an option for the lucky few.[17] A second option is a part-time, on-campus format, which may be feasible if the campus is within driving distance. Advantages include ability to pursue the degree at your own pace, availability of elective courses, and often in-state tuition. Disadvantages include the longer time required for the degree (up to 5 years) and the difficulty of fitting a regular university course schedule into an active medical practice.[17]

A third option is the executive format, which is designed to fit the schedule of the mid-career student who is employed on a full-time basis. As an example, the executive M.B.A. program at the University of South Florida meets all day Friday of one week and all day Saturday the next week for 2 years. Similar executive programs meet one weekend per month. Alternatively, the executive M.B.A. for physicians at the University of South Florida meets in six separate two-week blocks over the course of two years. The major advantages of the executive format are the ability to retain employment and an income stream during the program and the unified curriculum with one single class unit creating a bond for the entire group. Disadvantages of the various executive models include fragmentation of the academic experience, travel time and expense, relative lock-step nature of the program, limited availability of faculty between classes, and generally higher fees.[17] The course load in the executive format is constant and heavy, with significant pressure to keep up with the class. Time spent outside of class averages 20 hours per week.[16] This type of format may prove to be a grueling experience that often takes a toll on family and friends. A considerable amount of tension can develop among work demands, academic load, and family responsibilities.[17]

The decision about which specific college or university involves convenience, reputation, specific program content, and cost. Clearly, proximity to the class site is an important variable; however, programs that combine guided independent study with periodic in-resident sessions may minimize its importance. A program with a strong reputation adds value to the degree, but this factor may be less important for the mid-career physician who is more interested in an education than a credential. According to Lyons, "It doesn't matter where you get your MBA degree. Prospective employers are more interested in results and generally pay less attention to a top-name school, versus what you have been able to accomplish."[23] Specific program content may be an important variable. Education and training must fit with the career goals of the student. Program costs must be considered; they vary considerably among programs. Of the nine executive M.B.A. programs in Florida, the cost of tuition varies from $15,000–35,900 for the two-year program. Remember, however, that the direct costs pale in comparison to the indirect loss of income. Total direct and indirect costs can exceed $150,000 per year.[17]

SPECIFIC DEGREES

MASTER OF PUBLIC HEALTH (M.P.H.)

M.P.H. programs are generally located in schools of public health and are oriented toward public health administration. An M.P.H. may be obtained in one year or in the evening over several years. As an example, the traditional M.P.H. program at the University of South Florida requires the successful completion of five core courses consisting of 15 semester hours (biostatistics, epidemiology, health services organization and administration, environmental health, social and behavioral sciences). An additional 24 semester hours may be sought as electives to meet the 39-hour requirement for graduation from the various departments in the college (community and family health, epidemiology and biostatistics, environmental and occupational health, health policy and management).

The University of South Florida has recently developed an executive M.P.H. for physicians (Table 4). Class members progress through required courses over 20 months. Participants are expected to commit to the schedule of five, two-week resident sessions plus a minimum of 12–15 hours per week between resident sessions for program-related readings, case analyses, computer-based training, and other assignments. Additional requirements include completion of field experience, a written special project, and a comprehensive examination.

TABLE 4. Course Outline for the Executive M.P.H. for Physicians at the University of South Florida*

Session 1	Environmental and Occupational Health
	Social and Behavioral Science Applied to Health
	Biostatistics I
Session 2	Biostatistics II
	Principles of Health Policy and Management
	Epidemiology
Session 3	Epidemiology of Diseases of Major Public Health Importance
	Information Management in Public Health Settings I
	Introduction to Social Marketing
Session 4	Management of Public Health Programs
	Community Coalition Development and Advocacy
	Information Management in Public Health Settings II
Session 5	Seminar: Ethics, Policy, and Law in Public Health
	Seminar: Public Health Practice

---

* For more information, contact Executive MPH for Physicians Program, University of South Florida, College of Public Health, 13201 Bruce B. Downs Boulevard, MDC 56, Tampa, FL 33612-4799. Phone: 813-974-6606, fax: 813-974-4718.

In general, the M.P.H. curriculum does not include management material in great depth. The University of North Carolina, however, offers an M.P.H. in management. Subjects such as epidemiology and biostatistics may be more adequately covered in an M.P.H. program compared with other degrees.

MASTER OF HEALTH ADMINISTRATION (M.H.A.) AND MASTER OF SCIENCE IN HEALTH ADMINISTRATION (M.S.H.A.)

The M.H.A. degree often requires two full years of on-campus study. Accredited programs require an integrated series of courses that cover the following: (1) determinants of health and illness and measurement of health status; (2) economic, ethical, legal, political, and psychosociologic perspectives on the organization, financing, and delivery of health services; (3) management of organizations and their environments, including communication, conflict management, leadership, management of change, and negotiation; (4) financial, economic, and quantitative analysis, including accounting, finance, economics, cost/benefit analysis, and statistics; (5) information management; and (6) strategic management and marketing. Field work and an integrating thesis usually are required.[17]

Executive format programs are also available. The University of Colorado in Denver in cooperation with the Network for Healthcare Management offers an executive program in health administration (Table 5). This 25-month program includes five residential sessions totaling 7 weeks on campus. An average of 20 hours of study time per week is required at home. Approximately one-third of the class are physicians, one-third are from nursing and other allied health professions, and one-third are nonclinical managers. The University of North

---

TABLE 5. Course Outline for the Executive Master of Health Administration Program at the University of Colorado*

Management Accounting in Health Organizations	Management Information Systems
Organizational Theory and Design	Quantitative Methods
Statistics and Epidemiology	Marketing Management
Health Economics	Ethics and Health Law
Health Care Sociology and Medical Care Organization	General Systems Theory
	Competitive Strategy
Human Resources Management	Management of Health Care Institutions
Financial Management in Health Organizations	Microeconomics

---

* For more information, contact Executive Programs, University of Colorado, PO Box 480006, Denver, CO 80248-0006. Telephone: 303-623-1888, fax: 303-623-6228.

Carolina offers an executive master's program in health policy and administration. The program requires both annual on-site summer institutes and independent guided study.

MASTER OF SCIENCE (M.S.)

M.S. programs vary greatly with the specific nature of the degree. An example is the executive program in general management offered by Northwestern University's Kellogg Graduate School of Management, which leads to a Master of Management degree. Another example is the M.S. in administrative medicine from the University of Wisconsin. This 22-month program is divided into four semesters with six residential sessions for a total of 9 weeks on campus. The program recruits physicians and nurses who have administrative responsibilities or plan a career change into management. The course of study includes courses from the M.B.A. and M.H.A. programs (Table 6). Tulane University offers a Master of Medical Management degree program. Successful completion of the graduate program in medical management earned through the American College of Physician Executives and three one-week, on-campus modules are requirements for the degree. The curriculum includes key management skill areas such as financial management and decision making; strategy formulation and implementation; payment systems and risk management; organizational dynamics, marketing, health economics and policy; and human resource management.

MASTER OF BUSINESS ADMINISTRATION (M.B.A.)

The M.B.A. is generally offered by the college of business. The accreditation standards and guidelines for the M.B.A. are less specific; therefore, specific program content may differ. Foundation courses in accounting, economics, and statistics are encouraged. One year of instruction is required in the common body of knowledge in business administration, which includes production and marketing of goods and services; financing of business and other types of

TABLE 6. Course Outline for the Master of Science in Medical Administration Program at the University of Wisconsin*

Business and Management Fundamentals	Medical Management Applications
Health Accounting and Financial Management	Epidemiology/Outcomes Management
Organizational Behavior	Quality Measurement and Improvement
Strategic Planning	Medical and Managerial Ethics
Quantitative Methods in Management	Health Policy and Law
Health Economics	Technology Assessment
Principles of Insurance	Management of Health Care Professionals
Marketing	History of Medicine
Information Systems	Integrating Case Summary
Capital Budgeting	Executive Preceptorship
	Management Analysis Thesis

* For more information, contact Administrative Medicine Program, University of Wisconsin–Madison, 214 Bradley Memorial, 1300 University Avenue, Madison, WI 53706-1532. Telephone: 608-263-4889, fax: 608-263-4885.

organizations; economic, legal, and ethical environments pertaining to profit and nonprofit organizations; concepts and applications of accounting, quantitative methods and management information systems; organizational theory, behavior, and interpersonal communication; and study of administrative processes under considerations of uncertainty, including integrating analysis and policy determination at the management level.[17] The content of the advanced course work in the second year varies widely.

An executive-format example is the M.B.A. for physicians at the University of South Florida. This 21-month program includes six residential sessions for a total of 12 weeks on campus (Table 7). Additional examples include the executive M.B.A. in health services management at the Olin School of Business at Washington University in St. Louis. Classes meet every other weekend for 21 months. The University of California at Irvine offers a health care executive M.B.A. program. This two-year program allows practicing physicians, as well as other health care professionals, to attend classes once a month from Thursday night to noon on Sunday.

WHICH DEGREE?

The answer, of course, depends on various factors. The M.B.A. has the advantages of more courses in advanced business and analytic skills but often at the expense of applications to medical management.[17] Kindig and Sanborn estimated that for most physician executives, 30–40% of advanced business knowledge may be of limited usefulness.[17] Physicians should seek M.B.A. programs that offer electives or course work in health care finance, health care law, economics, epidemiology, ethics and values, management of health professionals, and health organization management.[17] Depending on the position sought,

---

TABLE 7. Program Outline for the Master of Business Administration for Physicians at the University of South Florida*

Session 1	Statistics for Managers
	Decision Support Tools
	Microeconomic Analysis for Managers
	Management Processes
Session 2	Financial Accounting for Managers
	Marketing Management
	Epidemiology
Session 3	Macroeconomic Analysis
	Administration of Human Resource Systems
	Managerial Accounting
Session 4	Financial Management I
	Management of Conflict and Bargaining Behavior
	Management Information Systems
	Service Operations Management
Session 5	Financial Management II
	Strategic Planning
	Legal Environment of Business
	Seminar in Organizational Change
Session 6	Risk Management
	Health Policy Analysis
	Total Quality Management

---

* For more information, contact The MBA Program for Physicians, College of Business Administration, University of South Florida, 4204 Fowler Avenue, BSN 3403, Tampa, FL 33620-5500. Telephone: 813-974-4876, fax: 813-975-6604.

the M.B.A. is likely to be the preferred credential. However, the softer management skills of effective communication, participatory leadership, team building, conflict resolution, and quality management are perhaps more important for the successful physician manager. In most formal M.B.A. programs, little time may be devoted to these core competencies.

The M.H.A. or M.S. programs offer a balance of business and health management courses. Prospective students should examine the specific programs carefully, however, to be sure that adequate business course work in finance, organization theory, marketing, and insurance concepts are covered by business school faculty.[17]

An M.B.A. or an M.H.A./M.S. is the most common management degree sought by physician executives. As a rule, the M.P.H. is directed at a specific area of medicine and is therefore not considered a general business or management degree.

CONCLUSION

Medicine is changing rapidly. Not long ago, the health care industry was truly different from other business enterprises, but this is no longer the case.

Medicine is now under the same intense pressures that trouble General Motors, IBM, and Bob's Bicycle Repair. Physicians undoubtedly will play an important role in shaping the health care system of tomorrow. Unfortunately, however, physicians will not be the only players and may not even be the major players. Nonphysician administrators may have more than their fair share of the influence. Although a sound educational background, significant clinical experience, and a solid reputation will continue to be important credentials, physicians who hope to influence or actively participate in the change will have to acquire and master a widening range of business and management skills.

Fortunately, there are several routes to acquiring these skills. On-the-job training and self-paced learning are common approaches but may not be sufficient or optimally efficient. Short-term seminars and workshops may provide the basics and may be sufficient for many situations. More formal programs, such as fellowships, sabbaticals, or certificate programs, offer advanced education and training within a limited time frame. A master's level degree program offers the most complete learning experience. The decision to pursue a graduate business and management degree requires significant thought and planning. Major time and resource factors must be considered. Successful completion of such a program, however, provides substantial career and personal growth benefits.

REFERENCES

1. Borzo G: Coping in the new world will take a new set of skills. Am Med News January 2, 1995, pp 3–5.
2. Leider HL, Bard MA: Leadership in managed care organizations: The role of the physician manger. In Nash DB (ed): The Physician's Guide to Managed Care. Gaithersburg, MD, Aspen Publishers, 1994, pp 63–94.
3. Rice JA: A new era of power: Doctors moving toward roles of 'statesmen,' managers. Modern Physician May:58–62, 1997.
4. Solomon RJ: Medical profession needs business training to survive. Am Med News April 24, 1995, p 19.
5. Tibbitts GM: Leadership education for medical students. Physician Exec 22(9):31–34, 1996.
6. Brooks JP: Suggestions for management training of residents. Physician Exec 22(3): 26–28, 1996.
7. Boyer MH: A decade's experience at Tufts with a four-year combined curriculum in medicine and public health. Acad Med 72:269–275, 1997.
8. Kirschman D: Physician executives share insights. Physician Exec 22(9):27–30, 1996.
9. Hay Management Consultants: Medical Management Compensation Survey—1995. Tampa, American College of Physician Executives, 1995.
10. Kurtz ME: The dual role dilemma. In Curry W (ed): The Physician Executive. Tampa, American College of Physician Executives, 1994, pp 81–88.
11. Kissick WL: Bridging the cultural gaps. Physician Exec 21(2):3–6, 1995.

12. Roth L: Life as a medical manager. In Hammon J (ed): Fundamentals of Medical Management. Tampa, American College of Physician Executives, 1993, pp 1–6.
13. Brown M, McCool BP: High-performing managers: Leadership attributes for the 1990's. Health Care Manage Rev 12:69–75, 1987.
14. Ottensmeyer DJ, Key MK: Lessons learned hiring HMO medical directors. Health Care Manage Rev 16:21, 1991.
15. Hillman AL, Nash DB, Kissick WL, Martin SP: Managing the medical-industrial complex. N Engl J Med 315:511–515, 1985.
16. Bloomberg M: Management training for the physician executive. Physician Exec 18(2): 10–14, 1992.
17. Kindig D, Sanborn A: Is there a master's degree in your future? Physician Exec 16(1): 15–18, 1990.
18. Cooksey J, Hand R: Training medical managers at the academic health center. In Minogue WF (ed): Managing in an Academic Health Care Environment. Tampa, American College of Physician Executives, 1992, pp 159–168.
19. Berman JI: Nondegree business education program may be the answer. Physician Exec 17(1):56–58, 1991.
20. Kindig D, Lastiri S: Administrative medicine: A new medical specialty? Health Affairs 5:146–156, 1986.
21. Anders G: A new breed of MD's add MBA to vitae. Wall Street J 1995, pp B1 and B10.
22. Grebenschikoff J, Kirschman D: Getting the third degree. Physician Exec 15(2):27–28, 1989.
23. Lyons MF: The MBA mystique. Physician Exec 22(11):39–41, 1996.

JOHN S. LLOYD, MBA, MSPH
MARY FRANCES LYONS, MD

19

From Medicine to Management: When Physicians Become Executives

As executive search consultants in the health care industry, we hear frequently from physicians who are considering a career change. Their desire is to move from working as a full-time clinician or teacher to a leadership role in administration or management in a health care organization. Although some have already embarked on a new course, enrolling in management classes or even full-time business degree programs, others are still testing the waters, unclear about their options. They feel unsure about the risks involved in leaving active work in the profession for which they spent so much of their lives preparing.

Our work also brings us into contact with experienced physician executives who have achieved success in many different situations—hospitals, systems, managed care organizations, insurance companies, pharmaceutical and medical device companies, agencies, and professional associations, among others. They have already made the challenging career change to full-fledged executive, demonstrating that for them, at least, the risks are worth the rewards.

At whatever stage of the decision-making process you may find yourself, take these words of encouragement and support from executive search consultants who are daily in the marketplace for senior executives: the opportunities in health care management have never been greater for physicians, and the need has never been more pressing for the unique combination of clinical insight and leadership that talented physician managers can provide.

Additional proof of the increasing importance of the physician executive, if any were needed, can be found in the stunning growth of the American College of Physician Executives (ACPE) from a small group in the 1980s to its current membership of more than 12,000. More evidence of burgeoning growth is the development of physician-specific M.B.A. programs. These, along with the broad range of business and management educational opportunities now available to physicians through many sources, attest to the national trend that is moving many from medicine to management.

A seasoned physician executive who is particularly positive about opportunities in the field is John C. Babka, M.D., FACP, FACPE, FACHE, vice president of medical affairs (VPMA) for Morton Plant Mease Health Care in Dunedin, Florida. He commented recently:

> This is the best time yet for entry-level physician executives. They can readily find starting positions in managed care companies and PHOs [physician-hospital organizations], where their medical skills are needed as much as their management abilities. Stronger management skills are needed to progress to the VPMA level, but there are plenty of places where one can begin.

According to Babka, the proliferation of physician executives comes at the right time for the health care industry:

> It is a dream of mine that one day soon we will see not-for-profit, provider-sponsored networks truly *managing* care for community health. And the leadership for those networks will come from those who know best how to care for patients while controlling costs—physician executives, who are ideally positioned to take on the challenge.

However, he warned young physician executives:

> This is not a job for everyone. If you're a person who places great value on the collegial aspects of your work, you'll need to rethink your career change from medicine to management. Because of ingrained distrust, physician executives essentially function without a supportive peer group and are not entirely accepted by either physicians or administrators.

SEARCHES DOUBLED IN ONE YEAR

Those who pursue a career in health care management are not guaranteed success, but the timing has never been better for qualified individuals. A review of our firm's search assignments for 1995 and 1996 shows that the number of physician executive search engagements has doubled in that time. That is remarkable growth.

Even more revealing: 1996 was the first year that the percentage of search assignments for physician executives (18% of the firm's total searches) was greater than search assignments for chief executive officers (CEOs) (14%). There can be no doubt that physician executives are in demand.

A combination of factors has led to the emerging need for physician executives, led perhaps by personal choice but also influenced greatly by national trends in health care. Examples include the impact of diagnosis-related groups (DRGs) and the consequent need for clinical expertise in senior management decision-making; integration of health care delivery and creation of better-managed large continuum models requiring savvy leadership; and cost-efficiency and quality questions posed by managed care and insurance companies.

We possess a unique perspective because it is our job to assist organizations to find precisely the right person with exactly the right combination of skills and character. When our clients—health care organizations of every size and configuration—began asking us to find physicians who have strong executive skills and experience, we knew that that a new trend had begun to unfold

A GLANCE BACKWARD

Only about 20 years have passed since significant numbers of physicians began to seek out (or be offered) administrative opportunities within the health care industry. Once having tasted the challenges and rewards of management in hospitals, first in appointed posts such as chief of staff or department chairperson and moving into part- or full-time medical director roles, some physicians began to relish the career growth and development opportunities offered by the evolving health care environment. However, they were still few and far between.

The need for clinically trained administrators who can assess quality of care and outcomes began to increase in health care organizations with the proliferation of Medicare-mandated payment schemes based on DRGs. As the health care industry became more competitive, individual organizations sought to downsize by creating leaner and more efficient administrative teams. This trend produced the climate in which the physician executive's breadth and depth—a combination of executive talent with clinical insight—suddenly was highly valued. In addition, genuine partnering with physicians by hospitals and systems became necessary; physician executives who can bridge the gap between physicians and nonphysician administrators became vital members of the senior management team. Another thrust came from the business community, which began to depend on physicians for guidance in achieving economies through the thickening maze of health care costs. In addition, the explosion of diversity in health care delivery systems that began in the 1980s led to new, more diverse career paths for physicians. When opportunities for physician executives opened in these new types of organizations, qualified individuals were ready to accept the challenges. A vital, dynamic career marketplace for physician executives has emerged swiftly.

WHY DO PHYSICIANS ENTER MANAGEMENT?

In 1996, our search firm, Witt/Kieffer, Ford, Hadelman, & Lloyd, conducted a national survey of physician executives employed in both provider and payor organizations. A total of 820 questionnaires was distributed, and 247 usable responses were received (response rate = 30%). The results were published in the magazine of the ACPE in the fall of 1996. In addition, a summary of the findings was published by the firm in early 1997.

When asked why they had entered medical management careers, physician executives gave positive and optimistic responses. Forty-five percent said that they had a desire to be part of the health care solution. Another 36% said that their interest in management/leadership challenges led to their decision. Other reasons cited by respondents included the following: waning of medicine's challenge over time; frustration with practicing in a managed care environment; desire to improve income; wish to enhance management skills; post-retirement opportunities; health or disability factors that curtail medical careers; and desire for more predictable schedules and defined hours.

This chapter focuses on issues that may arise when physicians decide to make a career change from medicine to management. Although the transition is not easy, according to those who have made the move, it is ultimately rewarding.

ROLE OF PHYSICIAN EXECUTIVES

Most health care provider organizations have (at the minimum) a vice president of medical affairs (VPMA) or equivalent physician executive whose job, in large part, is to mediate and communicate effectively between the employer and its physicians. Of course, physician executives in provider organizations hold many other roles and titles—in medical information service, practice development, and management of various treatment facilities, to name but a few. However, the VPMA is usually the most senior role specifically held by physicians in management and is typically a career goal of those who make the move from practitioner to executive.

The role of the VPMA is complex. The VPMA must be able to move easily between physicians and administrators and communicate effectively with both. In a crisis, however, although medical colleagues may wish to claim the VPMA's first loyalties, the VPMA is a member of administration whose priorities must encompass the good of the entire hospital or system. Executive leadership, not just clinical ability, is required.

In our 1996 national study findings, physicians in senior management considered the roles of physician, leader, and manager and ranked them as they view themselves today and five years ago (Table 1). The rankings indicated a major shift in the self-perceptions of physician executives. The percentage of those who view themselves first as physicians has declined, whereas perceptions of their role as leaders have risen markedly. A higher percentage of those in payor as opposed to provider organizations continue to view themselves first as physicians, perhaps because their positions have a greater clinical emphasis.

TABLE 1.   National Surveys of Physician Executives*

Role Ranked No. 1	Total (%)	Payors (%)	Providers (%)
Current rankings			
Physician	42	46	40
Leader	47	51	40
Manager	10	13	8
Rankings 5 years ago			
Physician	80	74	83
Leader	13	18	11
Manager	6	8	5

* Multiple responses may add to > 100%.
Source: Witt/Kieffer, Ford, Hadelman, & Lloyd

CAREER CHANGE CAVEATS

As executive search consultants, we speak daily with physicians at every stage of their careers (from new medical school graduates to seasoned practitioners); many are considering a change to management. Our experience includes hundreds of personal interviews each year with physician executives, and our firm recorded more than 60 successful senior executive searches for physician executives in 1996. This extensive background has shown us that the transition is not for everyone. Based on our experience in the field, we offer important points that will affect the success of your career change:

1. Mobility increases your marketability. Physicians often remain in a single locale throughout their careers because they like the familiarity and continuity. On the other hand, executives must be willing to go where the best opportunities exist, accepting career moves as necessary to success. Relocation is an issue that involves your family's needs and wishes as well as your own. You must be willing to move, and your family should be enthusiastic as well.

2. You must be thick-skinned. Executives must make many tough calls—e.g., closing services, downsizing, allocating limited resources—and be willing to accept the consequences. In contrast, physicians generally enjoy their status as healers and life-savers; they thrive on the emotional rewards that come with caring for patients when they are ill and vulnerable. In which mode are you more comfortable?

3. Compensation is more than money. Although the average earning power of physicians and senior health care executives is not so different, the method of payment certainly is. In medicine, physicians (especially in fee-for-service situations) are compensated directly for their work. Their annual earnings represent how many patients they see efficiently in a year's time, not how many return to health. However, executive compensation is more long-term and related to success, although the results may not be known for months or years. Thus, executive compensation, especially with incentives and bonuses, depends on the performance of many other people. Can you be comfortable with this method of compensation? (Current salary information is included in a later section.)

4. Tolerating new stresses. Physicians already know the stresses that come with making life-and-death decisions. As executives, they will experience other kinds of stressful situations, often caused by leading lengthy decision-making processes to influence and persuade others. The physician executive position was once considered a step toward retirement but not today. Unlike a physician, whose key decisions involve the diagnosis and treatment of patients, an executive faces problems that often have no single right answer. The result: a different kind of stress. Can you work well in a situation in which decisions always seem to be in process?

CAREER OPPORTUNITIES ABOUND

Assuming that you have not been deterred by the previous caveats, take a look at the many options. Diverse opportunities for physicians include both traditional and cutting-edge situations. The newest opportunities for physician executives are in information systems, whether for a data management company (e.g., HCIA, Inc., in Baltimore or the National Committee for Quality Assurance [NCQA] in Washington, D.C.) or as director of information systems at a health care organization, putting information technology at the service of medicine to make possible better diagnoses and treatment.

Other opportunities for physicians with management ability abound in health care systems, physician group practices, corporate offices of pharmaceutical firms and insurance companies, consulting firms, outcomes and quality management organizations, universities and medical schools, and hospitals. A physician who is an experienced, skilled executive can go far in a wide variety of health care and industry organizations.

WHAT SKILLS ARE NEEDED?

The basic skills portfolio of a physician entering a position in health care management is likely to include:

1. Human resources management. Managing people is an art, involving both learned skills and good natural instincts. To enhance a career transition to management, some physicians enroll in short-course business management programs or full M.B.A. degree programs; both are excellent ways to learn management techniques. However, positions that offer actual management responsibility should become your priority. Do not miss a chance to exercise management skills in your current employment and in professional or community activities.

Do not be passive or half-hearted about acquiring management skills. Those who do not genuinely wish to manage others will find it difficult, if not impossible, to succeed as physician executives.

2. Communication. An executive must be able to relate well with a wide range of people. Good communication requires strong listening, speaking, and writing skills. Effective communication can achieve the consensus sought by the process-oriented decision making of most health care organizations. Hierarchical systems have been replaced by empowerment and shared decision making, which depend on good communication skills.

3. Financial understanding. A solid understanding of the financial implications of issues is essential for physicians in management. Success is measured by whether an organization's books are balanced and its overall financial picture is healthy. An executive who can identify areas where cost-savings can be found or revenue expanded without sacrificing quality is in demand.

4. Strategic thinking. An executive must have a global perspective on issues and an increasingly sophisticated understanding of population-based health care scenarios. Openness to new concepts for health care delivery is vital.

5. Team play. An executive must listen to many points of view to formulate a planning strategy. Team leadership can be a challenge for physicians who are accustomed to planning and deciding alone.

6. Physician relations. It is unwise to assume that a physician executive is skilled in physician relations. The most credible physician relations skills are applicable in many settings, not just with old friends and trusted colleagues. The ability to generate credibility and establish rapport quickly greatly enhances the potential for success.

7. Specific skills for managed care. To be effective in managed care positions, a physician executive needs all of these skills and more. Managed care positions demand understanding of how physician efficiency translates into quality. Because some physicians believe that restrictions on their decision making can lower the quality of patient care, a physician executive in managed care must be able to explain the intricacies of payment methods while helping physicians appreciate managed care's virtues. To accomplish this goal, the physician executive has to understand both outcomes measurement methodology and outcomes management. Success is achieved by those who are able to cultivate respect and leadership. General skill areas utilized in managed care positions include *marketing and sales*. Often physicians in managed care settings are involved in making presentations—for example, in contract negotiations with business coalitions or meetings with consumer groups. Such public forums require thinking on your feet. Another key skill is *quantitative disease management*. Some progressive managed care organizations have moved away from traditional utilization review in favor of better care systems, using pathways and best practices as templates. Managed care also requires

---

TABLE 2. National Professional Groups

American College of Physician Executives (ACPE)
4890 W. Kennedy Blvd., Suite 200
Tampa, FL 33609
(813) 267-2000

American College of Healthcare Executives (ACHE)
One North Franklin Street, Suite 1700
Chicago, IL 60606-3491
(312) 424-2800

American Association of Health Plans (AAHP)
1129 20th Street, NW, Suite 600
Washington, DC 20036-3421
(202) 778-3200

---

skill in *outcome measurement*. Benchmarking results is a challenge in assessing effectiveness of care systems and requires knowledge of information systems, data capture, and analysis.

GETTING A START

If you are serious about making your move into management, begin by looking for opportunities in your current situation. Ask for responsibility, and learn everything you can in the process. Those enrolled in management courses, especially in a management degree program, will find advisors able to offer valuable suggestions and tips, but you have to ask them for assistance.

Look into opportunities offered by the ACPE as well as other national and regional professional groups, such as the American College of Healthcare Executives (ACHE) and the American Association of Health Plans (AAHP) (Table 2). Any or all may be an appropriate professional group for your interests and circumstances.

When you have achieved a reputation for outstanding executive ability, you can expect to hear from executive search firms, who will want to talk with you about how well your skills meet the needs of their clients. Do not call an executive search firm to find a job; they will call you. You should send a resume to one or more executive search firms and ask to be included in their databases of talented executives. Establish friendly relationships with executive search consultants whom you may meet at conferences or presentations or who may call you for a reference for someone else. Do not assume that you can call them for a job. Search firms work for their client organizations, not for individuals or candidates.

Most search consultants are willing to give you career advice, and they have fresh information to share. For example, because we work with so many clients and regularly conduct national studies, our firm has excellent data about physician executive compensation.

TABLE 3. 1996 Survey Findings: Average Salaries Analyzed by Key Factors

Key Factor	Total ($)	Payors ($)	Providers ($)
1–3 years in organization	155,000	146,000	166,000
4+ years in organization	187,000	167,000	193,000
Promoted as physician executive in current organization	186,000	162,000	200,000
Not promoted as physician executive	158,000	144,000	167,000
Worked as physician executive only in current organization	171,000	141,000	183,000
Worked in 2 or more organizations as physician executive	179,000	160,000	197,000
Career mentor	176,000	154,000	191,000
No career mentor	169,000	152,000	179,000
Mentored other physician executives	190,000	167,000	203,000
Has not mentored others	151,000	137,000	160,000
Currently in medical practice	177,000	148,000	185,000
Not currently practicing	167,000	154,000	181,000
Base is $150,000 or less	126,000	130,000	120,000
Base is $151,000–199,000	174,000	172,000	176,000
Base is $200,000+	246,000	219,000	252,000
Employed in health system	—	—	177,000
Employed in hospital	—	—	187,000
Employed in group practice	—	—	153,000
Employed in insurance company	—	147,000	—
Employed in managed care company	—	158,000	—

The firm's 1996 national survey of physician executives in both provider and payor organizations yielded key information about salaries of physician executives (Table 3). The average base salary of respondents was $172,000, ranging from under $100,000 to $500,000. The average salary for those in provider organizations (e.g., hospitals, systems, clinics) was $183,000; for those in payor organizations (e.g., managed care, insurance companies), the average was $153,000. Note that these are average salaries; above-average performers can command far higher salaries. A review of the firm's search assignments for the past year offered similar information for 1996 (Table 4).

TABLE 4. Salary Information from 1996 Search Engagements

Function	No. of Placements	Low ($)	High ($)	Average ($)
Physicians (M.D.s) (all)	62	70,000	350,000	178,677
Chief executive officers (all)	51	50,000	550,000	160,474

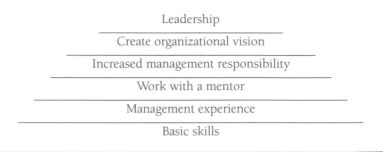

Leadership

Create organizational vision

Increased management responsibility

Work with a mentor

Management experience

Basic skills

FIGURE 1. Pyramid of health care leadership attainment.

GOING TO THE NEXT LEVEL

Whether you have just decided to enter the management ranks or embarked on that course some time ago, achieving proficiency in basic skills is the necessary first step. But you are likely to aspire to higher titles and greater responsibility as you acquire experience and seasoning.

As a practicing clinician, you may not have considered your next career move. You did not need to do so. You probably expected to remain in the same practice or location, dealing with patients (and their children and grandchildren) until you retired. An executive, in contrast, seeks to move up, to enhance his or her position, as skills are mastered. The question is how you will leverage basic skills and enthusiasm into administrative positions at higher levels. Competitive individuals will already have noted that nonphysician executives in health care organizations have a head start of 15 years or more.

Figure 1 demonstrates a physician executive's path to full exploration of his or her executive potential. Assuming that you have achieved competence in the basic skills through education and by seizing volunteer opportunities that came your way, you are ready to move on and up.

Management Experience. Ask for management responsibility; seize it if it is offered. There is no shortage of tasks to be performed, but often too few hands are ready to take them on. Have you served an elected term in your organization or taken your turn as head of a key committee? One young physician literally created his first management opportunity by persisting with requests until his CEO found him administrative work. Although the assignments he was given may have seemed humble, they were completed well and with good humor. In brief, he was launched. This is no time for false pride. You must prove yourself, just as when you were fresh out of residency. You may have to ask for a management internship, unpaid if need be, to get a foothold in the kind of organization that you want. Your unpaid status soon will be rectified if you can show that you have the ability to do the job.

Work with a Mentor.   The national research by Witt/Kieffer in 1996 showed that at least two in five active physician executives credited a mentor with playing "a pivotal role" in their careers. A mentor relationship can take many forms. Some mentors are role models, demonstrating their own management skills; others take a more advisory role. A mentor can offer encouragement, counsel, support, and feedback while also listening and giving direction. Your mentor need not be a physician executive. If you find a civilian senior executive who has an interest in your career, one with whom you can communicate easily, ask him or her to be your mentor and look no further. The 1996 survey data indicated that the average physician executive's mentor was a senior health care executive (75%). Rarely did a colleague at the same level (16%), a non-health care executive (3%), or other (7%) serve as a mentor. A good mentor can provide priceless grooming, polish, and style. There may be, in fact, no better or faster way to fine-tune your career than by working with a mentor.

Increased Management Responsibility.   This move upward can result from luck, skill, or a bit of both. One physician executive's mentor was named CEO of a system; the mentor subsequently recommended her for the presidency of one of the system's hospitals. Others have sought opportunities more directly, looking for organizations that offer new experiences to improve their skills. Sometimes that may require leaving the provider side entirely, either to a corporate managed care setting or into business or industry. The opportunities are definitely there, if you want them. Taking this step is not without its down side. Stepping up may involve real sacrifices for you and your family—moving far away or making other big changes in your lives. You must really want to reach the top if you are to get there—yet there are still no guarantees of success.

Creating a Vision.   This step seems almost inevitable, as it flows from the experience of greater responsibility. Leaders tire of having a boss; you will begin to want to *be* the boss. You will articulate your own operating style, and others will gravitate to your position. You are not attempting to create dissension, but when you see it occur, you bring cohesion. You are developing a leadership vision.

Leadership.   The apex of the pyramid is the place that some (but not all) physician executives aspire to reach. This is the place where the physician executive is able to exercise vision and move organizations, or even the whole country, forward. The charismatic leadership of David Kessler, M.D., at the Food and Drug Administration through two presidential administrations led the country to adopt a new, more critical perspective on nicotine and tobacco. His vision and leadership are inspirational for many others. Some day there will be cures for cancer, AIDS, and Alzheimer's disease—and physician executives, like Kessler and others, will be leading the way. And when new challenges arise, physician executives will continue to step up and provide the needed leadership. The future will be an exciting time for physician executives.

REFERENCES

1. Babka JC, personal interview, 1997.
2. Compensation Trends for Healthcare Executives in 1996: Compensation Report No. 3. Oak Brook, IL, Witt/Kieffer, Ford, Hadelman & Lloyd, 1997.
3. Lloyd JS, Lyons MF, Singer GR: The new physician executive. Physician Exec Fall, 1996.
4. The New Physician Executive: Leadership for the Future. Oak Brook, IL, Witt/Keiffer, Ford, Hadelman & Lloyd, 1997.

20

Going to Court

There is little doubt that we live in a litigious society. By nature of their profession in caring for people who have been injured or who have had complications from medical treatment, physicians must expect that during their careers they will become participants in the litigation process. This chapter explores the ways in which physicians are involved in litigation, either as fact witnesses, expert witnesses, or defendants in a medical malpractice case.

FACT WITNESS

Physicians should be aware of the possibility that every time they treat a patient who has been injured or is incapacitated, the circumstances giving rise to the injury or the consequences of the injury or incapacity may lead to litigation. The litigation may be criminal, civil, or administrative.

CRIMINAL LITIGATION

Many physicians' first experience with litigation occurs during residency, in the criminal court, as a result of providing emergency treatment. If a patient has been the victim of an assault, the criminal prosecution of the accused perpetrator often requires testimony from a physician about the nature and extent of injuries suffered by the patient. Almost without exception criminal trials of a sexual assault case involve testimony by a physician concerning the clinical findings at the initial examination.

As eager as physicians may be to see that the perpetrator of a vicious assault does not go unpunished, they must not ignore their legal obligations to the patient. Sometimes, particularly in domestic violence situations, the patient may not want a prosecution to go forward. Although the physician may strongly disagree with the patient's position, the patient does not usually waive her right to confidentiality by having been assaulted. Many states, however, require physicians who suspect that a patient has been abused (e.g., child abuse, elderly abuse, domestic assault, sexual assault) to report the case to either the police or a state social service agency. Physicians, particularly those whose practice involves a significant amount of emergency or primary care treatment, should be aware of their state's regulations. In the absence of a state statute that mandates reporting of suspected domestic abuse, the physician must be cautious when the prosecutor (usually an assistant district attorney or assistant state's attorney) telephones to discuss a patient who was possibly abused. The physician may not discuss any details about the patient's condition or care without the patient's express consent. In most instances, the patient is quite happy to have the physician review clinical findings with the prosecutor; thus, the patient's consent is obtained by the prosecutor without difficulty. However, if the patient wants the prosecution dropped, the physician risks being sued by the patient for breach of confidentiality if the physician speaks to the prosecutor or testifies without a court order compelling the testimony. Whenever they are contacted by an attorney on a matter involving litigation, physicians should consult either the legal department or risk management office at their hospital or their own attorney before giving out information or responding to a subpoena from a prosecutor to testify or to produce records.

The other side of the coin is when the patient is the target of the criminal justice system. For instance, after a physician treats the injured driver of an automobile, the police and prosecutor may seek the physician's opinion about whether the patient was intoxicated. This information is of particular importance if other parties to the accident have been seriously hurt or killed. Despite a possible natural inclination to see that justice is done, without a state statute authorizing or requiring physicians to report suspected intoxication to the police in such circumstances, physicians cannot violate the patient's confidentiality without a specific judicial order requiring them to testify.

CIVIL LITIGATION

Unlike criminal litigation, which involves a legal action brought by the state, usually seeking the imprisonment of the accused, civil litigation involves a lawsuit brought by an individual seeking monetary damages against another individual or corporation. The area of civil litigation that requires physician input is *tort*, or personal injury, law. The typical tort case is the result of an accident, such as an automobile accident or a fall, in which the patient claims that his or her injuries were caused by the negligence of another person. A patient usually needs at a minimum medical records from the physician to establish the nature and extent of his or her injuries. In some instances, the patient or the party that the patient has sued also may seek the testimony of the physician about the injuries. A physician is often made aware of the possibility of a tort suit on receipt of a letter from an attorney requesting a copy of the patient's records. The letter usually makes clear that the attorney is representing the patient in connection with the accident or injury. The letter should be accompanied by a document signed by the patient authorizing the physician both to provide the attorney a copy of the record and to speak to the attorney about care and treatment. Because the records are the patient's, the patient is entitled to have his or her attorney provided with a copy. The records cannot be released in response to a letter, however, unless the patient has signed an authorization. The physician can charge the attorney a reasonable copying fee for the records.

At some point after the records are sent, the attorney may call the physician to set up an appointment to talk about the case. Physicians are under no legal obligation to speak to the attorney and may so advise the attorney. Many physicians, however, believe that as part of their professional relationship with a patient, they should be willing to speak to the patient's attorney about the patient's care and treatment. However, a physician is entitled to be compensated for speaking with the attorney. Before the meeting, the physician should request a reasonable fee, usually based at a minimum on the amount of billing the physician would have generated if the time spent in meeting with the attorney had been spent seeing patients. To discourage attorneys from taking up their time or unnecessarily involving them in the litigation process, some physicians demand an hourly fee that will give pause to the attorney's request for their time.

There is no reason for physicians to feel that their fee for meeting the attorney should be reduced because the patient cannot afford it. The patient is referred to in civil litigation as the plaintiff, the allegedly injured party who brings the lawsuit. Most plaintiff attorneys have a "contingency fee" arrangement with their clients. Typically, if the patient receives monetary recovery by either a favorable judgment or a settlement, the attorney receives one-third of the judgment or settlement plus expenses. The expenses include, among others, court filing fees, medical records fees, deposition transcription fees, and physicians' or other witnesses' fees. If the plaintiff recovers nothing, the attorney receives no fee. (The plaintiff is legally obligated to pay the attorney the expenses, but plaintiff attorneys often waive or write off their expenses if there is no recovery.) The person who the patient claims caused the injury and from whom the patient is seeking monetary damages is called the defendant. The defendant in most tort cases is represented by an attorney whose fee is paid, usually at an hourly rate, by the defendant's insurance company. Unless the defendant has substantial personal assets, the true target of tort litigation is the company that insures that defendant. The insurance company—for example, the defendant's automobile insurer for an automobile accident or the defendant's home-owner's insurer for a visitor's slip and fall on the home-owner's walkway—is responsible for paying the plaintiff any judgment or settlement against the defendant up to the amount of the policy coverage limit.

DEPOSITION—FOR PRODUCTION OF RECORDS

In addition to receiving a letter from the patient's attorney, physicians may receive a subpoena, an official legal document that cannot be ignored without risking sanctions from the court. A subpoena is usually served at the physician's office by a court-appointed constable, but some jurisdictions permit service of a subpoena by mail. A subpoena should be examined carefully to determine whether it is for a deposition or a trial and whether it requires the physician to testify or just to produce the patient's records. The subpoena specifies the date, time, and location of the event for which the subpoena has been issued. If the location is an attorney's office, the subpoena is for a deposition; if the location is a courthouse, the subpoena is for a trial. The subpoena also should list the names of the parties to the lawsuit and the name, address, and telephone number of the attorney who issued the subpoena and which party the attorney represents. If the purpose of the subpoena is to obtain a copy of the patient's records rather than testimony by the physician, the subpoena usually is addressed to "Keeper of Records of Doctor John Jones" as opposed to "Doctor John Jones."

If the subpoena asks for a copy of the physician's records, it most likely was issued by the attorney representing the party sued by the patient. As explained above, the patient's attorney is entitled to the patient's records simply by mailing a letter and including an authorization signed by the patient. The defendant's attorney typically issues subpoenas to obtain the complete record from each physician who has treated the plaintiff. The physician's duty to respond to a subpoena for records depends on state law. Some states permit a defending party in a lawsuit to obtain the plaintiff patient's records by issuing a subpoena to the physician. Some states require the defending party to obtain judicial permission—that is, a court order—to obtain the plaintiff's records. Therefore, before complying with a subpoena or an apparent court order requesting a patient's records, physicians should consult the legal counsel or risk manager at their hospital or their personal attorney to find out whether they are legally required by the subpoena to produce the records.

In addition, before releasing records in compliance with a subpoena, a court order, or a request from a patient's attorney, the records should be scrutinized. If the records contain certain types of highly confidential information, such as information about mental health treatment, testing or treatment for HIV or sexually transmitted diseases, alcohol abuse or its treatment, or drug abuse or its treatment, release of these portions of the record may be prohibited without the patient's specific consent. The patient may have no qualms about disclosing such information. However, without the patient's specific consent authorizing disclosure, physicians risk a lawsuit for breach of confidentiality, even if they believe in good faith, albeit mistakenly, that they are legally required to produce the entire record. Again, physicians should check with their hospital's legal counsel or risk manager or their personal legal counsel if the records contain particularly sensitive information. Many hospitals, when the patient does not consent to the release of particularly sensitive information, respond to subpoenas by sending redacted records and indicating that disclosure of the redacted part of the record without the patient's express consent is prohibited by law or by hospital policy.

DEPOSITION—TESTIMONY

When the subpoena requires the physician to testify at a deposition, the physician should ascertain whether the date and time present a significant scheduling problem. Most attorneys are quite willing to reschedule a deposition as long as the physician gives them timely notice and alternative dates and times. Physicians also should expect to be compensated for travel time and time spent in the deposition. This fee is considered the responsibility of the attorney who issued the subpoena for the deposition. Assuming that the attorney represents the defendant, physicians should speak with colleagues in the area or their own legal counsel about the going rate for a deposition and then request a check for the entire amount before the deposition. However, because the payment of a fee to physicians for time spent testifying is generally not mandated by statute but is more a matter of custom and practice, no request should be unreasonable. An unreasonable request may cause the attorney who issued the subpoena to respond that he or she will pay nothing beyond the minimal witness and mileage fees that the law requires for every deposition witness.

Because of patient confidentiality, the physician cannot discuss care and treatment of the patient with the defending party's attorney before the deposition (unless state law specifically provides a waiver of privilege when a lawsuit has been brought). The patient's attorney usually requests a meeting with the physician before the deposition to review the case and prepare. The physician is not legally required to do so, but if he or she agrees, the patient's attorney is expected to compensate the physician for the meeting and any time spent reviewing records in preparation. Physicians are entitled to have their own attorney attend and represent them at the deposition, but this is usually unnecessary in the typical personal injury case. If there is any possibility that the treatment in question may lead to an allegation of malpractice against the physician or a colleague, the physician should promptly contact his or her malpractice insurer to request an attorney to assist in preparing for the deposition and to represent the physician at the deposition.

Depositions are usually held in a conference room in the attorney's office, but many attorneys are willing to accommodate a busy physician by conducting the deposition at the physician's office. The parties to the lawsuit may attend but frequently do not. Both parties, however, are represented at the deposition by their attorney. No judge is present. The deposition begins with the swearing in of the physician by the court reporter, who then records the testimony stenographically or by tape recording. The deposition has a question-answer format, and the physician's obligation is to answer each question that is asked. Physicians should rely on patient records to ensure the accuracy of their answers. Although the proceeding is not as formal as an actual trial, the physician should maintain a professional demeanor because any question and answer may be read into evidence at the trial.

In the typical personal injury case, the questioning of the physician focuses on the issues of causation and damages. In a civil case, the plaintiff must prove that the defendant was negligent, that negligence caused the plaintiff's injury, and that the plaintiff suffered legally compensable damages. Because the physician did not witness the accident, in most cases the physician can offer no opinion about the issue of negligence. In some cases—for example, when an emergency department physician treats a patient with a fractured leg immediately after an automobile accident—causation is not in dispute. However, in certain personal injury cases, the physician's testimony about causation of the injury is crucial. For instance, a mailman may go to his physician with a complaint of back pain and state that he has had the pain for three weeks since falling on an icy walkway. The mailman subsequently brings suit against the property owner. The physician should expect to be asked at the deposition whether a diagnosis of lumbar radiculopathy is consistent with falling on the icy walkway, as claimed by the patient; with long-standing degenerative disc disease; or with aggravation or exacerbation of a preexisting condition.

The physician's opinion about damage to the plaintiff is usually explored during the deposition. In addition to the obvious questions about the nature and extent of injury, prognosis is an important factor in determining the amount of monetary damages that the patient might recover. In a civil case, the amount available to the plaintiff is compensation for *special damages* (e.g., medical bills and lost wages) and *general damages* (commonly referred to as "pain and suffering"), including scarring, loss of function, or loss of use of any organ or limb. In the case of a fractured leg from an automobile accident, the physician's opinion about the prognosis—that the patient will have permanent sequelae such as a limp and inability to ski or jog again—is important to each party in assessing the settlement value and potential jury verdict. Therefore, the basis of the physician's opinion is the subject of detailed questioning at the deposition.

After the deposition, the physician is sent a copy of the transcript. The physician must read the transcript, make any corrections (usually nonsubstantive) on an errata sheet, and sign under oath a document verifying that the transcript is true and accurate. The physician should keep the transcript until the lawsuit is over, because if the case goes to trial, he or she will want to review the transcript before testifying.

TRIAL

Physicians who receive a trial subpoena should realize that scheduling for testimony is not as flexible as scheduling for a deposition. The court, not the attorneys, assigns trial dates. The selection of trial dates, however, is a hopelessly optimistic undertaking. Unlike elective surgery, which can be scheduled weeks in advance at a particular time (and then usually begins at that date and time), trial dates are frequently changed. Trials are continued (sometimes at the last minute) for any number of reasons. The most common are unavailability of one or more of the attorneys because of another trial or unavailability of the courtroom because a preceding trial is still ongoing or because another trial has been given priority. Thus a physician may receive a new subpoena each time that a trial is scheduled. Attorneys are usually willing to rearrange the order of witnesses to accommodate a physician's schedule. Nonetheless, even physicians who have been involved in only a few trials probably have kept their schedule open for a certain morning or afternoon in anticipation of being at the courthouse, only to be called the day before and told that the case has been continued or settled. Many states permit the trial testimony of a physician to be presented by videotape. Although trial lawyers believe that video testimony is less compelling than live testimony, videotaping eases the physicians' and lawyers' problems with the uncertainty of the trial schedule. Busy physicians should not hesitate to request testimony by videotape, particularly if they are scheduled to be away at the time of the trial.

At trial, physicians are most effective as witnesses if they are prepared and professional and understand that they are speaking to lay people. Before going to the courthouse, physicians should be intimately familiar with the contents of the patient's medical record so that they do not spend minutes—which feel like hours—thumbing through the record in front of the judge and jury, trying to answer when they first saw the patient. Physicians should review the deposition transcript so that their answers at trial do not contradict their sworn deposition testimony. If the trial answers are different, physicians suffer the embarrassment of being asked to read aloud to the jury the questions and answers in the deposition.

Physicians should not forget that their role at trial is as physicians. They do not enhance their credibility by coming across to the jury as obvious advocates for or against the patient. Advocacy is the attorney's function. Physicians' testimony is credible if they explain their findings and opinions, first in medical terms and then in lay terms, just as they do daily in speaking to patients and patients' families. Although perhaps feeling under attack during cross-examination, physicians should not alter their voice, facial expression, or demeanor from what they were on direct examination. If necessary, physicians should defend their opinions vigorously but always in a professional rather than a confrontational fashion.

MEDICAL MALPRACTICE CASES—PHYSICIAN AS WITNESS

Medical malpractice suits are tort or personal injury cases. A later section in this chapter addresses the litigation process when a physician becomes a defendant in a malpractice case. If a physician receives a deposition or trial subpoena for a medical malpractice case, the physician, as indicated earlier, should immediately contact his or her malpractice insurer to request an attorney. Because the law allows physicians to be added (or dropped) as defendants in a lawsuit during the course of discovery after a malpractice suit has been filed, a physician is foolhardy to assume that he or she is at no risk of being added to a malpractice case. The lawyer assigned by the malpractice insurer reviews the case in detail with the physician before the deposition and points out areas of potential legal vulnerability of which the physician should be mindful. The attorney also points out that the physician has no legal obligation to act as an expert witness for or against the patient or for or against the defendant physician.

Physician witnesses, whether or not they know the physician listed on the subpoena as the defendant, should not contact the defendant physician. At the deposition the physician witness will be asked to identify each person with whom he or she has discussed the patient from the beginning of treatment until the present. The physician is not required to testify about discussions with his or her attorney because they are obviously privileged. However, conversations with the defendant physician are not privileged, and the witness is required to testify about everything said between them concerning the patient or the lawsuit. Conversations with colleagues are also not privileged. If on receiving a deposition notice a physician reviewed the case with his or her department chief, the physician will be asked to recite that conversation. A deposition subpoena may be on its way to the department chief as soon as the physician's deposition has ended. For the same reasons, the physician witness should avoid discussing a malpractice lawsuit with the patient if the physician witness is still treating the patient at the time of receiving a subpoena. In the same vein, if the patient is no longer under treatment, the physician should not telephone the patient to talk about the case or to ask why he or she was subpoenaed.

ADMINISTRATIVE PROCEEDINGS

Administrative proceedings sometimes involve the testimony of physicians but more often require written reports or affidavits from a physician. For example, patients applying for Social Security disability benefits are required to submit a form affidavit from their physician certifying the nature and extent of disability. As much as a physician wants to maintain an amicable relationship with a patient, the physician must appreciate the seriousness of attesting to a disability, whether for Social Security, insurance, or any other purpose. Over a lifetime, depending on the patient's age, disability payments can total hundreds of thousands of dollars. In many cases, on receipt of a disability application, the Social Security Administration will have the patient examined by an independent physician. Disputed claims result in formal evidentiary hearings. In the case of Social Security disability applications, the hearings are held before federal administrative law judges. Physicians, therefore, should not attest in writing to a disability unless they are reasonably confident that they can explain and defend their opinion under oath in an administrative law proceeding.

EXPERT WITNESS

In general, an expert medical witness differs from a medical fact witness in that the expert has not treated the patient. The expert witness is hired by the attorney for one side in a tort case to review the case and give opinions about issues of negligence, causation, or damages. Tort cases, of course, are populated with all kinds of expert witnesses, not just physicians. For instance, in a so-called product liability case, it is customary for the plaintiff's attorney to retain an engineering expert in the hope of eliciting testimony that a particular product was designed so defectively that it presented an unreasonable risk of injury to the product's user, the plaintiff. The defendant manufacturer's attorney retains an engineer to determine whether testimony can be offered that the design of the product conformed to industry standards and that the injury was caused by the plaintiff's misuse of the product. In serious automobile accident cases, accident reconstruction experts are engaged by each side. In personal injury cases with permanent injuries to the plaintiff, forensic economists are retained to estimate the plaintiff's lost earning capacity.

Physicians with specialized training are asked to be expert witnesses in various kinds of tort cases. In particular, in so-called toxic tort cases, expert physician testimony is crucial to each side. Oncologists and epidemiologists are obviously needed by both sides to review claims that people living in certain areas allegedly had a higher incidence of cancer because of a company's allegedly improper disposal of a potential carcinogen in the area. In the ongoing breast implant litigation, the parties have sought the opinions of endocrinologists and infectious disease specialists about the question of a causal connection between certain systemic disorders and allegedly leaking silicone breast implants. In suits against keyboard manufacturers for alleged repetitive strain injuries, the opinions of orthopedic surgeons, physiatrists, and neurologists are sought by the attorneys for each side.

MEDICAL MALPRACTICE CASES

Physicians have no legal obligation to act as expert witnesses in a medical malpractice case. The House of Delegates of the American Medical Association (perhaps to fend off allegations from some plaintiff attorneys about physicians' "conspiracy of silence") has adopted a policy statement on expert witnesses: "Regarding expert witnesses in clinical matters, as a matter of public interest the AMA encourages its members to serve as impartial expert witnesses" (Policies of House of Delegates-I-96, AMA, H-265.994). Some hospitals have specific policies about staff physicians who become expert witnesses, such as requiring the consent of the department chief. Other hospitals, in an attempt to avoid disruption of patient care caused by the demands of a trial, require that staff physicians testify as experts only by videotape.

Although expert witnesses are obviously important in malpractice trials to both the plaintiff patient and the defendant physician, the plaintiff, almost without exception, cannot succeed at trial without testimony of a physician expert witness on his or her behalf. In a personal injury case, the plaintiff has the burden of proof and goes first at trial. If the plaintiff fails to introduce sufficient evidence of negligence and causation, the trial judge is required to enter a directed verdict in favor of the defendant even before the defendant has called any witnesses. To avoid a directed verdict, the plaintiff's attorney must call at least one expert physician witness willing to testify that in his or her opinion the treatment of the patient by the defendant physician fell below the standard of care expected of the average qualified physician practicing the defendant's specialty *and* that as a result of substandard treatment the patient was injured. Once the plaintiff's expert witness has given this opinion, the plaintiff has established a prima facie case. No matter what evidence the defendant offers on his or her own behalf, including the opinion of expert witnesses directly contradictory to the plaintiff's expert, the plaintiff has avoided a directed verdict and is entitled to have the jury decide the case.

The trial judge decides whether a person is qualified to give expert opinion testimony to the jury. In most instances, as long as the physician witness is board-certified in the same speciality as the defendant, the trial judge will not hesitate in ruling that the witness is qualified as an expert. The witness does not need to be recognized by medical colleagues as an expert or as an authority in the specialty. In fact, it is not required that the expert witness be board-certified in the defendant's specialty or even practice the defendant's specialty as long as the judge finds that the witness is qualified to give expert testimony. Medical malpractice trials are decided by lay jurors and not by a medical panel. The term *expert*, in the context of litigation, means that by reason of education, training, and experience in a particular field a person has knowledge beyond that possessed by lay people and is therefore qualified—in the judge's opinion—to render opinions in his or her area of specialty that may be helpful to the jury in deciding the issues in the trial. Judges always instruct juries, however, that simply because a witness has been allowed to give expert opinions, the jury is not bound by those opinions or the opinions of any other expert witness. The jurors are instructed that they should assess the testimony and credibility of each expert witness in the same way that they assess the testimony and credibility of all witnesses. The jurors are instructed (in the same manner as with all other witnesses) that they may accept as true all, some, or none of the opinions offered by each expert witness.

The AMA's House of Delegates has adopted a policy regarding the qualifications of expert witnesses:

> (a) The AMA believes that the minimum statutory requirements for qualification as an expert witness should reflect the following: (1) that the witness be required to have comparable education, training, and occupational experience in the same field as the defendant; (2) that the occupational experience include active medical practice or teaching experience in the same field as the defendant; and (3) that the active medical practice or teaching experience must have been within five years of the date of the occurrence giving rise to the claim (Policies of House of Delegates-I 96, AMA, H-265.994).

As indicated above, this policy is not binding on trial judges. Presumably it was enacted by the AMA in response to defendant physicians' concerns about the willingness of physicians who have no active practice or who practice a different specialty to testify about the standard of care to which a defendant specialist should be held. The AMA policy provides useful guidance on what credentials an expert witness should have to be able to persuade a jury that his or her opinions are valid. If an expert witness is not board-certified in the defendant's specialty or does not actively practice, these facts are impressed on the jury by the opposing attorney during cross-examination. Similarly, if a physician frequently appears in court as an expert witness or receives a large number of cases to review from organizations that advertise expert witness services or a significant portion of the physician's income is derived from expert witness testimony, these facts are elicited on cross-examination. The cross-examination implies that the witness is more interested in making money by testifying than in taking care of patients.

Physicians who agree to review a case, as a potential expert for either the plaintiff or the defense, should make sure that the attorney provides them with all of the relevant medical records before arriving at any conclusions. The physician should charge, on an hourly basis, for any time spent reviewing the records and meeting with the attorney. Physicians who realize that they know the defendant physician should immediately advise the attorney, because a jury may not accept their opinion as unbiased. After reviewing the records, physicians should not agree to become an expert witness unless they are prepared to give their opinions publicly and under oath. Physicians who write a letter to an attorney summarizing the case and their opinions about the defendant's compliance with or breach of the standard of care should realize (despite the attorney's possible assurances otherwise) that the letter may be made public at some stage of the lawsuit. They should understand and accept the time commitment of being an expert witness at trial, which may include having to testify at a deposition. An effective expert witness believes strongly either that the patient was injured because of substandard care or that, despite an unfortunate outcome, the care was the same as the average physician in this circumstance would have provided. An expert witness who has second thoughts about testifying, as trial approaches, may irreparably change the outcome of the trial. Well in advance of the trial, the attorney is required to advise the court in writing of the name of each expert witness and to provide a detailed summary of each expert's expected testimony. Judges are understandably reluctant to allow attorneys to change expert witnesses on the eve of a trial; thus, a balking expert witness can cause a party to lose the lawsuit.

The principles for effective trial testimony in the section about fact witnesses apply equally, if not more so, to expert witnesses in medical malpractice cases. Before testifying, the witness must spend time with the attorney, reviewing the questions that will be asked on direct examination and anticipating and preparing to answer the likely questions on cross-examination. Despite their credentials, the most renowned experts in the eyes of their peers will not be persuasive to a jury if they are arrogant or too technical. The expert who does not know the record well has little credibility. The expert who is not familiar with the literature (particularly recent peer-reviewed articles) about the medicine at issue is vulnerable on cross-examination, because the opposing attorney is probably in possession of and knowledgeable about literature that may raise questions about the expert's opinions. Experts who needlessly concede points on cross-examination rather than vigorously and reasonably defend their opinions do not help the party on whose behalf they have agreed to testify. Even if they have not published articles about the particular medical condition and even if they are not considered by peers to be the best specialist in their community, physicians can be persuasive witnesses if they have sufficient experience in treating patients with conditions similar to those for which the plaintiff was treated by the defendant. Effective expert witnesses convey to the jury by demeanor, tone of voice, and terminology that they want to explain the medicine so that the jury can understand it and truly believe their opinions.

MALPRACTICE CASE DEFENDANT

A physician is formally notified that he or she is a defendant in a malpractice case by being served with a summons and complaint. The complaint's caption identifies the name of the plaintiff and the name of the defendant or defendants; it is not unusual that two or more physicians are named as defendants in a malpractice case. The caption also lists the court in which the complaint has been filed. The complaint sets out, sometimes in detail but more often in legal generalities, the allegations against the physician and a demand for payment of damages. The complaint is signed at its conclusion by the plaintiff's attorney. The summons is a standard form legal document from the court advising the physician that the complaint has been filed and that the physician is required to serve an answer to the complaint within a specific time (usually 20 days after receipt).

As disheartening and upsetting as it is to be served with a malpractice complaint, every physician is exposed to the risk. Thousands of doctors are sued for malpractice every year in the United States. Many physicians (particularly those in high-risk specialties such as obstetrics) are sued several times in their careers. Thinking of the lawsuit more as part of the business of being a physician and less as a personal attack on one's professional abilities may ease the emotional trauma.

Physicians should immediately inform their malpractice insurer that they have been served with a complaint. The insurer assigns, at its expense, an attorney to represent the physician. Because of the insurer's obvious self-interest, the assigned attorney will be experienced in defending malpractice cases. The attorney's first order of business is to file with the court an answer to the complaint. In standard legal terms the answer denies the allegations of malpractice. As early in the process as possible, the physician should send a complete copy of the patient's records to the attorney. Once the attorney has examined the records, he or she will meet with the physician to review the course of treatment and allegations of malpractice.

Many states have enacted legislation giving physicians a procedural protection not available to other tort defendants. At the time of filing the lawsuit (or within a short time thereafter) the plaintiff's attorney is required to present to the court a letter from a physician attesting that he or she has reviewed the medical records and believes that malpractice has occurred. Some states require the letter to specify with some detail the basis for the opinions. This procedural protection is intended to reduce the number of malpractice cases by requiring plaintiff attorneys to screen potential cases with a physician before initiating a lawsuit. In addition, the letter provides defendant physicians and their attorneys some guidance as to what the plaintiff's attorney will contend are the specific negligent acts.

DISCOVERY

The *discovery* part of the case begins as soon as the answer is filed. An elaborate set of procedural rules allows each side in a tort case to discover (find out about) the opposing party's case. "Paper" discovery involves "interrogatories" and "requests for production of documents." Each side in the lawsuit makes use of these tools. The plaintiff's attorney will file a request for documents from the physician's attorney, including copies of all records, imaging studies, correspondence, calendar entities, computer records, or any other documents in the defendant physician's possession concerning the plaintiff patient.

As a practical matter, the plaintiff's attorney most likely obtained the physician's records before filing the lawsuit. Physicians should realize that they are potential targets of a malpractice suit whenever they receive a request from an attorney for the records of a patient who has had an unexpectedly poor outcome or significant complications from treatment. Therefore, physicians should notify their malpractice insurer at the time they receive any such request, because the lawsuit, depending on the state's statute of limitations, may not be filed until several years later.

The plaintiff's request for production of documents also includes a request for a copy of the physician's curriculum vitae (CV) and malpractice insurance policy. The plaintiff's attorney is interested in the CV for background information about the physician's education, training, and professional experience. In addition, the plaintiff's attorney scrutinizes the CV to see if the physician has authored publications about the medical subject at issue. If so, the attorney will obtain the publications. The plaintiff's attorney wants a copy of the insurance policy to find out the amount of coverage available to pay any judgment in the case.

The physician's attorney sends to the plaintiff's attorney a request for a copy of all of the plaintiff's medical records for the period before the treatment at issue up to the present. The physician's attorney requests a copy of all medical bills that the plaintiff contends were incurred because of treatment necessitated by the malpractice. If the plaintiff has made a claim for lost wages, the physician's attorney requests a copy of the plaintiff's income tax returns for at least five years before the treatment at issue.

Interrogatories are written questions, drafted by an attorney, that the opposing party must answer in writing and under oath. Answering the interrogatories and preparing for and attending the deposition are the two occasions during the discovery period that make a significant demand on the defendant physician's time. In the interrogatories, the plaintiff's attorney attempts to compel the physician to commit to writing a detailed account of his or her interaction with the patient during the relevant period. The interrogatories ask the physician for recollection of conversations with the patient and the patient's family as well as with colleagues and consultants about the patient's treatment. The physician is asked what treatment risks he or she specifically advised the patient about and what alternative treatments were known to the physician or discussed with the patient. The interrogatories ask what records and reports were available to the physician and which ones the physician relied on at the time of treatment. Moreover, the physician is asked about thought processes regarding treatment decisions, differential diagnoses, and reasons for instituting the treatment at issue. The interrogatories also ask the physician about any previous malpractice cases in which he or she has been a defendant or in which he or she has testified as a fact witness or an expert witness. If deposition or trial transcripts of the physician from previous cases are available, the plaintiff's attorney will obtain them. The answers to interrogatories can be read into evidence at the trial. The physician's attorney carefully reviews the physician's draft of his or her answers and suggests changes in wording that the attorney thinks are prudent for legal reasons before the answers are finalized and signed.

The physician's attorney sends out detailed interrogatories to be answered by the plaintiff. The attorney wants a detailed account from the plaintiff of interactions and conversations with the defendant. If the plaintiff claims that any of these conversations took place in the presence of others, the plaintiff is requested to provide the names and addresses of such persons. The plaintiff is asked to name every physician and medical facility that provided care for any of the medical problems at issue. If claiming lost wages, the plaintiff is asked to provide a detailed employment history. The physician's attorney carefully reviews the plaintiff's answers and sends a subpoena to obtain complete records from every physician and medical facility that has treated the plaintiff. All of these records are scrutinized to see whether they refer to other physicians or facilities not mentioned by the plaintiff in his or her answers. If so, those records will then be obtained. A subpoena for employment records will be served on the patient's most recent employers.

At some point after the interrogatories are answered, each side conducts depositions of the opposing party. The physician's attorney helps the physician to prepare for the deposition, which is obviously an important event in the case. The attorney usually has a checklist or form to go over with the physician about the do's and don't's of depositions. In general, physicians should have in mind two thoughts as they prepare for their deposition:

1. The deposition answers can be read by the plaintiff's attorney to the jury at trial; thus, the physician should keep in mind that the jury is the potential audience for the deposition. Before answering each question, physicians should consider how the words that they are about to say will sound if read aloud in the courtroom. If trial testimony differs from what physicians say during the deposition, the jury will hear the deposition answers and naturally be skeptical of trial testimony.

2. Physicians should not attempt to persuade the plaintiff's attorney that their treatment was not negligent. The plaintiff's attorney has made a business decision to spend time and resources pursuing the lawsuit. The attorney has already paid, at a minimum, for a review of the case by at least one physician. It is extremely unlikely that anything said by the defendant physician at the deposition will convince the attorney that he or she was wrong to file suit against the physician. Defendant physicians who do not follow their attorney's advice simply to answer the question that is asked inevitably talk too much. The more the defendant says at the deposition, the greater the opportunity for the plaintiff's attorney to find some language—often taken out of context—to throw back at the physician at trial. The plaintiff's attorney will be prepared for the deposition and will be thorough. Defendant physicians who speak too much not only invite further questioning at the deposition but also make themselves more vulnerable to impeachment with their own words at trial.

SETTLEMENT OR TRIAL

The physician's attorney and insurance company will have the case reviewed by physicians practicing the defendant's specialty. As discussed in the expert witness section, the question for potential expert witnesses is whether the defendant's treatment met the standard of care expected of a physician in this circumstance. The opinions of the reviewing physician play a major role in the insurance company's decision whether to attempt to settle the case or to take the case to trial. If the reviewing physicians believe that the defendant was negligent and that the negligence led to the plaintiff's injuries, the insurance company's claim representative or claim manager will likely begin the settlement process. On the other hand, if the expert reviews are positive and the reviewers are willing to testify, settlement probably will not be offered.

Additional factors are also considered in deciding whether to go to trial or to settle. Important considerations are the credibility, personality, and circumstances of the plaintiff. A five-year-old girl with cerebral palsy, particularly when her parents come across as sincere, hard-working people, is a plaintiff for whom any jury will have great sympathy. A forty-year-old married father of four, who has worked twenty years as a carpenter and became partially paralyzed after disc surgery, is likely to be a sympathetic plaintiff. People who have been chronically sick, who have not worked or managed a household in years, who have been plaintiffs in other lawsuits, and who frequently missed appointments or did not follow up on treatment recommendations are not likely to elicit much sympathy from the jury.

Potential exposure is another important factor in deciding whether to go to trial or settle. With a serious injury case in which the potential jury verdict if the plaintiff wins is high (even if the insurance company's representative thinks that the defense will probably win the case), a settlement may be proposed at a figure far below what the jury verdict may be. The plaintiff's attorney then has to weigh, with the plaintiff, whether to chance hitting the lottery with the jury or to settle for a guaranteed sum.

The defendant's opinion about whether to go to trial or to settle is also taken into consideration. Under the terms of the standard malpractice policy the insurance company has the right to settle any case, but malpractice insurers generally give some weight to the insured physician's thoughts about settlement. The possible benefit of settlement from the physician's point of view is that the case ends; thus there is no further demand on time, and the physician avoids the stress of a trial. Although physicians win a significant majority of malpractice cases that go to trial, a physician should realize the potential for media reporting of an adverse jury verdict. In most instances when a case is settled, there is no media reporting, and often the amount of the settlement is not even disclosed in the filings with the court. However, if a jury trial ends in a significant verdict against a physician, the physician should anticipate media coverage.

Another potential benefit of settlement is that the physician avoids the risk of personal financial liability from a jury verdict above insurance policy limits. A malpractice insurer is responsible to pay to the plaintiff any settlement or verdict up to the policy limit. The amount of a verdict above the policy limits is the physician's own liability. Although rare, such a verdict may lead to collection efforts that include real estate attachments and garnishment of wages. If the potential damages in a malpractice case are very high—typically situations involving a permanent, totally incapacitating injury or condition —the physician should consider retaining a personal attorney. The function of the personal attorney is not to defend the case in place of the attorney paid by the insurer but to counsel the physician about whether an attempt should be made to settle the case within the insurance policy limits. The physician's personal attorney may then write a letter to the insurance company on behalf of the physician. The letter "demands" that the insurance company attempt to settle within the policy limits. If the insurance company does not attempt to settle and a verdict is returned above the policy limits, the physician may maintain a "bad faith" failure to settle the claim against the insurance company for the amount for which the physician was personally liable.

Settlement of a malpractice case, however, is not without consequences to the physician. Federal law requires every malpractice insurer that makes a payment to a plaintiff after a settlement or after a verdict to report the matter to the National Practitioner Data Bank (NPDB) (42 U.S.C. §11131). The report by the insurer must include the physician's name, the amount of the payment, a brief description of the incident giving rise to the payment, and the name of any hospital with which the physician is affiliated. Federal law also requires that hospitals query the NPDB for each physician to whom it considers granting privileges. Once privileges are granted to a physician, the hospital must still query the NPDB every two years. In addition, most state medical licensing boards require physicians to report any malpractice settlements or verdicts against them. In 1996, Massachusetts, perhaps heralding a national movement, enacted legislation giving the public access to information about malpractice payments made in the previous 10 years on behalf of each physician licensed in the state. A physician applying to be authorized as a provider by various health insurers or HMOs must report any history of malpractice payments on the application. Given that the reporting requirements are for payments made either in settlement or after a jury verdict, many physicians try to convince their malpractice insurer that if they have a reasonable chance of winning, the case should go to trial.

THE TRIAL

If the decision is made not to settle, the case proceeds to trial. Trial begins with jury selection. Depending on the procedural rules of the state in which the trial is held, pretrial questioning of prospective jurors is done by either the attorneys or the judge. The purpose of the questioning is to determine whether prospective jurors may be biased for or against one side or the other. Prospective jurors (just as in every trial whether civil or criminal) are asked whether they know any of the parties, witnesses, or attorneys and whether they know or have heard anything about the case. They are asked whether they or family members have had the same condition or disease as the plaintiff, whether they or family members have been involved on one side or the other in a medical malpractice case, and whether they have any opinions about doctors who are sued in malpractice lawsuits that may make them less than impartial. The judge, on his or her own or in response to an attorney's request for a "challenge for cause," may disqualify a prospective juror as a result of the responses to the questioning. The attorneys for each side are allowed a certain number of peremptory challenges, for which no reason need be stated, of the remaining prospective jurors. The final number of trial jurors depends on state rules (the number varies nationally from six to twelve).

Once the jury is chosen, many judges start the trial by giving the jury a brief statement of legal principles that govern medical malpractice cases. The statement informs the jury that the burden of proof is on the plaintiff; that the plaintiff must prove his or her case by a "preponderance of the evidence" (as opposed to "beyond a reasonable doubt," which is the standard in criminal cases); that the plaintiff must prove that the care rendered by the defendant physician fell below the standard of care expected of the average physician in this circumstance; and that as a result of this substandard care, the plaintiff was injured.

The attorney for each side is permitted to make an opening statement. The plaintiff's attorney goes first. During the opening statement both attorneys outline their case to the jury, including the important evidence from their client's point of view. Because the opening statement of the plaintiff's attorney is the first public airing in detail of the allegation that the physician was negligent and injured the patient, the physician should not be caught unaware and react visibly to the allegation. Just as at any other point in the trial when a witness or the plaintiff's attorney alleges negligence, the physician should be seen by the jury to be attentive but impassive. Shaking the head, sighing, smirking, or even wiping away a tear will be seen by the jury as unprofessional.

After the opening statements, the plaintiff's case begins. There is no set order to the calling of witnesses, but at some point the plaintiff and the plaintiff's medical expert will be called as witnesses. If the plaintiff is a child, the suit is brought on the child's behalf by the parents, both of whom are likely to testify. If the patient is deceased, the suit is brought by the executor or administrator of the estate, who is usually a spouse, parent, or child of the deceased; the executor or administrator will testify. If the patient has been rendered mentally incapacitated by the alleged malpractice, the suit is brought by the patient's legal guardian, who is usually a close relative, and he or she will testify. When the injured person is too incapacitated to testify, the plaintiff's attorney may attempt to introduce a "day-in-the-life" videotape that depicts the plaintiff and the assistance needed by the plaintiff in eating, dressing, brushing teeth, combing hair, or other activities of daily living. Such videotapes are admitted into evidence if the judge, who views the tape before it is seen by the jury, finds that it is a fair and accurate representation of the plaintiff's daily existence.

During the testimony of the plaintiff's expert witness, the physician should be particularly attentive. It is often helpful to the physician's attorney for the physician to make notes about any factual errors or inaccurate medical conclusions voiced by the expert. The physician's attorney can review these notes in preparing to cross-examine the expert. As indicated previously, the defense attorney will be ready to elicit testimony about whether the expert is a "professional witness." Also, if medical literature contradicts the expert's opinion about standard of care or causation, the physician's attorney will cross-examine the expert about this literature. A favorite tactic for defense attorneys is to attempt to have the expert acknowledge that there are two schools of thought about the treatment of the condition at issue. If the expert does so, the defense argues that the physician was not negligent in following a particular course of treatment, despite the fact that the expert and some other physicians would have used the other course of treatment. Defendant physicians must realize that they may be wounded emotionally during the plaintiff's case. They will hear a fellow physician, the plaintiff's expert, castigate their care, and they will hear the plaintiff testify about how the injury caused by the treatment has devastated his or her life. Physicians must not despair of winning. Their own case has not started, and their own expert witness has yet to be heard.

Defendant physicians may be called to testify by the plaintiff's attorney during the plaintiff's case or by their own attorney during the defense case; sometimes they testify during both. Civil trial rules permit the plaintiff's attorney to call the defendant physician in the plaintiff's case. Some plaintiff attorneys take advantage of this strategy, particularly if they think that the physician will make concessions helpful to the plaintiff's case. If the physician is called by the plaintiff's attorney, the physician's attorney has the choice of when to question the physician: during the plaintiff's case, immediately after the plaintiff's attorney has finished his or her questioning, or after the plaintiff's case is concluded. Many defense attorneys prefer to defer their questioning of the physician until the plaintiff's case is concluded so that the physician will have heard all adverse evidence before having to complete his or her testimony. If the physician is not questioned by the defense attorney until the defense case begins, the plaintiff's attorney will have another opportunity to question the physician (immediately after questioning by the physician's attorney). However, this second round of questioning by the plaintiff's attorney is often limited by the trial judge, particularly if the questioning during the plaintiff's case was extensive.

Regardless of when the physician is called to testify, it is important that he or she come across as truthful and competent. Unlike a deposition, in which the content of what is said is all that matters, at trial how physicians speak and present themselves is as important as what they say. Physicians should remember that their audience is not the person asking the questions, the judge, or the people in the spectator's section of the courtroom. The jury is the only audience as far as physician defendants are concerned. Without staring at any one particular juror, physicians should focus their attention on the jury when responding to questions. Physicians should present themselves as wanting to share with the jury their thought processes in reaching treatment decisions. A physician whose voice is too low, who has a hand in front of the mouth, who never looks at the jury, or who conveys no interest in what he or she is saying will not be a persuasive or effective witness. Similarly, physicians who fight the plaintiff's attorney at the slightest provocation so that they sound more like a lawyer than a doctor, who have a more defensive or aggressive tone of voice on cross-examination than when questioned by their own attorney, or who come across as arrogant and dismissive of the allegations against them are not effective witnesses. Physicians who come across as informed, thoughtful, not condescending, knowledgeable about the contents of the medical records, and trying to explain the medicine in terms that jurors can understand present well. Defense attorneys believe that the physician most likely to win is a physician to whom the jurors would be willing to go themselves or to send a family member.

Part of the jury's determination of who is telling the truth is based on witnesses' demeanor. Some people are naturally more relaxed and better public speakers than others, and these qualities aid in projecting truthfulness. However, no matter how good or poor their public speaking ability, physicians can enhance their credibility by preparation. They must be intimate with the medical record, particularly all notes that they recorded. They also must know what they wrote in answers to interrogatories and what they testified at deposition. If on cross-examination the plaintiff's attorney can point out significant discrepancies between trial testimony and medical record, written answers, or deposition transcript, the jury will doubt the physician's credibility. If there are no such discrepancies to exploit, the damage that the plaintiff's attorney can inflict on cross-examination will be limited. The physician's attorney prepares the physician not only for direct testimony but also for questions that should be expected on cross-examination. Hearing such questions before taking the witness stand helps to lessen the intimidation of hearing them asked in an accusatory fashion in the courtroom.

The defense case at trial includes the defendant physician's testimony and the testimony of the defense expert witness. The defense attorney, as well as the plaintiff's attorney, also may call as witnesses other physicians who treated the patient before or after the defendant. Assuming that the defense expert is experienced, has impressive credentials, and presents well, the defense attorney is likely to call him or her as the final witness. Many attorneys believe that when jurors deliberate, they struggle to recall the testimony of numerous witnesses and may give more weight to a persuasive final witness whose testimony is fresh in their minds.

After the evidence is concluded, both attorneys give a closing argument or summation to the jury. Closing arguments attempt to weave the testimony into a pattern most favorable to their client's position. The arguments of plaintiff's attorneys are often emotional and subtly or not so subtly ask the jurors to allow the patient some recompense for the injury or disability that has so transformed his or her life. Defense attorneys often point out the physician's experience and the severity and complexity of the plaintiff's presenting condition in arguing that the jurors should not let their sympathies overcome the allegedly minimal evidence of negligence. Despite the attorneys' best rhetoric, most cases are won or lost not in the closing arguments but in the testimony of the witnesses as it is heard and assessed by the jurors.

The final words that the jury hears before deliberations are the judge's instructions on the law. The judge explains the legal definition of malpractice and tells the jury that the burden of proof is with the plaintiff. The judge also instructs the jury about the damages that it may award if it finds malpractice. The trial judge makes it clear to the jury that the verdict is theirs and that the judge has no personal preference for one side or the other. As distressing as it may be to have the appropriateness of their professional care reviewed and ruled upon by lay people in the emotionally charged forum of a public trial, *physicians win the majority of cases decided by jurors.* Although sometimes taken aback by an apparently inexplicable jury verdict, lawyers generally agree that for the most part jury verdicts are fair.

The insurance company's decision to go to trial does not mean that a settlement will not occur after trial starts. The insurance company usually has a representative in the courtroom watching the entire trial. The representative probably has monitored many malpractice trials and has a good sense of when a case is going well or poorly. The representative assesses whether the respective parties' witnesses did as well as had been expected before trial and, just as the lawyers do, tries to "read" the jurors to see if they appear interested in the case and sympathetic to the plaintiff. Until the time the jury returns to the courtroom to announce its verdict, the case may be settled if the plaintiff's attorney and the insurance company representative reach an agreement on an amount.

APPEALS

Although each side has the right to appeal the jury's verdict, most appeals are not successful, and the verdict stands. Appeals must be based on the claim of legal error made by the judge during trial. The typical appeal alleges that the judge's instructions to the jury misstated the law of malpractice to the detriment of the losing party or that the judge erred in admitting or excluding certain evidence or testimony. Appeals are decided by an appellate court, which usually consists of three or more judges who decide the appeal based on their review of the trial transcript and the legal briefs and arguments of the attorneys. If an appeal is successful, the usual remedy is the ordering of a new trial. The new trial jury is not informed of the results of the earlier trial. In rare instances, judgments are entered on appeal for the physician if the appellate court finds that there was insufficient evidence of malpractice for the case even to have been submitted to the jury.

ALTERNATIVE DISPUTE RESOLUTION

The expense and time involved in malpractice litigation have led some plaintiff attorneys, defense attorneys, physicians, and insurers to agree to binding arbitration or "alternative dispute resolution" forums to resolve malpractice complaints. The typical arbitration involves a private screening before an arbitrator, often a retired judge, agreed upon by both sides. The arbitrator hears the evidence in a similar but less formal fashion than a trial and then issues a decision that is binding on the parties. Arbitration proceedings are quicker and less costly to the parties than a jury trial. Physicians usually find them less emotionally stressful than public trials. The physicians' insurer is required to notify the NPDB of any arbitration finding requiring payment to the plaintiff. Some health insurers and HMOs attempt to mandate arbitration of malpractice claims. The mandated arbitration may be before a nonmedical arbitrator or an impartial panel of physicians. Trial attorneys' organizations have opposed most legislative proposals for mandatory arbitration or any restriction on a plaintiff's right to trial by jury. Physicians, therefore, should anticipate that medical malpractice trials will continue and that they may find themselves participating at some point in their careers.

CONCLUSION

Physicians, particularly those inexperienced with litigation, should be aware of the responsibilities and potential hazards created by any type of involvement in the litigation process. Physicians should not hesitate to make use of available resources—the hospital's legal counsel and risk manager, their malpractice insurer, and their personal attorney—for information and advice whenever they are invited or compelled to enter the litigation arena.

WILLIAM B. HOWARD, JR., BBA, ChFC, CFD

21

Planning for Your Personal Financial Success

Financial security is the big motivator for working long and hard hours. Achieving financial success does not just happen. You need an understanding of the key areas pertinent to your fiscal health. Just as you follow procedures in analyzing your patients' health, you can follow the financial planning process to identify your personal goals and objectives in the key areas of your financial health: insurance, investments, college funding, income tax, retirement, and estate planning. The first step is committing the time to get organized. In my 19 years of advising clients, the biggest hurdle that many busy physicians have to clear is making the time to go through the financial planning process. Procrastination is tough to defeat, but you can do it.

GETTING ORGANIZED

GATHER DATA

A personal financial statement is the foundation of getting organized. It tells you what you are worth as of a particular date. What you own (assets) less what you owe (liabilities) equals your net worth (equity). Your net worth is the bottom line. To determine the value of your assets, you should gather the most recent statements from all bank accounts, investment accounts, and retirement plans. Table 1 offers a checklist of items needed for financial planning.

Divide your investment assets into liquid, marketable, and nonmarketable. Liquid assets, such as checking accounts and certificates of deposit, are stable in price. Marketable assets, such as stocks and bonds, convert easily into cash, but their value may be more or less than your purchase price. Nonmarketable investments are more difficult to value. Examples include an interest in a medical practice, real estate, or limited partnerships. You should also include personal

---

TABLE 1. Items Needed for Financial Planning

---

1. **Cash and equivalents**
   The latest statements on each of the following:
   - ☐ Checking account statement
   - ☐ Savings account statement
   - ☐ Credit union statement
   - ☐ Money market account statement
   - ☐ Certificates of deposit

2. **Notes receivable**
   A copy of the note, record of payments received, and the current balance if available for any loans that you have made to others.

3. **Securities**
   The latest statements for all investment accounts; copies of securities if held personally and a purchase/confirmation statement showing how the securities were acquired and the cost (or other basis if gift or inheritance) for each of the following:
   - ☐ Bonds
   - ☐ Stocks
   - ☐ Mutual funds
   - ☐ Unit investment trusts
   - ☐ Variable annuities
   - ☐ Variable life insurance

4. **Limited partnerships**
   Prospectuses, documentation of purchase prices, number or units, and current value if known.

5. **Insurance contracts**
   Policy numbers, coverage amounts, and any current policy statements/reports for each of the following, if applicable:
   - ☐ Single premium annuities
   - ☐ Flexible premium annuities
   - ☐ Single premium life insurance
   - ☐ Universal life insurance
   - ☐ Homeowner's or renter's insurance
   - ☐ Professional liability
   - ☐ Whole life insurance
   - ☐ Term life insurance
   - ☐ Medical insurance
   - ☐ Disability insurance
   - ☐ Automobile insurance
   - ☐ Umbrella liability

6. **Personal assets**
   Provide documentation showing the original purchase price, closing papers (if applicable), and current market value for each of the following:
   - ☐ Primary residence
   - ☐ Second residence
   - ☐ Rental real estate
   - ☐ Automobiles (copy of auto title)
   - ☐ Boats (copy of boat title)
   - ☐ Personal property such as home furnishings, jewelry, art

7. **Liabilities**
   Provide the original document setting forth the liability as well as statements showing the most recent balance for each of the following:
   - ☐ Mortgages
   - ☐ Personal notes
   - ☐ Credit cards and lines of credit

8. **Retirement plans**
   The most recent statements and beneficiary information from the following retirement plans, if applicable:
   - ☐ IRA
   - ☐ IRA/rollovers
   - ☐ Keogh
   - ☐ SEP
   - ☐ Thrift plan
   - ☐ Profit sharing plan
   - ☐ ESOP or PAYSOP
   - ☐ Stock purchase plan
   - ☐ Pension plan

9. **Tax, personal, and business documents**
   - ☐ Personal tax returns for past 3 years
   - ☐ Business tax returns for past 3 years
   - ☐ Retirement plan tax returns for past 3 years
   - ☐ Payroll stubs showing current earnings
   - ☐ Current will(s)
   - ☐ Current trust agreements
   - ☐ Divorce decree(s)
   - ☐ Prenuptial agreement(s)
   - ☐ Business interests
   - ☐ Buy/sell agreements
   - ☐ Deferred compensation
   - ☐ Stock options/bonus plan

property such as your home, automobile, and jewelry. List the value at which they could realistically be sold. Include life insurance cash values or the accumulation of funds inside a life insurance policy (the amount that you would receive if you were to cash in the policy). Be sure to list the loans against each policy, if you have any. Identify liabilities such as student loans, auto loans/auto leases, credit card debts, lines of credit, and mortgages on your residence and other real estate.

Your financial statement also should include a breakdown of your income, date of your will, and personal information. A few hours of self-evaluation reveal a lot about your current fiscal health and provide the foundation for achieving financial security. Although a personal financial statement takes time, it is well worth the effort.

According to Stanley and Danko, authors of *The Millionaire Next Door*,[10] physicians do not tend to be wealth accumulators. Their research found that among all major high income-producing occupations, physicians have a significantly low propensity to accumulate wealth.

DEVELOP A BUDGET

As a physician who is interested in accumulating wealth, you need to commit to developing a budget. Being frugal is the cornerstone of wealth building.[10] To analyze your finances, divide your cash flow among the following five areas: income, savings, taxes, insurance, and standard of living. The math is simple. Spend less than what you bring in, and you have a surplus to allocate for your financial goals and objectives. Millionaires live well below their means.[10] Spend more than you make, and you have a deficit. Table 2 is an example of a cash flow analysis form.

The biggest percentage of income usually goes toward paying the home mortgage. The traditional 30-year mortgage is popular because of lower payments compared with a 15-year mortgage. The following is an example of how you can save substantial dollars even if you go for the 30-year mortgage instead of the 15-year mortgage:

> Dr. Jones recently purchased a $300,000 house and made a $30,000 down payment. Long-term rates are at 8%. His monthly payment, exclusive of taxes and insurance, is $1,981.16. He wants to know if there is a way to pay off the 30-year mortgage early so that he will not have a mortgage at his retirement in 25 years. Assuming that his mortgage allows prepayment of principal without penalty, he could make biweekly payments vs. monthly payments and the net effect would be an extra payment on principal each year. This would save him approximately $126,794 in interest payments over the life of the mortgage. In addition, Dr. Jones would be mortgage-free by age 63 (Table 3).

Try to keep your mortgage payment (including taxes and insurance) at 28–35% of your pretax income. In addition, paying 20% of the sales price as a

TABLE 2. Cash Flow Analysis Form

Description	Monthly	Other	Period
Income			
Wages, salaries			
Taxable interest income			
Tax-exempt interest income			
Dividend income			
Taxable refunds, credits			
Alimony received			
Business income or loss			
Capital gain or loss			
Other gains or losses			
Total IRA distributions			
Total pensions or annuities			
Rents, royalties, partner, estates, trusts			
Social Security benefits			
Other income			
Total income			
Savings and investments			
Savings accounts			
Money market fund			
IRA			
Pension plan or TSA			
Profit sharing plan			
401 (K) plan			
Simplified employee pension plan (SEP)			
Mutual funds			
Stocks and bonds			
Other savings and investments			
Total savings and investments			
Taxes			
Federal income tax			
State income tax			
Social Security tax			
Medicare tax			
Property tax			
Other taxes			
Total taxes			
Insurance			
Homeowner's/renter's insurance			
Automobile insurance			
Life insurance			
Medical insurance			
Disability insurance			
Excess liability insurance			
Professional liability insurance			
Other insurance			
Total Insurance			

(Continued on facing page.)

TABLE 2. Cash Flow Analysis Form *(Continued)*

Description	Monthly	Other	Period
Standard of living			
Mortgage/rent			
Utilities			
Telephone			
Cable television			
Home maintenance/repairs			
Yard maintenance/repairs			
Pool maintenance/repairs			
Household furnishings/improvements			
Automobile maintenance and repairs			
Fuel and oil			
Food, groceries			
Personal care			
Clothing			
Cleaners/laundry			
Education			
School needs			
Child care			
Allowances			
Lessons (e.g., music, dancing)			
Professional dues			
Club dues			
Entertainment			
Dining out			
Sports, hobbies			
Books, subscriptions			
Gifts			
Vacations			
Charitable contributions			
Medical			
Dental			
Drugs/medical supplies			
Legal fees			
Nonreimbursed business expenses			
Tax preparation fee			
Bank charges and credit card fees			
Safe deposit box			
Child support			
Alimony			
Loans or notes payable			
(1)			
(2)			
Other expenses			
(1)			
(2)			
Miscellaneous			
Total standard of living			
Total expenses			

TABLE 3. Mortgage Analysis Comparison*

	Monthly Mortgage Payments	Biweekly Mortgage Payments
Principal	$270,000	$270,000
Annual rate	8%	8%
Payment amount	$1,981.16	990.58
Duration of mortgage	30 years	22 years, 10 months
Total interest paid	$443,217.60	$316,423.36

* Assumes interest compounding monthly, no prepayment penalties, payment in arrears (you get the money before payments are due), and regular amortization.

down payment avoids costly mortgage insurance required by the lender. Dr. Jones must pay an extra $230 per month because he was not able to pay 20% down. Another area of major expense is automobiles. Consider your options to lease versus purchase. In general, if you are going to trade in your auto every 3 years, leasing makes sense. On the other hand, if you drive your car until the wheels fall off, purchase works in your favor. Before making the decision, ask your advisor to prepare a comparison.

DEFINE GOALS AND OBJECTIVES

With the financial statement and cash flow analysis complete, the next step is defining your specific goals and objectives. If you do not know where you are going, how will you know if you ever get there? People do not plan to fail; rather, they fail to plan. Your goals should be clearly identified and written down. They should be realistic and quantifiable. How does one rank the goals? Take this simple quiz. Rank from 1 through 8 the following financial planning goals:

____ Financial independence (retirement) planning	____ Insurance planning
____ Education planning	____ Estate planning
____ Home/second home purchase	____ Income tax planning
____ Investment planning	____ Other

Answers vary not only from physician to physician but also within your own lifetime. Once your children have completed their education, for example, all of the other goals will shift. Therefore, it is important to reanalyze your goals periodically.

INSURANCE PLANNING

Before investing, make sure that you have adequate insurance protection, including life insurance for the person producing the wages for the family and disability insurance to protect the income of the wage earner. Other coverage, such as health, auto, homeowner's, and personal liability, is also part of insurance planning. You can reduce premiums with higher deductibles. Work with an agent who represents various companies, and ask for a cost–benefit analysis and comparison each year.

PROTECTING YOUR FAMILY'S STANDARD OF LIVING

Life insurance provides financial security for dependents in the event of the wage earner's premature death. It provides a means to pay off the home mortgage, to fund education expenses, to pay off liabilities, to provide an income stream to the surviving spouse for the family's standard-of-living needs, and to meet any other financial obligations for which you are responsible. Life insurance also provides money to pay estate taxes and facilitates the transition of practice value to a decedent's family. Although sorting through the maze of insurance plans and options is confusing, life insurance is necessary to make sure that your family can reach its financial goals after your death. Determine your life insurance needs before making a quick decision to buy life insurance.

Although your needs may vary, keep your insurance plan simple. You can rent your insurance, or you can own it. Term insurance is cheaper at first but in the long term usually costs more because you pay more as you get older. You do not own the coverage, and at some point the cost becomes prohibitive. Permanent insurance, such as whole life, carries fixed costs throughout the life of the insured. This type of insurance also builds equity or cash value. Other types include variable life, universal life, variable universal life, and mix life insurance with investment options.

View your life insurance policy as a means to provide death benefits—not as an investment vehicle. You can purchase the products from a licensed insurance agent or directly from the insurance company. By going with a low-load insurance carrier, you can significantly reduce your acquisition costs, especially if you buy permanent insurance. For example, eliminating the sales commission cuts distribution costs to 5–10% over the life of the policy.[11] Traditional policies often pay more than 100% of the first year's premium in commissions and 20–25% of the total premiums paid over the life of the policy.[12] However, the company's financial stability should come first. You want to make sure that the company can pay your death claim. Some low-load companies carry the highest scores from rating services such as Moody's, Standard and Poors, and A.M. Best. Request the most recent ratings before you purchase the coverage.

In most cases, if you are at an early stage in your medical career, you will want to go with term insurance. You should monitor your needs and purchase additional coverage to meet your family's needs. If you are an older and more established physician who has estate tax liquidity needs, you should consider permanent coverage, usually a policy that insures both you and your spouse and pays a death benefit at the second spouse's death (known as "second-to-die" life insurance).

PROTECTING YOUR MEDICAL PRACTICE

Business protection or continuation is another reason to consider life insurance. The death of a partner in a medical group can wreak havoc in the practice. A properly drafted buy-sell agreement mitigates much of the possible financial confusion surrounding the decedent's interest in the practice. Just as an individual's will specifies how property is to be distributed at death, a buy-sell agreement sets the parameters for liquidating an interest in the practice. It establishes the value of each interest and can function as the will for the practice. Major provisions of a buy-sell agreement include the following:

- **Statement of conditions of the buy-out.** The agreement should name the parties involved and the period for the purchase and describe any special provisions.
- **Price.** The agreement establishes the framework for determining the value of the practice and also states under which circumstances or time frame the buy-sell agreement price will be reevaluated and adjusted.
- **Method of funding the buy-sell.** Without a method of funding, the buy-sell agreement may be worthless.
- **Name a trustee.** The agreement should specify an impartial third party who will carry out the terms of the agreement, often the group's attorney or accountant.

There are two types of plans. In the first type, the corporation or the partners are the focus of the plan. If the agreement centers on the corporation, it is known as a *stock redemption plan*. Under this agreement, the corporation agrees to purchase the deceased shareholder's interest from his or her estate. The estate receives cash equal to the value of his or her interest in the practice. The value of each surviving shareholder's interest increases accordingly. The second type of plan is a *cross-purchase agreement*. The surviving physicians agree to purchase the interest from the estate of the deceased physician. The interest of the surviving partners depends on the number of shares that they purchase rather than on the value of the shares that they currently own. Numerous factors must be considered before choosing between a cross-purchase or stock redemption agreement. Tax issues are first on the list. The number of shareholders and their ages are also important.

Most agreements are funded with life insurance. It is usually the most economical way to provide money for the individual or corporation to purchase the deceased physician's interest. Split-dollar insurance can be used in conjunction with funding buy-sell agreements. Split-dollar insurance is not a particular type of insurance; rather, it is a method of sharing premiums, death benefits, and sometimes cash values between an employer and an employee.

A buy-sell agreement can also provide terms for the purchase of a disabled shareholder's interest. A disability buy-out agreement provides that, after a reasonable length of time, the disabled physician's interest will be purchased by the remaining partners or redeemed by the corporation. The price paid to the disabled owner is the amount agreed upon in advance based on a predetermined formula. Many groups allow accounts receivable to fund the agreement; however, this approach may not be appropriate in all cases. Above all, remember that buy-sell agreements are essential documents for a smooth redistribution of ownership in a medical practice.

DISABILITY INSURANCE

Protecting Your Income

Your greatest asset is your ability to earn a living, and unless you have socked away plenty of money, you need disability insurance. Disability can destroy a financial plan if the risk is not covered. Disability insurance is designed to pay a monthly benefit if you become disabled. The best policies provide an *own occupation* definition of disability: if you cannot perform the important duties of your own occupation, you are considered totally disabled. For example, if a thoracic surgeon has a policy that defines his specialty exclusively as a thoracic surgeon and back problems do not allow him to stand throughout long operations, he is considered disabled even if he can practice in another area of medicine. Some policies define disability as it relates to a *loss of earnings*. Because of underpricing of policies sold in the 1980s,[9] disability insurance is more restrictive. The amounts of monthly coverage that companies are willing to issue has dropped, the definition of disability has been altered, and the premiums have increased. Despite these changes, you should still get coverage.

Types of Coverage

Get as much long-term coverage (insurance that pays benefits to age 65) as you can qualify for and find a policy that insures you in your specialty. Short-term coverage may be added to your long-term benefits, if it is available. Generally short-term coverage pays benefits for less than 2 years and does not provide an *own occupation* definition of disability. Many policies base the definition of disability on *loss of earnings* (not your occupation). For example, if you earn $10,000 a month, but because of a disability your earnings drop to $4,500, you would receive 55% of the disability benefit. Make sure to get a policy that carries the definition of disability that meets your needs. Have your insurance agent compare policies and select a financially sound company.

INVESTMENT PLANNING

DEFINE YOUR GOALS AND OBJECTIVES

Investing is a major topic of conversation for many physicians, especially in the doctors' lounge. The stories are generally about the stock that tripled—not the investments that failed. Your money must grow if you are going to fund college for your children, reach financial independence or retirement goals, provide financial security for you and your family, or purchase a vacation house. Your age, time horizon for meeting goals, tolerance for risk, tax bracket, health, and income are just a few of the factors that must be considered in designing an investment portfolio. Define your goals and objectives before you make any investments. You would not dare treat a patient without knowing his or her medical history. Give yourself the same courtesy; know what you are trying to accomplish before investing any money.

DETERMINE YOUR TIME HORIZON

As an investor, your time horizon greatly influences the types of risks that you want to take. For example, if you are saving money to buy a new house in the next 2 years, your main concern is that the money be available. A money market fund is an appropriate vehicle. It is safe, and you do not have to worry about the principal value going down. On the other hand, the stock market is a risky investment for 2 years. You stand the chance of losing principal and having no return on your funds. The threat of volatility in the stock market overrides the possible loss of purchasing power from inflation by investing in a money market fund (Table 4).

The longer your time frame for investing, the more of a threat inflation is to your financial security. Over the long term—typically 5 years or longer—volatility is actually your ally. It provides an opportunity to earn higher rates of

TABLE 4. Highest, Lowest, and Average Annual Returns, 1926–1966

	Highest Return (%)	Lowest Return (%)	Average Return (%)
Inflation*	18.2	−10.3	3.2
Cash and equivalents	14.7	0.0	3.8
U.S. intermediate term government bonds	29.1	−5.1	5.4
U.S. large company stocks	54.0	−43.3	12.7
U.S. small company stocks	142.9	−58.0	17.7

* With inflation, the higher the return equates to a larger loss of purchasing power; i.e., the higher the return, the worse off you are.
From Ibbotson Associates: Stocks, Bonds, Bills, and Inflation 1997 Yearbook. Chicago, Ibbotson Associates, 1997.

TABLE 5. The Effect of Inflation on $100,000*

	What $100,000 Would be Worth			Future Amount Required to Equal $100,000 Today			
Age (yr)	Amount ($)	Age (yr)	Amount ($)	Age (yr)	Amount ($)	Age (yr)	Amount ($)
40	100,000	70	38,879	40	100,000	70	249,896
45	85,432	75	33,215	45	116,491	75	291,107
50	72,986	80	28,376	50	135,702	80	339,115
55	62,353	85	24,242	55	158,081	85	395,039
60	53,269	90	20,710	60	184,151	90	460,186
65	45,509	95	17,693	65	214,519	95	536,076

*Assuming inflation at 3.1% per year.

return for the level of risk that you are assuming. For example, a physician and his wife, both age 40, are planning to retire in 25 years with $100,000 in today's dollars (assume that inflation averages 3.1%). They have an average remaining life expectancy of 49 years, according to the joint and life expectancy table in IRS Publication 590. At age 65 they need $214,519 to keep the same standard of living required at age 40 (Table 5). Obviously, the sooner you start investing the better. Compound interest over extended periods has a huge effect on the money that is accumulated (Table 6).

DIVERSIFY YOUR ASSETS

Selecting asset classes or investments that have similar characteristics comes after you have a good understanding of your goals and the time horizon to meet them. Examples of asset classes include cash and equivalents, bonds, and stocks. Diversification is a buzzword synonymous with successful investing. The concept of "not putting all your eggs in one basket" is easy to understand. But *it ain't gonna work like it's supposed to unless you select the right baskets.* The driving factor that reduces volatility and improves return is the correlation or relationship between the investments in your basket.

TABLE 6. Accumulated Values Saving $10,000/Year at 8%

Starting Age (yr)	Accumulated Value ($) at Age 65	Starting Age (yr)	Accumulated Value ($) at Age 65
25	2,797,810	45	494,229
30	1,861,021	50	293,243
35	1,223,459	55	156,455
40	789,544	60	63,359

TABLE 7. Intermediate Bonds and Stocks During Declining Stock Markets

Stock Market Down Years Since 1973*	Decline of U.S. Stocks (%)	Performance of Intermediate Bonds (%)
1973	14.7	4.6
1974	26.5	5.7
1977	7.2	1.4
1981	4.9	9.5
1990	3.2	9.7

* Stock market declines in 1953, 1957, 1962, 1966, and 1967 were accompanied by positive returns for bonds in all years except 1969, when bonds declined 0.7%.
From Ibbotson Associates: Stocks, Bonds, Bills, and Inflation 1997 Yearbook. Chicago, Ibbotson Associates, 1997.

Ideally, you want both bonds and stocks, because they generally behave differently over the same period. For example, when stocks retreat, intermediate bonds usually go forward. They have a negative or imperfect correlation—they tend to move in opposite directions. As a result, they create stability when combined in a portfolio in proper proportion. Table 7 illustrates the relationship between intermediate bonds and stocks during declining stock markets.

Adding international bonds and stocks to an all-domestic portfolio also enhances diversification. In 1960 the U.S. Capital Markets represented 73.3% of the worldwide capital markets; in 1980, 51.0%. As of December 31, 1996, U.S. Capital Markets accounted for 45.9% of the world's available securities. (Capital markets are defined as the universe of public traded securities such as money market instruments, bonds, and stocks.) International investing carries both currency and political risks, thus making it riskier than U.S. markets; however, combining domestic and international securities has historically reduced risk and increased performance. With the opportunity to invest in global markets, it is no longer a question of whether to invest internationally. Rather, the question is how much should be allocated outside the United States. A diversified portfolio with international stocks added to U.S. stocks and bonds generally limits volatility. Table 8 illustrates various portfolio mixes and compares best and worst calendar year performance. Note that the portfolio of three assets earned almost as much as an all-U.S. stock portfolio with substantially less volatility. Of course, past performance does not guarantee future results. Table 9 shows the performance of these portfolios in declining stock markets.

Because studies indicate that asset allocation accounts for over 90% of the return,[1,2] selecting the right mix is an essential element of diversifying a portfolio. The return of the entire portfolio rather than the individual bond and stock components should be your measure for performance. The benefit of diversification is that the portfolio as a whole is actually safer than the individual investments.

TABLE 8. Asset Mixes

	Best Calendar Year (%)	Compound Annual Return (%)	Worst Calendar Year (%)
100% intermediate bonds	29.10	9.60	1.40
40% U.S.stocks 10% international stocks* 50% intermediate bonds	30.40	11.20	–9.40
80% U.S. stocks 20% international stocks	40.50	12.20	–24.50
100% U.S. stocks	37.20	11.60	–26.50

* As represented by the Morgan Stanley Capital International EAFE (Europe, Asia, and Far East) Index.
Source: Morgan Stanley Capital International, Ibbotson Associates, Inc., and Sanford C. Bernstein & Co., Inc.

MONITOR YOUR PROGRESS

Measuring your return is a must if you want to know how your investments are doing. The total return is the amount of income generated in the form of dividends or interest added to the increase or decrease in value. For example, one may compute total return for three basic asset classes: cash and equivalents, bonds, and stocks. Cash and equivalents, which include certificates of deposit, treasury bills, and money market accounts, earn interest or dividends and do not have the potential to grow in value; their total return equals their income. If a CD earns 5%, its total return is the same.

Bonds pay interest, but you also have the opportunity for change in market values, depending on the direction of interest rates. When you invest in a bond, you loan your money to a government or corporation in return for a stated interest payment and principal amount at maturity, when the issuer returns the amount you invested. The issue may call the bond before maturity. The direction of interest rates, maturity, and credit ratings influence the change in market values. For example, if a long-term bond has a yield of 8% and interest

TABLE 9. Stock Market Down Years Since 1973

	1973 (%)	1974 (%)	1977 (%)	1981 (%)	1990 (%)
100% intermediate bonds	4.6	5.7	1.4	9.5	9.7
40% U.S.stocks 10% international stocks* 50% intermediate bonds	–4.3	–9.4	–1.1	–2.4	–1.8
80% U.S. stocks 20% international stocks	–13.2	–24.5	–3.5	–4.7	–6.1
100% U.S. stocks	–14.7	–26.5	–7.2	–4.9	–3.2

* As represented by the Morgan Stanley Capital International EAFE (Europe, Asia, and Far East) Index.
Source: Ibbotson Associates, Inc., Morgan Stanley Capital International, and Bernstein as cited in Sanford C. Bernstein & Co: Gaining the global edge. Investment Planning in the Global Era, July, 1994.

rates drop 1%, it may increase 10–15% in value. On the other hand, if rates go up by 1%, the bond's value may plummet.

Stocks generally give you the opportunity for the highest return but also involve more risk. For example, if a stock pays a 4% quarterly dividend and the share value increases by 5%, the total return is 9%. History has shown that stocks provide better returns after taxes and inflation than cash equivalents and bonds.

Cash and equivalents such as certificates of deposit are safe from volatility risk, but taxes and inflation hit them hard. For your real rate of return, you have to subtract inflation and taxes. For example, a $100,000 CD earning 5% generates $5,000 in income but forfeits $1,550 in taxes (at a 31% tax bracket: 0.31 × $5,000) and loses $3,000 to inflation at a 3% rate. The net gain after taxes and inflation is $450 (0.45%). *Taxes and inflation must be considered when determining your allocation and return* (Table 10).

Mutual funds allow investors with common investment objectives to pool their dollars and get professional money management with instant diversification. Purchasing shares in mutual funds is one of the easiest ways to invest; however, making the selection is a bit more difficult with over 8,000 funds to choose from. A mutual fund is an investment company that pools money from many investors and is run by a manager who invests that money in various stocks, bonds, and money market instruments. A mutual fund has an investment objective stated in its prospectus or disclosure document. Some funds state their objective clearly, whereas others are vague. Table 11 lists mutual fund objectives used by Morningstar, an industry watch-dog.

Do not throw darts at various funds to make your selection. Consider the following facts before you invest:

- **Performance record.** Compare total return with other funds that have the same investment objective and own the same types of underlying securities. You want to compare apples to apples. Once again, a solid

---

TABLE 10. After-tax and Inflation-adjusted Returns*

Compound Annual Returns,[†] 1926–1996	Before Taxes and Inflation (%)	After Taxes (%)	After Taxes and Inflation (%)
U.S. large company stock	10.7	8.2	4.9
Long-term municipal bonds	4.1	4.1	1.0
Long-term government bonds	5.1	3.6	0.4
Treasury bills	3.7	2.1	–1.0

* Federal income tax calculated on a monthly basis using the actual marginal tax rates for a single taxpayer earning $75,000 in 1989 dollars every year. This annual income is adjusted using the Consumer Price Index to obtain the corresponding income level for each year. No state income taxes are included. Taxes are paid monthly, and no capital gains taxes on municipal bonds are assumed. Assumes reinvestment of income and no transaction costs. Past performance is no guarantee of future results.
† From Ibbotson Associates: The Asset Allocation Decision. Chicago, Ibbotson Associates, 1997.

TABLE 11.   Mutual Fund Classes and Categories

Large growth	Specialty: real estate	Intermediate-term government bonds
Mid-cap growth	Specialty: communication	Short-term government bonds
Small growth	Specialty: unaligned	Long-term domestic bonds
Large blend	Domestic hybrid	Intermediate-term domestic bonds
Mid-cap blend	Convertibles	Short-term domestic bonds
Small blend	Foreign stock	Ultra-short domestic bonds
Large value	World stock	High yield (a.k.a. junk) bonds
Mid-cap value	Europe stock	Multisector bonds
Small value	Diversified Pacific/Asia stock	International bonds
Specialty: precious metals	Pacific/Asia ex-Japan stock	Muni bonds: national long
Specialty: natural resources	Japan stock	Muni bonds: national intermediate
Specialty: technology	Diversified emerging markets	Muni bonds: single state long
Specialty: utilities	Latin America stock	Muni bonds: single state intermediate
Specialty: health	International hybrid	Muni bonds: short
Specialty: financial	Long-term government bonds	

track record is no guarantee of future results. Make sure that the manager of the fund with the good performance is still running the show.

- **Beta measure.** A fund's beta measure compares its fluctuations with the Standard & Poors 500 Index. This number is a measure of volatility. For example, the S&P 500 has a beta of 1.00. If the fund you select carries a beta of 0.80, your fund is more conservative than the market and should be 20% less volatile.
- **Turnover ratio.** Turnover ratio is a gauge to measure the fund's trading activity. A low turnover ratio is generally associated with low-risk funds.
- **Expenses and commissions.** The expense ratio includes operating, marketing, and management expense. The lower the better. Many funds sold through brokers carry sales commissions ranging from 4–8.5% or "back-end" sales charges. The commission is calculated based on the amount of money invested in the fund. For example, on a $100,000 contribution to a fund that has a 4% sales charge, $4,000 is deducted and only $96,000 goes to the fund for investment. Pure "no-load" funds do not add a sales charge, and 100% of your contribution goes toward your savings. Always request a prospectus. Read it carefully to analyze all costs associated with the fund.

EXPECT MARKET VOLATILITY

Volatility in the financial markets is real, and unless you know your threshold for pain or how you will react when your investments decline in value, investing in stocks is a nerve-wracking experience. Fear and greed are tough

TABLE 12. The Market Made Up Its Losses Fairly Quickly—But Not for Those Who Sold Out

Bear Market	Total Months	Total Return (%) (S&P 500)	First Year after Decline Total Return (%)	Months to Break-even (from End of Bear Market)
07/48–05/49	11	9.6	42.4	4
01/53–08/53	8	8.7	35.0	5
08/57–12/57	5	14.9	43.4	7
01/60–10/60	10	8.4	32.6	2
01/62–09/62	6	19.4	31.7	7
02/66–09/66	8	15.6	30.6	6
12/68–06/70	19	29.2	41.9	9
01/73–09/74	21	42.6	38.1	21
01/77–02/78	14	14.1	16.6	5
12/80–07/82	20	16.9	59.4	3
09/87–11/87	3	29.5	23.2	18
Average	**11**	**19.3**	**35.9**	**8**

Source: Ibbotson Associates and Bernstein.

emotions for an investor to handle. If you have the chance to earn higher rates of return, you had better be prepared to weather some ups and downs in your portfolio. Be aware that investors are generally used to rising domestic stock prices and have not had to endure a significant decline since the period from July to mid October in 1990. But do not panic. Although your stock portfolio may plummet at any time, savvy investors know that if you hang on to your stocks, the values come back (Table 12).

Timing the market—trying to pick the best times to own stocks or be on the sidelines—seems impossible. The stock market has increased on average about 1% per month since 1925. In the best 60 months—only 7% of the total period—the average return was approximately 12% per month. If you missed the surge in stock prices, your returns languished (Table 13). The penalty for

TABLE 13. Dangers of Market Timing—S&P 500 Returns, 1926–1996*

	Percent of All Months	Average Monthly Return (%)
852 months	100	1.01
Best 60 months	7	11.89
All other months	93	0.19

* Being out of the stock market during its best gains—usually sudden—meant missing almost all of the long-term growth.
Source: Ibbotson Associates and Bernstein. Computed using data from Ibbotson Associates: Stocks, Bonds, Bills, and Inflation 1996 Yearbook. Chicago, Ibbotson Associates, 1996.

TABLE 14. Missing a Few Good Days Substantially Reduces Return*

1980–1989	S&P 500 Annualized Returns (%)
All 2,528 trading days	17.5
Minus 10 best days	12.6
Minus 20 best days	9.3
Minus 30 best days	6.5
Minus 40 best days	3.9

* Figures assume that when not invested in stocks, assets were earning interest at the average rate of 30-day treasury bills over the 1980–1989 period.
Source: Datastream, Ibbotson Associates, and Sanford C. Bernstein & Co.

missing best performing days in the market can be substantial, as indicated by Tables 14 and 15.

Trying to time the market by switching asset allocations among cash, bonds, and stocks has a low probability of success. *It is time, not timing, that counts most.* The surges in stock prices tend to come in short, powerful bursts. If you are not invested, it is too late to participate. A buy-and-hold strategy does not take into account rebalancing or selling when the prices are high and reallocating based on an asset allocation model. The asset allocation is driven by the investment criteria mentioned earlier. For example, Dr. McCarthy is a 40-year-old physician who is saving for retirement and has a moderate risk profile. Her portfolio may be allocated in the following manner: 5% cash and equivalents, 25% U.S. bonds, 20% U.S. large company stocks, 15% U.S. small company stocks, 20% international stocks, and 15% real estate. As the percentages change in her allocation by 10% or more in any class, the change should set off

TABLE 15. The Difficulty of Timing Market Moves

1991 Market Performance	S&P 500 Appreciation (%)	No. of Trading Days
Entire year	26.3	253
January 16–February 13	17.6	21
Last 7 days	9.0	7
Rest of 1991	−1.5	225
1989–1994	**S&P Annualized Returns (%)**	
All 1,275 trading days	10.30	
Minus 10 best trading days	4.28	
Minus 20 best trading days	0.14	
Minus 30 best trading days	−3.29	
Minus 40 best trading days	−6.56	

From Evensky HR: Wealth Management. Dubuque, IA, Times Mirror Higher Education Group, 1997.

a trigger to rebalance the portfolio. It forces her to sell assets when they have gone up in value and allocate the proceeds to the areas in the portfolio that are underperforming. Portfolio allocations vary according to investment criteria of the individual. There are no shortcuts for building financial security. If the investment sounds too good to be true, it probably is.

COLLEGE FUND PLANNING

College tuition is escalating faster than the rate of inflation.[4] Unfortunately, some parents do not plan for college expenses until they are faced with their first semester cost. According to Barron's, parents typically start saving about 10 years before their first child matriculates. Tuition usually comes from current earnings or is financed with loans. Scholarships are available in some cases. Prefunding or saving before tuition comes due is obviously the most economical path to follow. Why? Because the sooner you start saving, compound interest can lower your real cost (Table 16).

Various planning strategies are available. Once the appropriate method is finalized, investments can be selected. Administration expenses vary according to the method and should be reasonable. Structure, flexibility, property control, and tax ramifications are essential issues to discuss with your advisor.

EDUCATION PLANNING TOOLS

Parents and grandparents can integrate estate planning strategies with education planning tools. Trusts and custodianships can be created as receptacles of gifts for a child's benefit. The gift must satisfy the present interest requirement to avoid gift tax and can be up to $10,000 per year. For substantial gifts over several years, trusts come in handy. A husband and wife may each donate $10,000 or $20,000 per year free of gift tax to the trust. Include two grandparents, and you may see $40,000 per year escaping gift tax. Income and principal distributions as well as the life of the trust vary depending on the type of trust selected.

TABLE 16.   College Savings at Birth vs. at Child's Age 10 Years

	Start at Birth ($)	Wait until Age 10 ($)
Present annual cost	15,000	15,000
Projected cost of 4 years' attendance*	187,300	187,300
Single payment needed to fund cost	46,872	101,192
Annual payments needed to fund cost	4,631	16,305

* At $15,000/yr after 18 years of inflation.

Charitable Remainder Trust. If you own highly appreciated property that would realize substantial taxes if you sold it and you are interested in benefiting charity and need to provide education expenses, a charitable remainder trust may be the appropriate tool. After the property is transferred to the trust, it may be sold without tax. The proceeds may be reinvested to provide income or education expenses for a specified number of years or for the life of the beneficiary. The individual transferring the property is entitled to an income tax deduction. The property passes to charity upon termination of the trust term.

Custodianship for Minors. A simple tool often used is custodianship for minors. Gifts qualify for the annual gift tax exclusion; however, they lack the flexibility offered by trusts. If the donor serves as custodian and the minor dies during the term, the account value will be included in the donor's estate. The custodial property is transferred to the minor at age of majority. Think twice about allowing an 18-year-old to control his or her college tuition money. An 18-year-old may decide to use it for another purpose.

Direct Tuition Payments. Grandparents can make tuition payments directly to the institution. This approach avoids the annual gift tax exclusion rules, and there is no limit on the amount that can be paid for tuition. But the check must be paid directly to the school.

After the funding method is selected, time frames, risk tolerance, and income needs should be determined and matched with suitable investments. Contact several likely colleges that your child may attend and request present tuition cost. Use these data to project future costs and to calculate how much you should save, assuming a conservative investment return.

INCOME TAX PLANNING

Have you ever wondered why we have a federal income tax? If you are like most taxpayers, you think about it only in April and try to forget it the rest of the year. Taxes are a sobering fact of life and are subject to constant change. Since its inception over 80 years ago, our tax system has undergone massive overhauls.

Americans were first introduced to federal income taxes in 1862 because of the costs of the Civil War. However, ten years after the war, the system lapsed. Congress adopted an income tax again in 1894, but the Supreme Court ruled in the Pollock case that it was unconstitutional because the tax was neither uniform nor apportioned among the states. In 1909 Congress adopted the Sixteenth Amendment, which serves as the foundation for the income tax law. It authorizes Congress to establish and collect taxes on income. By 1913, 75% of the states had ratified the income tax. On February 25, 1913, the Sixteenth Amendment became part of the constitution. Ten months later, it became law.

At that time, Woodrow Wilson was president, women could not vote, and horse and buggy carriages were on their way out.

The federal income tax system serves four purposes:

1. Generation of money to operate the federal government. Producing revenue for the federal government is the major function. Tax collection represents 75% of the government's net receipts.

2. Management of the nation's economy. Higher taxes result in less consumer spending, thus lowering inflation if government spending remains level. Lower tax rates and tax incentives reward consumers with more cash. The surplus can be directed toward increased spending, saving, and investing.

3. Regulation. Income tax discourages corporations from accumulating too much cash in excess of their reasonable needs. Expensive tax penalties are assessed under certain circumstances.

4. Social function. The income tax can be used to achieve government policy. Because the tax is progressive, your tax bill increases more than proportionately as your taxable income increases. The higher your income, the higher your income tax rate. The government funnels tax dollars to help lower income taxpayers. Congress attempts to balance the need for funds and, at the same time, to be fair to taxpayers.

METHODS TO REDUCE TAXES

Move Investments. Be on the look out for ways to cut your taxes. Simple moves reduce taxable income. For example, make a move from a taxable investment to one that is tax-free. If you have savings in a taxable money market fund, you may want to consider a tax-free money market fund. Alternatively, if you have taxable bonds, you may substitute municipal bonds. To see if the move is worthwhile, simply work through this formula: divide the tax-free return by 1 minus your bracket. The answer tells you if you are better off in a tax-free investment. For example, if you are considering a tax-free investment paying 6% and you are in a 36% tax bracket, divide 0.06 by (1–0.36). The answer is 9.375%. Unless you are earning more than the 9.375% before taxes, a move may be worthwhile.

Tax Deferral. Tax deferral occurs when you postpone the income you earn today to a future date. For example, you can buy short-term securities such as treasury bills and defer the income into the next year. A pension or profit-sharing plan shelters the earnings from taxes until distributions begin. You can combine both tax reduction and tax deferral through your retirement plan. This is generally the best way to save money and reduce taxes at the same time.

Income Shifting. Income shifting is the transfer of income-producing property to someone, such as a family member, in a lower tax bracket. For example, you can shift the ownership of dividend-paying stock to your 15-year-old child. The dividends will be taxed at his or her bracket. Earnings up to $1,300 from property transferred to children under age 14 are taxed at the child's bracket. Any amount over $1,300 is taxed at the parent's rate. Custodial accounts are commonly used to save for college and to shift earnings to a lower bracket. *But remember that any funds placed in a custodial account may not end up the way you planned.* The child ultimately decides how to spend the money. Maybe college—maybe not.

Investment Losses. Your investment portfolio is a good place to start looking for ways to trim your tax bill. If you have taken capital gains, you can offset those gains dollar for dollar against capital losses. Look for investments with paper losses to sell and reduce the gains. You can also offset ordinary income up to $3,000 from losses that exceed the gains.

Take a dry run. Project estimated income taxes, and review the impact that any moves would have on your tax bill.

RETIREMENT PLANNING

The specter of financial insecurity weighs heavily on physicians' minds these days. Haunted by the uncertainty of health care reform and what it may mean for their reimbursements, many physicians are turning their thoughts to retirement. Indeed, many of my physician clients ask me, "How soon can I retire?"

FUNDAMENTAL PRINCIPLES FOR FINANCIAL INDEPENDENCE

Planning for financial independence is essentially no different from setting any other financial planning goal. The same fundamental rules apply. They can be summarized in a few simple points:

- Retirement planning should be part of one's entire financial plan, which should be reviewed periodically to see that strategies are on target to meet stated goals.
- The earlier you start, the easier it will be.
- Saving for retirement is a discipline. As one shoe company puts it, "Just do it."

A physician may have an adequate concept of his or her financial goals and plans, but that is not enough. Emotional stress is inherent in retirement planning. For example, a physician and spouse may live another 30 years—approximately one-third of their life—in the golden years of retirement. Will their capital last? This fear can be addressed by incorporating retirement capital projections into planning. These analyses consider various financial factors. Although financial planning involves more than simply listing assets, liabilities, and insurance policies on a sheet of paper, the list is a key step.

The answer to the bottom-line question, "How soon can I retire?," is "It depends." People who feel an urgent need to retire probably need to make some sacrifices to save more now and perhaps will need to continue a leaner standard of living during retirement. On the other hand, people who will settle for nothing less than a similar standard of living must either save more now or continue to work longer. Other options to consider are trying to increase the rate of return on investments—or continuing to work part time. The retirement planning process is separated into two stages: accumulation and distribution.

ACCUMULATION STAGE

The accumulation stage involves setting goals such as a target retirement age and the amount of annual income needed to maintain your standard of living. The rate of return on your investments and the amount you need to save to accumulate adequate capital to provide retirement income are essential components for a solid savings foundation. There are two methods to save—before tax and after tax.

Before-tax Saving Method
Before-tax savings are more valuable because of the higher tax rates. For example, a $30,000 contribution to a pension and profit-sharing plan costs a taxpayer in the 36% bracket only $19,200. Tax savings total $10,800 ($30,000 × 36% = $10,800). The Internal Revenue Service shares in the contribution. *For retirement, save as much as you can before tax.*

The power of pretax savings can fuel an explosive advantage over methods of inferior after-tax savings. For example, a 40-year-old physician who saves $30,000 annually before tax for 25 years will accumulate $2,193,178 if the capital grows at 8%. The same dollars saved after tax total only $19,200 annually to invest, assuming a 36% tax bracket; taxes consume $10,800. The after-tax portfolio will have a balance of only $931,667 at age 65, a net difference of $1,261,511. The pretax accumulates into a larger, more secure retirement.

After-tax Saving Method
Methods of after-tax savings are tax-free, tax-deferred, and taxable investments. Municipal bonds, fixed and variable annuities, stocks, and government and corporate bonds are examples of after-tax saving vehicles. Higher taxes combined with the uncertainty of medicine require a disciplined approach to accumulating capital for retirement. The financial planning process removes the guesswork and provides a system for establishing and monitoring progress during the accumulation phase.

You can control such variables as spending and rates of return; however, inflation and taxes follow their own course. Together these components play a major role in setting your standards of living during your retirement years and are the driving force behind how long your retirement capital will last. The variables must be monitored frequently so that adjustments can be made as warranted.

Selecting investments to sustain your income needs is an area that requires more than a "seat-of-the-pants" approach and is a critical part of each phase. Investment mistakes can be overcome during your earning years, but once you rely on your capital, investment errors can devastate your golden years. If you do not have the expertise or have not taken the time to acquire money management skills, do not risk the do-it-yourself approach. It may come back to haunt you. Many tax, legal, financial, and nonfinancial issues must be considered in making the transition from the accumulation phase to the distribution phase.

DISTRIBUTION STAGE

The distribution stage of retirement planning involves monitoring distributions from your retirement plans, checking the performance of your investments, and keeping an eye on your spending. Retirement plans carry tax advantages. However, if you take your money out too soon or too late or if you take out too little, you may be hammered with penalty taxes. Planning in advance may prevent these expensive and often avoidable penalties from zapping your retirement funds.

Too-soon Penalty Tax

A distribution before age $59\frac{1}{2}$ years from a qualified retirement plan is subject to a 10% penalty tax on the taxable portion. There are certain exceptions to the penalty: distributions made to a beneficiary, distributions received due to the participant's disability, distributions that are part of a series of substantially equal periodic payments received not less than annually and made over the life expectancy of the participant (or life expectancies of the participant and his or her beneficiary), and distributions received after separation from service under a plan's early retirement provision [Internal Revenue Code Section 72(+)].

For example, a $100,000 premature distribution would be reduced by a $10,000 penalty tax ($100,000 × 10%) and $31,000 in regular income tax ($100,000 × 31% or 41%). A less expensive way to withdraw retirement plan funds is to have payments spread over your life expectancy. This payout method escapes the penalty.

Too-late Penalty Tax

A participant must receive minimum distributions from his or her retirement plan by April 1 of the year following the year in which the participant attains age $70\frac{1}{2}$. The minimum distribution for each subsequent year must be made no later than the last day of the year. The Small Business Job Protection Act of 1996 postpones the required distribution for an employee who owns 5% or less of the business with respect to the plan year ending in the calendar year in which the employee attains age 70½.

The penalty tax for tardy distribution is a hefty 50% tax on the shortfall that should have been withdrawn by April 1 after the year in which the participant attained age 70½. Of course, this tax is in addition to regular income taxes.

Too-little Penalty Tax

The minimum required distribution is based on the total balance of all IRAs and qualified retirement plans. It is calculated according to the life expectancy of the participant and beneficiary, if applicable. For example, a husband and wife, both age 71, have retirement plan values of $1,500,000. Their joint life expectancy is 19.8 years. The required minimum distribution (based on annual recalculation method) is $75,758 ÷ 19.8). If they withdraw $50,000, they are $25,758 short of the required minimum and face a "too-little" penalty tax of $12,879 ($25,758 × 50%).

If you are near the magic age, be certain that you are meeting the guidelines for the distribution amounts. The IRS may waive the penalty under certain circumstances if the minimum distribution shortfall was a result of reasonable error and reasonable steps are taken to correct it. But doing it right the first time is a much better guarantee that you will not be unduly penalized.

Both the timing and amounts of distributions from retirement plans should be evaluated in light of meeting your income needs and avoiding unnecessary penalty taxes. Be sure to follow the rules in withdrawing retirement funds. It can save you a bundle.

No More Success Tax

The Taxpayer Relief Act of 1997 repealed the 15% excise tax that applied to excessive distributions from retirement plans. It also repealed the 15% tax that applied to decedents who had accumulated too much in their retirement plan as of their date of death. As a result, you do not have to worry about paying triple taxes on retirement plan benefits. Estate taxes and income taxes take a bite out of these plans, but they still remain an attractive means to accumulate wealth.

Caveat: Do not pay estate taxes with retirement plan assets. Use life insurance or assets held outside the plan. It costs approximately 40 cents on the dollar if you use retirement plan assets to pay your estate tax bill.

Minimum Distribution Rules

Minimum distribution rules come into play when a participant in a retirement plan dies before reaching the required beginning date. The required beginning date is April 1 of the calendar year after the calendar year in which the participant reached or would have reached age 70½. These rules also affect distributions when a participant reaches the required beginning date and withdraws funds during his or her lifetime. The rules are different for each period. The beneficiary designation is an essential factor in calculating how the funds are distributed to the participant. It also sets the parameters for the payout period to the beneficiary after the participant's death

Distributions before the Required Beginning Date

If a participant dies before reaching the required beginning date, a spouse beneficiary generally can choose to receive benefits annually over his or her life expectancy beginning by December 31 of the year in which the participant would have reached age 70½. Another option for the spouse is to roll the benefits into an IRA and treat it as his or her own. The surviving spouse names a new beneficiary and is subject to minimum distribution rules. The rollover feature is available only for a surviving spouse. Distributions to a nonspouse beneficiary are paid in annual installments over the life expectancy of the nonspouse beneficiary beginning by December 31 of the year after the year in which the participant died. If the estate of the participant is named as beneficiary, the benefits have to be distributed within five years after death. Generally, the estate is not a recommended selection because the beneficiaries forego substantial tax deferral and are hit hard with income taxes.

Distributions at the Required Beginning Date

Profit-sharing plans, pension plans, 401(k) plans, 403(b) plans, and IRAs are subject to the required minimum distribution rules. The minimum distribution rules require you to take a minimum distribution by your required beginning date. In general, the required minimum withdrawal is based on the participant's life expectancy; the joint life expectancy of the participant and the participant's spouse; or the joint life expectancy of a participant and a nonspouse beneficiary. If a nonspouse beneficiary is more than 10 years younger than the participant, the minimum distribution is calculated as if the beneficiary were only 10 years younger than the participant, applying a special divisor [Proposed Treas. Regs. 1.401(a)(9)-2]. The minimum distribution incidental benefit rule (MDIB) prevents a participant from minimizing required distributions.

For example, if the surviving spouse, age 72, names her 42-year-old son as beneficiary, the minimum payout is calculated as if the son were 10 years younger. However, at his mother's death the MDIB divisor will be terminated. Moreover, the payout stream will be based on the adjusted original actual joint life expectancy divisor (1 less each year his mother had lived after the rollover was set up). Thus the son can receive benefits over his remaining life expectancy. The actual life expectancy of the mother and child is 40.9 years, but the MDIB rules shortens it for distribution purposes to 24.4. If the mother lives for 5 years, the son can take distributions over 35.9 years.

Beneficiary Designations

Many financial and nonfinancial factors must be considered before selecting a beneficiary. The financial needs of the account holder and spouse as well as their present health should be weighed before making a selection. Grand-children are candidates for beneficiaries if the account holder is in poor health, the spouse and children have sufficient income and/or assets, and the child of the IRA owner is in a high estate tax bracket and high income tax bracket.

For example, a 70-year-old physician may name his 5-year-old grand-daughter as beneficiary of his IRA. If the proper trust agreements are in place, at his death she will be able to take out distributions over her life expectancy. She will subtract one year for each year that withdrawals were made by the account holder and continue receiving distributions over her life expectancy. A trust qualifies as a designated beneficiary if the following conditions [Proposed Treas. Regs. 1.409(a)(9)-7, D-5A(a)] are met:

1. The trust is irrevocable.

2. The trust is valid under state law or would be but for the fact that there is no principal.

3. A copy of the trust is provided to the custodian.

4. The beneficiaries are identifiable from the trust instrument.

5. No person has the power to change the beneficiaries of the trust.

6. Each noncontingent beneficiary is an individual.

Be careful not to leave more than $1 million to grandchildren to avoid generation-skipping transfer tax, which is a hefty 55%. The generation-skipping tax applies to transfers of property that skip a generation.

Distribution Elections

Participants may elect to receive their distributions over a fixed term or period certain. The most common method in calculating distributions is recalculation. A participant with a spouse beneficiary can elect to receive distributions over their joint life expectancy. For example, if the two people are age 70 and 65, the benefits can be paid out over 23.1 years. The single life expectancy of a 70-year-old is 16 years. Each year a new life expectancy is recalculated under this method. If the beneficiary predeceases the participant, the participant can continue to withdraw funds based on the participant's life expectancy. However, at the participant's death, the beneficiaries have to withdraw the benefits within one year. Thus, the children, if named beneficiary, will not be able to stretch the payout period. Because the order of deaths is uncertain, generally the participant should elect the recalculation method and the spouse should elect to receive installments over a fixed period or term certain. This hybrid method affords the children the option of receiving the benefits over the remaining balance of the term certain period that the spouse originally elected if any remain after the participant's death. The hybrid method is available only for married couples.

In most instances, it is best for the wife to elect an IRA rollover if the husband predeceases. She can name a new beneficiary and begin withdrawals once she reaches age 70.5. At her death, the benefits can be paid out over the children's life expectancies. If she keeps the benefits in her husband's IRA, at her death the children must withdraw all benefits within one year of her death.

Selecting the distribution option from your retirement plans is one of the most important decisions you will make. Financial and nonfinancial factors must be considered before making any elections. Proceed with caution. I advise my clients to get a receipt from the retirement plan administrator or IRA custodian acknowledging receipt of the beneficiary distributions and the payout option selected.

ERISA GUIDELINES FOR RETIREMENT PLAN INVESTMENTS

Physicians are acutely aware of the potential liability arising from medical mal practice suits. However, many are unknowingly exposed to significant liability risks by directing the investments in their qualified retirement plans. Just as insurance can soften the blow of malpractice claims, following Employee Retirement Security Act of 1974 (ERISA) guidelines for pension and profit-sharing plans establishes a solid basis for protection if you are deemed a plan fiduciary and sued by an unhappy participant.

ERISA established standards for managing retirement plan assets and was enacted to protect money invested for participants and their beneficiaries. ERISA defines a fiduciary as a person who (1) exercises discretionary authority or control over plan management or any authority or control over management or disposition of plan assets, (2) renders investment advice for a fee or other compensation regarding plan assets, or (3) has discretionary authority or responsibility in plan administration [ERISA Sec. 3(21)(A)]. For example, any physician who selects investments for the practice's/group's retirement plan or is a member of a committee that recommends an investment advisor or a consultant to manage plan assets is considered a fiduciary. This roles carries tremendous responsibility to all plan participants.

Are you a fiduciary? If so, test yourself and determine if you are following prudent steps in managing your plan's assets. ERISA outlines the following procedures for a plan fiduciary to follow:

- **Establish an investment policy.** The policy should be in writing and contain information such as the plan's return objectives (e.g., achieving a rate of return of 4% over the Consumer Price Index). The policy specifies asset classes (e.g., type of stocks, bonds) that are consistent with the plan's risk level. The process for making investment decisions and selecting specific managers (mutual funds and/or private money managers) is defined. The investment policy statement serves as a foundation for making investment decisions.

- **Diversify plan assets.** Asset allocation or diversification plays a dominant role in the overall performance of plan assets. It reduces risk, mitigates volatility, and may increase potential return. Do not put all your eggs in one basket.
- **Make investment decisions with the skill and care of a prudent expert.** Owning all CDs in a retirement plan is not prudent. In fact, it is a direct violation of ERISA. Retirement plan assets must be diversified. If you choose to transfer investment decisions to a money manager, you still must use prudent standards in selection of an investment advisor.
- **Monitor performance.** The investment policy sets the standards to measure performance, which should be analyzed frequently and compared with indices such as the rate of inflation, treasury bills, and S&P 500.
- **Control investment expenses.** Expenses reduce the bottom-line return and vary according to the types of investments selected for your plan. Each year evaluate and review all commissions, execution costs, management fees, and custodian fees that are applicable. As plan assets grow, you should be able to negotiate reduced costs.
- **Avoid prohibited transactions.** This complex area is beyond the scope of this chapter. In general, avoid situations that seem to be a conflict of interest between the plan, the fiduciary, and any person dealing with plan assets.

If you are in doubt about your role as a fiduciary, seek advice immediately. Consult with your advisors, and determine whether you are following ERISA guidelines. It may save you many headaches and protect you in the event of a lawsuit from a disgruntled participant. Besides, it is a good common sense approach to investing.

ESTATE PLANNING

The verbiage in wills and trusts often makes these documents appear as if they are written in a foreign language. Review the following terms before meeting with an estate-planning lawyer.

Annual gift exclusion: $10,000 per calendar year per donee or $20,000 per year per donee in case of a married couple. Gifts that meet these guidelines escape gift tax.

Ascertainable standard: distributions made strictly to provide for the support, health, or education of a specific beneficiary.

Community property: both husband and wife are accorded status of equals because of the actual contribution that each makes to the marriage and the marital partnership. Eight states have community property systems: Texas, Washington, Idaho, New Mexico, California, Louisiana, Arizona, and Nevada.

Crummey power: allows each beneficiary of an irrevocable life insurance trust to be considered receiving a gift of present interest—the prerequisite to the annual exclusion rule.

Direct skip: an outright transfer of property that skips a generation.

Election against the will: the basic right under state laws of a surviving spouse to claim a specific share of the estate even if left out of a deceased spouse's will.

Five and five rule: provides that 5% of the corpus (the principle of a trust) or $5,000 (whichever is greater) can be allowed to lapse each year with no adverse gift or estate tax consequences.

General power of appointment: a power over property that may be considered to be actual ownership or control over the underlying property.

Gross estate: includes all property interests owned by the decedent at the date of death.

Incidents of ownership: ability to change beneficiary, power to assign the policy, make loans on the policy, or surrender the policy; criteria used for determining inclusion of a life insurance policy in the insured's estate.

Intestacy: dying without a will. If you die without a will, state laws control the distribution of your estate.

Irrevocable life insurance trust: a trust designed to keep life insurance out of the estate of the policy owner. Terms and provisions cannot be amended or changed.

Joint tenancy with right of survivorship: applies to jointly titled assets with a survivorship feature between joint owners.

Revocable trust: a trust in which the grantor reserves the beneficial employment of the transferred property and the power to change any part of the arrangement at any time.

Second to die policy: a life insurance policy that insures two lives and pays a death benefit at the second death.

Stepped-up basis: the cost of property acquired from a decedent is the fair market value of the property at the date of death.

Tenancy in common: each cotenant has an undivided interest in the property with no survivorship feature.

Unified credit: for decedents dying after December 31, 1986, a credit of $192,800 is allowed to be taken from the federal estate tax liability. Estates of $600,000 or less will not incur any federal estate tax liability.

OVERVIEW OF ESTATE PLANNING

A will is just the starting point in sound estate planning. In fact, if you have not created your own will, the government has an estate plan for you. Unfortunately, it will be dictated by your state of residence, and the state does not consider your wishes, timing of distributions, or special needs of your family. Once an estate breaks $600,000 for individuals or $1,200,000 for couples, the minimum federal estate tax rate kicks in at 37% and keeps climbing to a maximum rate of 55%.

The Taxpayer Relief Act of 1997 gradually increases the $600,000 exemption until it reaches $1,000,000 in 2006. For decedents dying in 1998, the unified credit will provide an effective exemption of $625,000; $650,000 in 1999; $675,000 in 2000 and 2001; $700,000 in 2002 and 2003; $850,000 in 2004; $950,000 in 2005; and $1,000,000 in 2006. The $600,000 amount applies to decedents who die before January 1, 1998.

Basic Issues

Most physicians have some sort of an estate plan—a will, power of attorney documents, and a trust or two. These documents alone will not solve all of your estate-planning concerns. Documents must be coordinated with title to property and distribution objectives. A will directs to whom and how your assets will be distributed upon your death. Is your will up to date? Do you own enough property in your name to take advantage of each spouse's $625,000 exemption? A will cannot control property titled as joint tenants with rights of survivorship because property passes directly to the surviving owner. Furthermore, passing property by joint tenancy may not work with your estate-planning objectives. The unlimited marital deduction works well if you want to pass all of your estate to your spouse tax-free. However, the marital deduction only postpones taxes until the surviving spouse's death. But what if you have children from a previous marriage for whom you want to provide? What if your spouse remarries after your death? Without adequate planning, a large portion of your estate may go to the new partner's family.

Retirement plan assets usually account for a large part of a physician's estate. These benefits pass to a named beneficiary at death. The surviving spouse is usually designated as beneficiary because of favorable income tax advantages. The funds can be rolled over to an IRA and postpone any income tax. However, it may prove costly if the spouse does not have financial experience or a team of advisors. Making investment decisions can be overwhelming without preparation.

Annual Gifts

Giving money away during your lifetime can lower your estate tax bite. For example, a person can give up to $10,000 annually in cash, property, securities, or any other asset to a designated beneficiary. The amount doubles if your spouse joins the giving. For example, if you have two children and each child has two children, you can give away tax-free $120,000 per year. It not only removes the property from your estate but also any future appreciation on the gift. For someone in the 43% tax bracket, one year of giving $120,000 will cut estate taxes by $51,600. After 1998, the $10,000 annual exclusion will be indexed for inflation.

ESTATE-PLANNING STRATEGIES

The high cost of dying can be minimized with various estate-planning strategies. Grieving the loss of a loved one is difficult, but planning ahead will relieve your family of the burden of inheriting an estate in financial disarray.

Using Trusts in Your Estate Plan

Legal documents, such as trusts, play a vital role in reducing estate taxes, managing assets for family members, and making tax-free gifts. A trust has three key positions: the creator(s), the trustee(s), and the beneficiary (ies).

1. The **creator** is also referred to as the settlor or grantor and is the person who establishes the trust. The creator appoints the trustee, names the beneficiaries, and defines the frequency of distributions to the beneficiaries.

2. The **trustee** is the person or institution responsible for managing the property in the trust according to the terms and provisions of the trust. The trustee is also responsible for all of the record keeping involved, such as preparing and filing income tax returns and distributing income and/or principal to the beneficiaries.

3. A **beneficiary** is the person or organization that receives distributions from the trust. A trust becomes operative when the creator transfers legal title of property to the trustee to manage the property for the beneficiary.

If you create a trust in your will, it is referred to as a *testamentary trust*. A testamentary trust takes effect and becomes irrevocable upon your death. If you create a trust during your lifetime, it is referred to as a *living* or *inter vivos trust*. A living or inter vivos trust operates during your lifetime and may be revocable or irrevocable. The terms and provisions of revocable trusts can be changed, but an irrevocable trust cannot be altered.

Reducing Estate Taxes

Testamentary trusts can save substantial taxes provided that your property can be distributed according to the provisions of your will. For example, if you and your spouse own all property jointly (with rights of survivorship), upon the first spouse's death all of the property goes outright to the survivor, regardless of what the will states. A will cannot control jointly owned property with rights of survivorship; thus, no property can be placed in the trust(s), and unnecessary taxes may be due at the surviving spouse's death. To avoid this common mistake, each spouse should title $625,000 of their joint property in their respective names. Individual ownership of property can be controlled with a will. If the will includes a bypass trust, up to $625,000 of property will avoid being taxed in the surviving spouse's estate.

A bypass trust allows each spouse to use his or her $625,000 federal estate tax exemption. The surviving spouse will receive all income payable at least annually and has the right to withdraw principal. If each spouse takes advantage of his or her $625,000 exemption, a combined estate of $1,250,000 can be transferred with no federal estate tax. Without proper planning, the same estate will pay approximately $235,000 in federal estate tax at the second spouse's death.

Irrevocable life insurance trusts should be considered for estates that exceed $1.2 million. If drafted correctly, these trusts will prevent life insurance policies from being included in the estate and from being taxed. If you transfer an existing policy to a trust and die within three years of the transfer, the life insurance policy will be included in your estate. If additional insurance is needed to pay estate taxes, let the trustee purchase the insurance and you will not have to worry about the three-year rule.

Managing Assets for Family Members

A trust can provide income and/or principal distributions to the beneficiaries at various ages and at regular intervals. They are excellent management vehicles for a surviving spouse who does not have money management skills. If your will provides for a qualified terminable interest property trust (Q-Tip trust), you can provide a lifetime income for your spouse, control the ultimate disposition of the property, and also have it qualify for the unlimited marital deduction. The Q-Tip property will be in the estate of the surviving spouse and may be subject to estate taxes.

Revocable living trusts are not considered tax-saving instruments but often are used to manage assets for someone who is legally incapacitated or incompetent. These trusts have been touted as miraculous medicine to avoid the hassles of administering a decedent's estate. Make sure that you understand how it works before you set one up.

Making Tax-free Gifts

People may give up to $10,000 per year to an unlimited number of recipients or $20,000 with a spouse's consent without any gift tax. For example, a husband and wife with two children can give $40,000 per year. Gifts can be made to one of several types of minor's trusts and later used to fund a college education or meet other objectives.

Summary

Trusts should be considered as one of the tools used in any solid estate plan. Stay away from the do-it-yourself trust kits. Trusts can be complicated and (when set up incorrectly) may lead to financial disaster. Instead, work with your legal advisor to tailor a trust to fit your specific needs.

TIPS FOR GETTING YOUR ESTATE IN ORDER

Financial organization is something that many physicians put off. "There just doesn't seem to be enough time to get it done" is the reason I hear most often.

Yet, when it comes time to make important financial decisions, you must know where you stand financially before you can make a prudent decision. Otherwise, you are just "winging it," and the decision may come back to haunt you.

One of the first steps in getting organized is establishing specific goals. A college education for your children, a comfortable retirement, and a solid estate plan are a good start, but the goals must be quantified so that you have a way to measure your progress. Estate planning is the most intricate and potentially hazardous part of the equation. The following nine rules of thumb cover most estate-planning basics:

1. Get a tax-wise will. Make sure that your will is drafted to save estate taxes. Ideally, work with an attorney who specializes in estate planning.

2. Reallocate property. If possible, each spouse should own $625,000 of property individually. A will designed to save estate taxes will not work unless property can be distributed according to the will. For example, if all property is owned jointly with right of survivorship, it will not be distributed according to the terms of your will. Thus, your will and title to your property must be coordinated to maximize estate tax savings.

3. Inform your spouse. Make sure that your spouse knows where your will is and vice versa. If you have granted your spouse or another individual power of attorney, make sure that he or she knows where all legal papers are located. If the documents are kept in a bank lock box, be sure that he or she knows which bank and where the keys are.

4. Consolidate accounts. If you have multiple IRAs or several retirement plans scattered around, try to consolidate them as much as possible. The goal is to simplify record keeping. It is not necessary to do so if consolidation means taking a loss.

5. Set up investment files. When you open an investment account, set up a file. Any purchases, statements, reports, letters, or other correspondence goes directly into the file. Even if you do not have the time to read each document when it arrives, a simple folder will keep the information easily accessible.

6. Update wills. Be sure that wills are kept up to date. A change in family relationships (such as a divorce or birth of a child), economic circumstances, or property disposition objectives or relocation to another state necessitates an update. This review should be part of your annual fiscal exam.

7. Update insurance. Insurance policies need to be kept current. Providing adequate liquidity to support your family in case of your death and leaving them enough money to pay estate taxes are good uses for life insurance. Irrevocable trusts are recommended to keep life insurance out of the estate.

8. Draft living wills/powers of attorney. Have living wills (if you desire them) in place before you need them. Likewise, be sure that powers of attorney are in place for health care.

9. Review beneficiary designations. All retirement plans, life insurance policies, and annuity contracts should list primary and contingent beneficiaries. The beneficiaries should be consistent with your estate distribution objectives.

Getting organized takes a commitment, but it is well worth the effort—especially for your family members.

CONCLUSION

Planning for your personal financial security is a lifelong process. You should monitor your fiscal condition periodically. Make an appointment for an annual fiscal exam each year to review your progress and to evaluate goals and objectives. Just as your annual physical examination is important, so is an annual review of your fiscal health. A little preventive medicine goes a long way.

ACKNOWLEDGMENTS The author thanks his staff members—Sheila C. Akin, Shannon L. Mock, Christopher D. Pack—for their assistance in preparing this chapter.

REFERENCES

1. Brinson GP, Hood LR, Beebower GL: Determinants of portfolio performance. Financial Analysis Journal, July–August, 1986.
2. Brinson GP, Singer BD, Beebower GL: Determinants of portfolio performance. II: An update. Financial Analysis Journal, May–June 1991.
3. Donlan TG: The price of education. Barron's, 23 December 1996.
4. Evensky HR: Wealth Management. Dubuque, IA, Times Mirror Higher Education Group, 1997.
5. Sanford C. Bernstein & Co: Gaining the global edge. Investment Planning in the Global Era, July 1994.
6. Ibbotson Associates: The Asset Allocation Decision. Chicago, Ibbotson Associates, 1997.
7. Ibbotson Associates: Stocks, Bonds, Bills, and Inflation Year-End Summary Report 1996. Chicago, Ibbotson Associates, 1997.
8. Ibbotson Associates: Stocks, Bonds, Bills, and Inflation 1997 Yearbook. Chicago, Ibbotson Associates, 1997.
9. Katt PC: Be wise about disability insurance. Journal of Financial Planning, June 1997.
10. Stanley TJ, Danko WD: The Millionaire Next Door. Atlanta, Longstreet Press, 1996.
11. Weber D: How to save big on life insurance commissions. Medical Economics 20 January 1992.
12. Wray AM III, Howard WB Jr: Fee insurance benefits clients and planners. Journal of Financial Planning, October, 1992.

INDEX

Page numbers in **boldface type** indicate complete chapters.